M000074539

THE PEDIATRIC CARDIOLOGY HANDBOOK

fourth
EDITION

THE PEDIATRIC CARDIOLOGY HANDBOOK

MYUNG K. PARK, MD, FAAP, FACC

Professor Emeritus (Pediatrics)
University of Texas Health Science Center
San Antonio, Texas

Clinical Professor of Pediatrics
Health Science Center
College of Medicine, Texas A&M University
College Station, Texas

Attending Cardiologist
Driscoll Children's Hospital
Corpus Christi, Texas

With a Contribution by

MEHRDAD SALAMAT, MD, FAAP, FACC

Clinical Assistant Professor of Pediatrics
Health Science Center
College of Medicine, Texas A&M University
College Station, Texas

Attending Cardiologist
Driscoll Children's Hospital
Corpus Christi, Texas

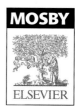

MOSBY

ELSEVIER

1600 John F. Kennedy Blvd.
Ste 1800
Philadelphia, PA 19103-2899

THE PEDIATRIC CARDIOLOGY HANDBOOK, FOURTH EDITION   ISBN: 978-1-4160-6443-5
Copyright © 2010, 2003, 1997, 1991 by Mosby, Inc., an affiliate of Elsevier Inc.

Notice

Knowledge and best practice in this field are constantly changing. As new research and experience broaden our knowledge, changes in practice, treatment and drug therapy may become necessary or appropriate. Readers are advised to check the most current information provided (i) on procedures featured or (ii) by the manufacturer of each product to be administered, or to verify the recommended dose or formula, the method and duration of administration, and contraindications. It is the responsibility of the practitioner, relying on their own experience and knowledge of the patient, to make diagnoses, to determine dosages and the best treatment for each individual patient, and to take all appropriate safety precautions. To the fullest extent of the law, neither the Publisher nor the Author assumes any liability for any injury and/or damage to persons or property arising out or related to any use of the material contained in this book.

The Publisher

Library of Congress Cataloging-in-Publication Data
Park, Myung K. (Myung Kun), 1934-
   The pediatric cardiology handbook / Myung K. Park ; with a contribution by Mehrdad Salamat.—4th ed.
     p. ; cm.
   Includes bibliographical references and index.
   ISBN 978-1-4160-6443-5
   1. Pediatric cardiology—Handbooks, manuals, etc. I. Title.
   [DNLM: 1. Cardiovascular Diseases—Handbooks. 2. Child. 3. Infant.
WS 39 P236p 2010]
   RJ421.P38 2010
   618.92'12--dc22

                                                                    2008053210

Acquisitions Editor: James Merritt
Developmental Editor: Andrea Vosburgh
Project Manager: Bryan Hayward
Design Direction: Louis Forgione
Marketing Manager: Courtney Ingram

Printed in China

Last digit is the print number: 9 8 7 6 5 4 3 2 1

Working together to grow
libraries in developing countries

www.elsevier.com | www.bookaid.org | www.sabre.org

ELSEVIER   BOOK AID International   Sabre Foundation

Dedication

To my loving wife, Issun

Preface

Since the publication of the third edition of *The Pediatric Cardiology Handbook* in 2003, important advances have been made in both the diagnosis and treatment of children with congenital and acquired heart diseases. These advances make it necessary to update the handbook. Although extensive updating and revisions have been made throughout the book, the handbook maintains its original goal of providing practitioners with fundamental and practical information for the management of children with cardiac problems.

Special emphasis was placed in the area of cardiac surgery, in which not only have new procedures been introduced but also the timing of old procedures has changed to earlier ages, making some previous descriptions of surgical management no longer appropriate for certain conditions. Although every topic and chapter has been updated, certain topics received more extensive revision, including cyanotic heart defects, infective endocarditis, Kawasaki disease, long QT syndrome, and ventricular arrhythmias. New sections on palpitation, athletes with cardiac problems, and preventive cardiology have been added. The revision includes the addition of many new figures of surgical procedures and diagrams of surgical options for most cyanotic heart defects. For the chapter on electrocardiography, new normative data are presented based on the recently revised fourth edition of *How to Read Pediatric ECGs* (which I coauthored with Dr. Warren G. Guntheroth). The number of two-dimensional echocardiographic diagrams has been increased. The Appendixes have been expanded to include normal values of both M-mode and 2D echocardiography and blood pressure standards.

I wish to acknowledge the contributions of the following individuals in the revision. My colleagues at the Driscoll Children's Hospital provided constructive suggestions. In particular, I am deeply indebted to Mehrdad Salamat, MD, attending cardiologist at the Driscoll Children's Hospital and clinical assistant professor at Texas A&M University Health Science Center, for his enthusiastic support and important contributions in the revision. Dr. Salamat has updated the chapter "Management of Cardiac Surgical Patients." Dr. Salamat was instrumental in updating drug dosages with newer drugs that are used in the practice of pediatric cardiology. He also contributed to Chapter 2 with the addition of magnetic resonance imaging and computed tomography. Paula Scott, PhD, MLS, librarian at the Driscoll Children's Hospital, has helped me with literature searches throughout the project. Linda Lopez, a cardiac sonographer and the manager of Driscoll's McAllen Cardiology Clinic, has provided me with valuable suggestions on the echocardiographic illustrations. Most of all, I thank my wife for her understanding during my long period of preoccupation with this project.

I believe this handbook will be an important companion to cardiology fellows, pediatricians, family practitioners, house staff, and medical students. The handbook may prove to be very useful even to practicing cardiologists because it makes the basic and advanced information in the practice of cardiology available instantly.

Myung K. Park, MD, FAAP, FACC

Frequently Used Abbreviations

AR	Aortic regurgitation
AS	Aortic stenosis
ASD	Atrial septal defect
AV	Atrioventricular
BAH	Biatrial hypertrophy
BBB	Bundle branch block
B-T shunt	Blalock-Taussig shunt
BVH	Biventricular hypertrophy
CAD	Coronary artery disease
CHD	Congenital heart disease or defect
CHF	Congestive heart failure
COA	Coarctation of the aorta
CPB	Cardiopulmonary bypass
CVD	Cardiovascular disease
CXR	Chest x-ray
DORV	Double-outlet right ventricle
ECD	Endocardial cushion defect
Echo	Echocardiography
HCM	Hypertrophic cardiomyopathy
HDL	High-density lipoprotein
HLHS	Hypoplastic left heart syndrome
HOCM	Hypertrophic obstructive cardiomyopathy
HT	Hypertension
IE	Infective endocarditis
IHSS	Idiopathic hypertrophic subaortic stenosis
IVC	Inferior vena cava
LA	Left atrium or left atrial
LAD	Left axis deviation
LAE	Left atrial enlargement
LAH	Left atrial hypertrophy
LBBB	Left bundle branch block
LDL	Low-density lipoprotein
LICS	Left intercostal space
LLN	Lower limit of normal
LLSB	Lower left sternal border
LPA	Left pulmonary artery
LPL	Left precordial lead
L-R shunt	Left-to-right shunt
LRSB	Lower right sternal border
LSB	Left sternal border
LV	Left ventricle or left ventricular
LVH	Left ventricular hypertrophy
LVOT	Left ventricular outflow tract
MLSB	Mid-left sternal border

MPA	Main pulmonary artery
MR	Mitral regurgitation
MRSB	Mid-right sternal border
MS	Mitral stenosis
MVP	Mitral valve prolapse
PA	Pulmonary artery
PAC	Premature atrial contraction
PAPVR	Partial anomalous pulmonary venous return
PAT	Paroxysmal atrial tachycardia
PBF	Pulmonary blood flow
PDA	Patent ductus arteriosus
PFO	Patent foramen ovale
PH	Pulmonary hypertension
PR	Pulmonary regurgitation
PS	Pulmonary stenosis
PV	Pulmonary vein or pulmonary venous
PVC	Premature ventricular contraction
PVM	Pulmonary vascular marking
PVOD	Pulmonary vascular obstructive disease
PVR	Pulmonary vascular resistance
RA	Right atrium or right atrial
RAD	Right axis deviation
RAE	Right atrial enlargement
RAH	Right atrial hypertrophy
RBBB	Right bundle branch block
RICS	Right intercostal space
R-L shunt	Right-to-left shunt
RPA	Right pulmonary artery
RPL	Right precordial lead
RV	Right ventricle or right ventricular
RVE	Right ventricular enlargement
RVH	Right ventricular hypertrophy
RVOT	Right ventricular outflow tract
S1	First heart sound
S2	Second heart sound
S3	Third heart sound
S4	Fourth heart sound
SBE	Subacute bacterial endocarditis
SEM	Systolic ejection murmur
S-P shunt	Systemic-to-pulmonary shunt
SVC	Superior vena cava
SVR	Systemic vascular resistance
SVT	Supraventricular tachycardia
TAPVR	Total anomalous pulmonary venous return
TG	Trigylcerides
TGA	Transposition of the great arteries
TOF	Tetralogy of Fallot
TR	Tricuspid regurgitation

TS	Tricuspid stenosis
ULN	Upper limit of normal
ULSB	Upper left sternal border
URSB	Upper right sternal border
VSD	Ventricular septal defect
VT	Ventricular tachycardia
WPW	Wolff-Parkinson-White (preexcitation or syndrome)

Contents

Routine Cardiac Evaluation in Children

Initial evaluation of children with possible cardiac problems includes (1) history taking, (2) physical examination, (3) electrocardiographic (ECG) evaluation, and (4) chest x-ray (CXR). The weight of information gained from these techniques varies with the type and severity of the disease.

I. HISTORY TAKING

Prenatal, perinatal, postnatal, past, and family histories should be obtained.

A. GESTATIONAL AND PERINATAL HISTORY

1. Maternal infection: Rubella during the first trimester of pregnancy commonly results in PDA and PA stenosis (rubella syndrome, Table 1-1). Other viral infections early in pregnancy may be teratogenic. Viral infections (including human immunodeficiency virus) in late pregnancy may cause myocarditis.

2. Maternal medications: The following is a partial list of suspected teratogenic drugs (with reported CHDs). Amphetamines (VSD, PDA, ASD, and TGA), phenytoin (PS, AS, COA, and PDA), trimethadione (fetal trimethadione syndrome: TGA, VSD, TOF, HLHS; see Table 1-1), lithium (Ebstein anomaly), retinoic acid (conotruncal anomalies), valproic acid (various noncyanotic defects), and progesterone or estrogen (VSD, TOF, and TGA) are highly suspected teratogens. Warfarin may cause fetal warfarin syndrome (TOF, VSD, and other features such as ear abnormalities, cleft lip or palate, and hypoplastic vertebrae; see Table 1-1). Excessive maternal alcohol intake may cause fetal alcohol syndrome (in which VSD, PDA, ASD, and TOF are common; see Table 1-1). Cigarette smoking causes intrauterine growth retardation but not CHD.

3. Maternal conditions: Maternal diabetes increases the incidence of CHD (TGA, VSD, and PDA) and cardiomyopathy (see Table 1-1). Both maternal lupus erythematosus and collagen diseases have been associated with congenital heart block in the offspring. History of maternal CHD may increase the prevalence of CHD in the offspring to as much as 15%, compared with 1% in the general population (see Appendix A, Table A-2).

B. POSTNATAL AND PRESENT HISTORY

1. Poor weight gain and delayed development may be caused by congestive heart failure (CHF), severe cyanosis, or general dysmorphic conditions. Weight is more affected than height.

TABLE 1-1

MAJOR SYNDROMES ASSOCIATED WITH CARDIOVASCULAR ABNORMALITIES

DISORDERS	CV ABNORMALITIES: FREQUENCY AND TYPES	MAJOR FEATURES	ETIOLOGY
Alagille Syndrome (Arteriohepatic Dysplasia)	Very common (85%); peripheral PA stenosis with or without complex CV abnormalities	Peculiar facies (95%) (consisting of deep-set eyes; broad forehead; long, straight nose with flattened tip; prominent chin; small, low-set, malformed ears); paucity of intrahepatic interlobular bile duct with chronic cholestatis (91%), hypercholesterolemia; butterfly-like vertebral arch defects (87%); growth retardation (50%) and mild mental retardation (16%)	AD Chromosome 22q11.2
Carpenter Syndrome	Frequent (50%); PDA, VSD, PS, TGA	Brachycephaly with variable craniosynostosis, mild facial hypoplasia, polydactyly and severe syndactyly ("mitten hands")	AR
CHARGE Association	Common (65%); TOF, truncus arteriosus, aortic arch anomalies (e.g., vascular ring, interrupted aortic arch)	**C**oloboma, **h**eart defects, choanal **a**tresia, growth or mental **r**etardation, **g**enitourinary anomalies, **e**ar anomalies, genital hypoplasia	Unknown
Cockayne Syndrome	Accelerated atherosclerosis	Senilelike changes beginning in infancy, dwarfing, microcephaly, prominent nose and sunken eyes, visual loss (retinal degeneration) and hearing loss	AR
Cornelia De Lange (De Lange) Syndrome	Occasional (30%); VSD	Synophrys, hirsutism, prenatal growth retardation, microcephaly, anteverted nares, downturned mouth, and mental retardation	Unknown; AD?
Cri Du Chat Syndrome (Deletion 5p Syndrome)	Occasional (25%); variable CHD (VSD, PDA, ASD)	Catlike cry in infancy, microcephaly, downward slant of palpebral fissures	Partial deletion, short arm of chromosome 5

cont'd

Syndrome	Cardiac defect	Features	Etiology
Crouzon Disease (Craniofacial Dysostosis)	Occasional; PDA, COA	Ptosis with shallow orbits, premature craniosynostosis, maxillary hypoplasia	AD
DiGeorge Syndrome	Frequent; interrupted aortic arch, truncus arteriosus, VSD, PDA, TOF	Hypertelorism, short philtrum, down-slanting eyes, hypoplasia or absence of thymus and parathyroid, hypocalcemia, deficient cell-mediated immunity	Microdeletion of 22q11.2 (overlap with velocardiofacial syndrome)
Down Syndrome (Trisomy 21)	Frequent (40%-50%); ECD, VSD	Hypotonic, flat facies, slanted palpebral fissure, small eyes, mental deficiency, simian crease	Trisomy 21
Ehlers-Danlos Syndrome	Frequent; ASD, aneurysm of aorta and carotids, intracranial aneurysm, MVP	Hyperextensive joints, hyperelasticity, fragility and bruisability of skin, poor wound healing with thin scar	AD
Ellis-van Creveld Syndrome (Chondroectodermal Dysplasia)	Frequent (50%); ASD, single atrium	Short stature of prenatal onset, short distal extremities, narrow thorax with short ribs, polydactyly, nail hypoplasia, neonatal teeth	AR
Fetal Alcohol Syndrome	Occasional (25%-30%); VSD, PDA, ASD, TOF	Prenatal growth retardation, microcephaly, short palpebral fissure, mental deficiency, irritable infant or hyperactive child	Ethanol or its by-products
Fetal Trimethadione Syndrome	Occasional (15%-30%); TGA, VSD, TOF	Ear malformation, hypoplastic midface, unusual eyebrow configuration, mental deficiency, speech disorder	Exposure to trimethadione
Fetal Warfarin Syndrome	Occasional (15%-45%); TOF, VSD	Facial asymmetry and hypoplasia, hypoplasia or aplasia of the pinna with blind or absent external ear canal (microtia), ear tags, cleft lip or palate, epitubular dermoid, hypoplastic vertebrae	Exposure to warfarin

TABLE 1-1—cont'd
MAJOR SYNDROMES ASSOCIATED WITH CARDIOVASCULAR ABNORMALITIES

DISORDERS	CV ABNORMALITIES: FREQUENCY AND TYPES	MAJOR FEATURES	ETIOLOGY
Friedreich Ataxia	Frequent; hypertrophic cardiomyopathy progressing to heart failure	Late-onset ataxia, skeletal deformities	AR
Glycogen Storage Disease II (Pompe Disease)	Very common; cardiomyopathy	Large tongue and flabby muscles, cardiomegaly; LVH and short PR on ECG, severe ventricular hypertrophy on echo; normal FBS and GTT	AR
Goldenhar Syndrome (Oculoauriculovertebral Spectrum)	Frequent (35%); VSD, TOF	Facial asymmetry and hypoplasia, microtia, ear tag, cleft lip/palate, hypoplastic vertebrae	Unknown; usually sporadic
Holt-Oram Syndrome (Cardio-limb Syndrome)	Frequent; ASD, VSD	Defects or absence of thumb or radius	AD
Homocystinuria	Frequent; medial degeneration of aorta and carotids, atrial or venous thrombosis	Subluxation of lens (usually by 10 yr), malar flush, osteoporosis, arachnodactyly, pectus excavatum or carinatum, mental defect	AR
Infant of Diabetic Mother	CHDs (3%-5%); TGA, VSD, COA; cardiomyopathy (10%-20%); PPHN	Macrosomia, hypoglycemia and hypocalcemia, polycythemia, hyperbilirubinemia, other congenital anomalies	Fetal exposure to high glucose levels
Kartagener Syndrome	Dextrocardia	Situs inversus, chronic sinusitis and otitis media, bronchiectasis, abnormal respiratory cilia, immotile sperm	AR
LEOPARD Syndrome (Multiple Lentigines Syndrome)	Very common; PS, HOCM, long PR interval	Lentiginous skin lesion, ECG abnormalities, ocular hypertelorism, pulmonary stenosis, abnormal genitalia, retarded growth, deafness	AD

cont'd

Long QT Syndrome: Jervell And Lange-Nielsen Syndrome	Very common; long QT interval on ECG, ventricular tachyarrhythmia	Congenital deafness (not in Romano-Ward syndrome), syncope resulting from ventricular arrhythmias, family history of sudden death (±)	AR
Romano-Ward Syndrome			AD
Marfan Syndrome	Frequent; aortic aneurysm, aortic and/or mitral regurgitation	Arachnodactyly with hyperextensibility, subluxation of lens	AD
Mucopolysaccharidosis Hurler Syndrome (Type I)	Frequent; aortic and/or mitral regurgitation, coronary artery disease	Coarse features, large tongue, depressed nasal bridge, kyphosis, retarded growth, hepatomegaly, corneal opacity (not in Hunter syndrome), mental retardation; most patients die by 10 to 20 years of age	AR
Hunter Syndrome (Type II)			XR
Morquio Syndrome (Type IV)			AR
Muscular Dystrophy (Duchenne Type)	Frequent; cardiomyopathy	Waddling gait, "pseudohypertrophy" of calf muscle	XR
Neurofibromatosis (von Recklinghausen Disease)	Occasional; PS, COA, pheochromocytoma	Café au lait spots, multiple neurofibroma, acoustic neuroma, variety of bone lesions	AD
Noonan Syndrome (Turner-like Syndrome)	Frequent; PS (dystrophic pulmonary valve), LVH (or anterior septal hypertrophy)	Similar to Turner syndrome but may occur in phenotypic male and without chromosomal abnormality	Usually sporadic; apparent AD?
Osler-Weber-Rendu Syndrome (Hereditary Hemorrhagic Telangiectasia)	Occasional; pulmonary arteriovenous fistula	Hepatic involvement, telangiectases, hemangioma, or fibrosis	AD

TABLE 1-1—cont'd
MAJOR SYNDROMES ASSOCIATED WITH CARDIOVASCULAR ABNORMALITIES

DISORDERS	CV ABNORMALITIES: FREQUENCY AND TYPES	MAJOR FEATURES	ETIOLOGY
Osteogenesis Imperfecta	Occasional; aortic dilation, aortic regurgitation, MVP	Excessive bone fragility with deformities of skeleton, blue sclera, hyperlaxity of joints	AD/AR
Pierre Robin Syndrome	Occasional; VSD, PDA; less commonly ASD, COA, TOF	Micrognathia, glossoptosis, cleft soft palate	In utero mechanical constraint?
Progeria (Hutchinson-Gilford Syndrome)	Very common; accelerated atherosclerosis	Alopecia, atrophy of subcutaneous fat, skeletal hypoplasia and dysplasia	Unknown; occasional AD or AR
Rubella Syndrome	Very common (>95%); PDA and PA stenosis	Triad: deafness, cataract, and CHDs; others include intra-uterine growth retardation, microcephaly, microphthalmia, hepatitis, neonatal thrombocytopenic purpura	Maternal rubella infection during the first trimester
Rubinstein-Taybi Syndrome	Occasional (25%); PDA, VSD, ASD	Broad thumbs or toes; hypoplastic maxilla with narrow palate; beaked nose, short stature, mental retardation	Sporadic; locus at 16p13.3
Smith-Lemli-Opitz Syndrome	Occasional; VSD, PDA, others	Broad nasal tip with anteverted nostrils, ptosis of eyelids, syndactyly of 2nd and 3rd toes, short stature, mental retardation	AR
Thrombocytopenia-Absent Radius (TAR) Syndrome	Occasional (30%); TOF, ASD, dextrocardia	Thrombocytopenia, absent or hypoplastic radius, normal thumb; "leukemoid" granulocytosis and eosinophilia	AR
Treacher Collins Syndrome	Occasional; VSD, PDA, ASD	Defects of lower lids, malar hypoplasia with down-slanting palpebral fissure, malformation of auricle or ear canal defect, cleft palate	Fresh mutation; AD

Syndrome	Cardiac Defects	Clinical Features	Etiology
Trisomy 13 Syndrome (Patau Syndrome)	Very common (80%); VSD, PDA, dextrocardia	Low birth weight, central facial anomalies, polydactyly, chronic hemangiomas, low-set ears, visceral and genital anomalies	Trisomy 13
Trisomy 18 Syndrome (Edwards Syndrome)	Very common (90%); VSD, PDA, PS	Low birth weight, microcephaly, micrognathia, rocker-bottom feet, closed fist with overlapping fingers	Trisomy 18
Tuberous Sclerosis	Frequent; rhabdomyoma	Triad of adenoma sebaceum (2-5 yr of age), seizures, and mental defect; cystlike lesions in phalanges and elsewhere; fibrous-angiomatosis lesions (83%) with varying colors in nasolabial fold, cheeks, and elsewhere	AD
Turner Syndrome (XO Syndrome)	Frequent (35%); COA, bicuspid aortic valve, AS; hypertension, aortic dissection later in life	Short female; broad chest with widely spaced nipples; congenital lymphedema with residual puffiness over the dorsum of fingers and toes (80%)	XO with 45 chromosomes
VATER association (VATER/VACTERL Syndrome)	Common (>50%); VSD, other defects	**V**ertebral anomalies, **a**nal atresia, congenital heart defects, **t**racheoesophageal (TE) fistula, **r**enal dysplasia, **l**imb anomalies (e.g., radial dysplasia)	Sporadic
Velocardiofacial Syndrome (Shprintzen Syndrome)	Very common (85%); truncus arteriosus, TOF, pulmonary atresia with VSD, interrupted aortic arch type B), VSD, and D-TGA	Structural or functional palatal abnormalities, unique facial characteristics ("elfin facies") with auricular abnormalities, prominent nose with squared nasal root and narrow alar base, vertical maxillary excess with long face), hypernasal speech, conductive hearing loss, hypotonia, developmental delay and learning disability	Unknown; chromosome 22q11.2 (probably the same disease as Di-George syndrome)
Williams Syndrome	Frequent; supravalvular AS, PA stenosis	Varying degree of mental retardation, "elfin" facies (with upturned nose, flat nasal bridge, long philtrum, flat malar area, wide mouth, full lips, widely spaced teeth, and periorbital fullness), hypercalcemia of infancy?	Sporadic; AD?

cont'd

TABLE 1-1—cont'd
MAJOR SYNDROMES ASSOCIATED WITH CARDIOVASCULAR ABNORMALITIES

DISORDERS	CV ABNORMALITIES: FREQUENCY AND TYPES	MAJOR FEATURES	ETIOLOGY
Zellweger Syndrome (Cerebrohepatorenal Syndrome)	Frequent; PDA, VSD, or ASD	Hypotonia, high forehead with flat facies, hepatomegaly, albuminuria	AR

From Park MK: *Pediatric cardiology for practitioners*, ed 5, Philadelphia, 2008, Mosby.

AD, autosomal dominant; AR, autosomal recessive; AS, aortic stenosis; ASD, atrial septal defect; CHD, congenital heart disease; COA, coarctation of the aorta; CV, cardiovascular; ECD, endocardial cushion defect; ECG, electrocardiogram; FBS, fasting blood sugar; GTT, glucose tolerance test; HOCM, hypertrophic obstructive cardiomyopathy; LVH, left ventricular hypertrophy; MR, mitral regurgitation; MVP, mitral valve prolapse; PA, pulmonary artery; PDA, patent ductus arteriosus; PPHN, persistent pulmonary hypertension of newborn; PS, pulmonary stenosis; TGA, transposition of the great arteries; TOF, tetralogy of Fallot; VSD, ventricular septal defect; XR, sex-linked recessive; ±, may be present.

2. Cyanosis, squatting, and cyanotic spells suggest TOF or other cyanotic CHD.

3. Tachycardia, tachypnea, and puffy eyelids are signs of CHF.

4. Frequent lower respiratory tract infections may be associated with large L-R shunt lesions.

5. Decreased exercise tolerance may be a sign of significant heart defects or ventricular dysfunction.

6. Heart murmur. The time of its first appearance is important. A heart murmur noted shortly after birth indicates a stenotic lesion (AS, PS). A heart murmur associated with large L-R shunt lesions (such as VSD or PDA) may be delayed. Appearance of a heart murmur in association with fever suggests an innocent murmur.

7. Chest pain. Ask if chest pain is exercise related or nonexertional; also ask about its duration, nature, and radiation. Nonexertional chest pain is unlikely to have cardiac causes. Cardiac causes of chest pain are usually associated with exertional pain and are very rare in children and adolescents. The three most common causes of nonexertional chest pain in children are costochondritis, trauma to chest wall or muscle strain, and respiratory diseases (see Child with Chest Pain in Chapter 6).

8. Palpitation may be caused by paroxysms of tachycardia, sinus tachycardia, single premature beats; rarely hyperthyroidism or mitral valve prolapse (MVP) (see Chapter 6).

9. Joint pain. Joints involved, presence of redness and swelling, history of trauma, duration and migratory or stationary nature of the pain, recent sore throat, rashes, family history of rheumatic fever, or the diagnosis of rheumatoid arthritis are important.

10. Neurologic symptoms. Stroke may result from embolization of thrombus from infective endocarditis, polycythemia, or uncorrected or partially corrected cyanotic CHD. Headache may be associated with polycythemia or, rarely, with hypertension. Choreic movement may result from rheumatic fever. Fainting or syncope may be due to vasovagal responses, arrhythmias, long QT syndrome, epilepsy, or other noncardiac conditions (see "Syncope" in Chapter 6).

11. Note medications, cardiac and noncardiac (name, dosage, timing, and duration).

12. Syndromes and diseases of other systems with associated cardiovascular abnormalities are summarized in Table 1-1.

C. FAMILY HISTORY

1. Certain hereditary diseases may be associated with varying frequency of cardiac anomalies (see Table 1-1).

2. CHD in the family. The incidence of CHD in the general population is about 1% (8 to 12 per 1000 live births). When one child is affected, the risk of recurrence in siblings is increased to about 3% (see Table A-1 in Appendix A). However, the risk of recurrence is related to the incidence of particular defects: Lesions with high prevalence (e.g., VSD) tend to have a

high risk of recurrence, and those with low prevalence (e.g., tricuspid atresia, persistent truncus arteriosus) have a low risk of recurrence (see Appendix A, Table A-1). The probability of recurrence is substantially higher when the mother, rather than the father, is the affected parent (see Appendix A, Table A-2). Tables A-1 and A-2 can be used for counseling.

II. PHYSICAL EXAMINATION

A. INSPECTION

1. Assess general appearance: happy or cranky, nutritional state, respiratory status (tachypnea, dyspnea, or retraction may be signs of serious CHD), pallor (vasoconstriction from CHF or circulatory shock or severe anemia), and sweat on the forehead (seen in CHF).
2. Inspect for any known syndromes or conditions (see Table 1-1).
3. Malformations of other systems may be associated with varying frequency of CHD (Table 1-2).

TABLE 1-2

INCIDENCE OF ASSOCIATED CHDs IN PATIENTS WITH OTHER SYSTEM MALFORMATIONS

ORGAN SYSTEM AND MALFORMATION	FREQUENCY (%)	SPECIFIC CARDIAC DEFECT
Central Nervous System		
Hydrocephalus	6	VSD, ECD, TOF
Dandy-Walker syndrome	3	VSD
Agenesis of corpus callosum	15	No specific defect
Meckel-Gruber syndrome	14	No specific defect
Thoracic Cavity		
TE fistula, esophageal atresia	21	VSD, ASD, TOF
Diaphragmatic hernia	11	No specific defect
Gastrointestinal System		
Duodenal atresia	17	No specific defect
Jejunal atresia	5	No specific defect
Anorectal anomalies	22	No specific defect
Imperforate anus	12	TOF, VSD
Ventral Wall		
Omphalocele	21	No specific defect
Gastroschisis	3	No specific defect
Genitourinary System		
Renal agenesis		
Bilateral	43	No specific defect
Unilateral	17	No specific defect
Horseshoe kidney	39	No specific defect
Renal dysplasia	5	No specific defect

Adapted from Copel JA, Kleinman CS: Congenital heart disease and extracardiac anomalies: association and indications for fetal echocardiography, *Am J Obstet Gynecol* 154:1121-1132, 1986.
ECD, endocardial cushion defect; TE, tracheoesophageal. Other abbreviations are listed on pp. xi-xii.

4. Acanthosis nigricans (a dark pigmentation of skin crease on the neck) is often seen in obese children and those with type 2 diabetes and may signify the presence of hyperinsulinemia.

5. Precordial bulge, with or without actively visible cardiac activity, suggests chronic cardiac enlargement. Pectus excavatum may be a cause of a heart murmur. Pectus carinatum is usually not a result of cardiomegaly.

6. Cyanosis usually signals a serious CHD. A long-standing arterial desaturation (usually more than 6 months), even of a subclinical degree, results in clubbing of the fingers and toes.

B. PALPATION

1. Precordium

a. A hyperactive precordium is characteristic of heart diseases with high volume overload, such as L-R shunt lesions or severe valvular regurgitation.

b. A thrill is often of real diagnostic value. The location of the thrill suggests certain cardiac anomalies: upper left sternal border (ULSB), PS; upper right sternal border (URSB), AS; lower left sternal border (LLSB), VSD; suprasternal notch, AS, occasionally PS, PDA, or COA; over the carotid arteries, AS or COA.

2. Peripheral pulses

a. Check the peripheral pulse for the rate, irregularities (arrhythmias), and volume (bounding, full, or thready).

b. Strong arm pulses and weak leg pulses suggest COA.

c. The right brachial artery pulse stronger than the left brachial artery pulse may suggest COA or supravalvular AS.

d. Bounding pulses are found in aortic runoff lesions (e.g., PDA, AR, large systemic AV fistula).

e. Weak and thready pulses are found in CHF and circulatory shock.

C. BLOOD PRESSURE

Every child should have blood pressure (BP) measurement as part of the physical examination whenever possible. To determine if the obtained BP level is normal or abnormal, BP readings are compared with reliable BP standards. Unfortunately, there have been problems and confusion regarding the correct method of measuring BP and the reliable normative BP values for children. Arm length–based BP cuff selection methods recommended by two NIH Task Forces (1977 and 1987) are scientifically unsound, and they have contributed to the lack of reliable normative BP standards for decades. Although the Working Group of the National High Blood Pressure Education Program (NHBPEP) has recently corrected the BP cuff selection method, its normative BP data are scientifically and logically unsound (see the following).

1. The following are currently recommended BP measurement techniques.

a. The width of the BP cuff should be 40% to 50% of the circumference of the arm (or leg) with the cuff long enough to completely or nearly completely encircle the extremity.

b. The NHBPEP recommends Korotkoff phase 5 (K5) as the diastolic pressure, but this is debatable. Earlier studies indicate that K4 agrees better with true diastolic pressure for children ≤12 years.

c. The average of two or more readings should be obtained.

d. The child should be in a sitting position with the arm at the heart level.

2. The normative BP standards recommended by the Working Group are not evidence based and are impractical for use by busy practitioners.

a. The Working Group's BP data have been derived from the methodology that is discordant with the Working Group's own recommendations; that is, the BP values are derived from currently invalid methods of NIH Task Force-1987 (with BP cuff width selected by the arm length). In addition, they are single measurements rather than averages of multiple readings, as currently recommended.

b. Rationale for checking BP values according to age and height percentile is statistically and logically unsound. Partial correlation analysis in the San Antonio Children's Blood Pressure Study (SACBPS) shows that when auscultatory (as well as oscillometric) BP levels were adjusted for age and weight, the correlation coefficient of systolic BP with height was very small ($r \equiv 0.070$), whereas when adjusted for age and height, the correlation of systolic pressure with weight remained high ($r \equiv 0.318$). Thus, there is no rationale to use both age and height percentile to express children's BP standards. These findings indicate that the contribution of height to BP levels is negligible. The apparent contribution of height to BP levels may reflect its close correlation with weight ($r \equiv 0.86$). Although weight is a very important contributor to BP, weight cannot be used as a second variable because this would interfere with detection of high BP in obese children. Therefore, we recommend children's BP values be expressed as a function of age only as has been done earlier by NIH Task Forces.

c. Recommendation of requiring additional computational steps to classify the level of a child's BP is unwise because BP levels obtained in a doctor's office are highly variable and not reproducible, unlike weight or height measurement.

3. Normative percentile curves from the San Antonio study are the only standards obtained according to the currently recommended methodology, including that of the NHBPEP (Figs. 1-1 and 1-2). BP values are the averages of three readings. In using these percentile curves, one should consider the patient's weight status before making the diagnosis of hypertension (BP levels ≥ 90th percentile). If the BP level is higher than the 90th percentile for the age and gender on three occasions, hypertension can be diagnosed, but the extent this abnormality is associated with weight should be considered before any presumption of organic disease is made. Percentile values of auscultatory systolic and diastolic pressures for children 5 to 17 years old are presented in Appendix B (Tables B-3 and B-4). Although BP standards recommended by the NHBPEP are

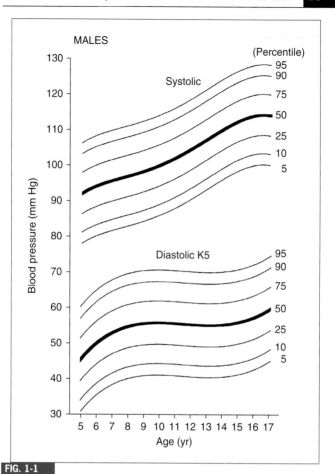

FIG. 1-1

Age-specific percentile curves of auscultatory systolic and diastolic (K5) pressures in boys 5 to 17 years of age. BP values are the averages of three readings. The width of the BP cuff was 40% to 50% of the circumference of the arm. The percentile values for the graph are shown in Appendix B, Table B-3. *(From Park MK, Menard SW, Yuan C: Comparison of blood pressure in children from three ethnic groups,* Am J Cardiol 87:1305-1308, 2001.)

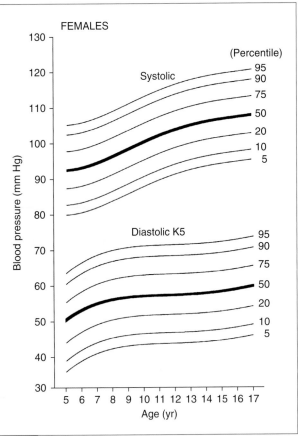

FIG. 1-2

Age-specific percentile curves of auscultatory systolic and diastolic (K5) pressures in girls 5 to 17 years of age. BP values are the averages of three readings. The width of the BP cuff was 40% to 50% of the circumference of the arm. The percentile values for the graph are shown in Appendix B, Table B-4. *(From Park MK, Menard SW, Yuan C: Comparison of blood pressure in children from three ethnic groups, Am J Cardiol 87:1305-1308, 2001.)*

unscientific, they are presented in Tables B-1 and B-2 for the sake of completeness.

4. **Oscillometric blood pressure values.** It should be noted that BP readings by the auscultatory method and the currently popular oscillometric devices are not interchangeable. In the San Antonio Children's Blood

Pressure Study, BP measurements were obtained using both the auscultatory and Dinamap (model 8100) methods. BP levels obtained by the Dinamap were on average 10 mm Hg higher than levels obtained by the auscultatory method for the systolic pressure and 5 mm Hg higher for the diastolic pressure. Therefore, one should use different normative BP standards when BP is obtained by the Dinamap method. Dinamap-specific BP standards for children 5 through 17 years of age are presented in Tables B-5 and B-6. Normative BP standards by Dinamap for neonates and children up to 5 years of age are presented in Table 1-3.

5. The following are additional comments regarding BP measurements in children and adolescents.

a. **How to interpret arm and leg BP values.** Four-extremity BP measurements are often obtained in neonates and children to rule out COA. Even with a considerably wider cuff used for the thigh, the Dinamap systolic pressure in the thigh or calf is about 5 to 10 mm Hg higher than that in the arm. This reflects in part the peripheral amplification of systolic pressure (see the following). If the systolic pressure is lower in the leg, COA may be present. The peripheral amplification is not seen in the neonate, probably due to the presence of normal isthmic narrowing in this age group.

b. **The concept of peripheral amplification of systolic pressure.** Many physicians incorrectly think that peripherally measured BP, such as that measured in the arm, is the same as the central aortic pressure. The peripheral systolic pressure, obtained by either direct or indirect method, is not always the same as the central aortic pressure. In fact, arm systolic pressures are in general higher than central aortic pressures and are much higher in certain situations. This phenomenon is called peripheral amplification of systolic pressure (Fig. 1-3). The systolic amplification increases as the site of BP measurement moves distally. The following summarizes key points of the phenomenon.

   (1) The amplification is limited to the systolic pressure (not in the diastolic pressure).

   (2) The systolic amplification is greater in children (with more reactive arteries) than in older adults who may have degenerative arterial disease.

TABLE 1-3

NORMATIVE BLOOD PRESSURE LEVELS [SYSTOLIC/DIASTOLIC (MEAN)] (IN MM HG) BY DINAMAP MONITOR (MODEL 1846 SX) IN CHILDREN UP TO AGE 5 YEARS

AGE	MEAN BP LEVELS	90TH PERCENTILE	95TH PERCENTILE
1-3 days	64/41 (50)	75/49 (59)	78/52 (62)
1 mo-2 yr	95/58 (72)	106/68 (83)	110/71 (86)
2-5 yr	101/57 (74)	112/66 (82)	115/68 (85)

Adapted from Park MK, Menard SM: Normative oscillometric blood pressure values in the first five years in an office setting, *Am J Dis Child* 143:860-864, 1989.

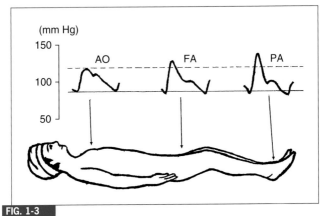

FIG. 1-3
Schematic drawing of pulse wave changes seen at different levels of the systemic arteries.
(From Park MK: Pediatric cardiology for practitioners, ed 5, Philadelphia, 2008, Mosby.)

    (3) Pedal artery systolic pressures are higher than the radial artery pressures.
    (4) The amplification is more marked in vasoconstricted states.
        (a) Patients in impending circulatory shock (with a high level of circulating catecholamines) may show normal peripheral artery systolic pressure when the central aortic pressure is abnormally low. Monitoring the mean arterial and diastolic pressures should be more useful in this situation.
        (b) Subjects receiving catecholamine infusion or other vasoconstrictors may show much higher peripheral systplic pressure than central aortic pressure.
        (c) A child in congestive heart failure (in which peripheral vasoconstriction exists) may exhibit an exaggerated systolic amplification.
        (d) Arm systolic pressure in subjects running on treadmill can be markedly higher than the central aortic pressure.

D. AUSCULTATION

Systematic attention should be given to heart rate and regularity; intensity and quality of the heart sounds, especially the second heart sound; systolic and diastolic sounds (ejection click, midsystolic click, opening snap); and heart murmurs.

1. Heart sounds
a. The first heart sound (S1) is associated with closure of the mitral and tricuspid valves and is best heard at the apex or LLSB. Splitting of the S1 is uncommon in normal children. Wide splitting of the S1 may be found in right bundle branch block (RBBB) or Ebstein anomaly.

b. The second heart sound (S2), which is produced by the closure of the aortic and pulmonary valves, is evaluated in the ULSB (or the pulmonary area) in terms of the degree of splitting and the relative intensity of the P2 (the pulmonary closure sound) in relation to the intensity of the A2 (the aortic closure sound). Although best heard with a diaphragm, both components are readily audible with the bell as well.

  (1) The degree of splitting of the S2 normally varies with respiration, increasing with inspiration and decreasing or becoming single with expiration (Fig. 1-4).

  (2) Abnormal S2 may take the form of wide splitting, narrow splitting, single S2, abnormal intensity of the P2, or, rarely, paradoxical splitting of the S2 (see Box 1-1 for summary of abnormal S2).

c. The third heart sound (S3) is best heard at the apex or LLSB (Fig. 1-5). It is commonly heard in normal children, young adults, and patients with dilated ventricles and decreased compliance of the ventricles (e.g., large-shunt VSD, CHF).

d. The fourth heart sound (S4) at the apex, which is always pathologic (Fig. 1-5), is seen in conditions with decreased ventricular compliance or CHF.

e. Gallop rhythm generally implies pathology and results from the combination of a loud S3 or S4 and tachycardia. It is common in CHF.

2. Systolic and diastolic sounds

a. An ejection click sounds like splitting of the S1 but is best heard at the base rather than at the LLSB (Fig. 1-5). The ejection click is associated with stenosis of the semilunar valves (e.g., PS at 2LICS and to 3LICS, AS at 2RICS or apex) and enlarged great arteries (e.g., systemic hypertension, pulmonary hypertension, and TOF).

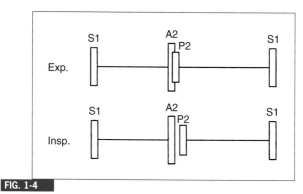

FIG. 1-4

Relative intensity of the A2 and P2 and the respiratory variation in the degree of splitting of the S2 at the ULSB (pulmonary area). *(From Park MK:* Pediatric cardiology for practitioners, *ed 5, Philadelphia, 2008, Mosby.)*

BOX 1-1

SUMMARY OF ABNORMAL S2

ABNORMAL SPLITTING

1. **Widely split and fixed S2**
   a. Volume overload (ASD, PAPVR)
   b. Pressure overload (PS)
   c. Electrical delay (RBBB)
   d. Early aortic closure (MR)
   e. Occasional normal child
2. **Narrowly split S2**
   a. Pulmonary hypertension
   b. AS
   c. Occasional normal child
3. **Single S2**
   a. Pulmonary hypertension
   b. One semilunar valve (pulmonary atresia, aortic atresia, persistent truncus arteriosus)
   c. P2 not audible (TGA, TOF, severe PS)
   d. Severe AS
   e. Occasional normal child
4. **Paradoxically split S2**
   a. Severe AS
   b. LBBB

ABNORMAL INTENSITY OF P2

1. Increased P2 (pulmonary hypertension)
2. Decreased P2 (severe PS, TOF, tricuspid stenosis)

---

b. A midsystolic click with or without a late systolic murmur is heard near the apex in patients with MVP (Fig. 1-5).
c. Diastolic opening snap is audible at the apex or LLSB in mitral stenosis (MS) (Fig. 1-5).

3. Heart murmur. Each heart murmur should be analyzed in terms of intensity, timing (systolic or diastolic), location, transmission, and quality (e.g., musical, vibratory, blowing).

a. Intensity of the murmur is customarily graded from 1 to 6.
   (1) Grade 1, barely audible
   (2) Grade 2, soft but easily audible
   (3) Grade 3, moderately loud but not accompanied by a thrill
   (4) Grade 4, louder and associated with a thrill
   (5) Grade 5, audible with the stethoscope barely on the chest
   (6) Grade 6, audible with the stethoscope off the chest

b. Classification of heart murmurs. Heart murmurs are classified as systolic, diastolic, or continuous.

c. Systolic murmurs

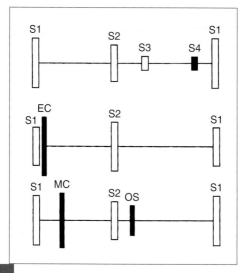

FIG. 1-5

Relative position of the heart sounds, ejection click *(EC),* midsystolic click *(MC),* and diastolic opening snap *(OS).* Filled bars show abnormal sounds. *(From Park MK: Pediatric cardiology for practitioners, ed 5, Philadelphia, 2008, Mosby.)*

(1) A systolic murmur occurs between S1 and S2. Systolic murmur was initially classified by Aubrey Leatham in 1958 into two types, ejection or regurgitant, depending on the timing of the onset, not the termination, of the murmur in relation to the S1. Recently, Joseph Perloff proposed a new classification into four types according to the time of *onset* and *termination:* midsystolic (ejection), holosystolic, early systolic, and late systolic.

    (a) Ejection systolic murmur (also called stenotic, diamond shaped, or Perloff's midsystolic) has an interval between S1 and the onset of the murmur and is crescendo-decrescendo. The murmur may be short or long (Fig. 1-6, *A*). These murmurs are caused by the flow of blood through stenotic or deformed semilunar valves or increased flow through normal semilunar valves and are therefore found at the base or over the midprecordium. These murmurs may be pathologic or innocent.

    (b) Regurgitant systolic murmur begins with the S1 (no gap between the S1 and the onset of the murmur) and usually lasts throughout systole (pansystolic or holosystolic) but may be decrescendo ending in middle or early systole (Fig. 1-6, *B*). Perloff's holosystolic and early systolic murmurs are regurgitant

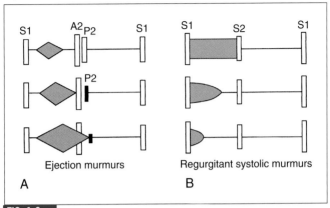

S1   A2 P2   S1   S1   S2   S1

P2

Ejection murmurs   Regurgitant systolic murmurs

A   B

FIG. 1-6

Ejection and regurgitant systolic murmurs. **A,** An ejection systolic murmur is audible in pulmonary valve stenosis (and other conditions). With mild stenosis the apex of the diamond is in the early part of systole *(top).* With increasing severity of obstruction to flow, the murmur becomes longer and its apex moves toward S2 *(middle).* In severe PS the murmur may last beyond A2 and the P2 is sometimes too soft to be audible *(bottom).* **B,** Regurgitant systolic murmur starts with S1. Most regurgitant systolic murmur in children is due to VSD and is holosystolic, extending all the way to S2 *(top).* In some children, especially those with small VSDs, and some neonates with VSD, the regurgitant systolic murmur may be decrescendo and ends in middle or early systole (not holosystolic) *(middle, bottom),* but never crescendo-decrescendo.

murmurs. These murmurs are always pathologic and are associated with only three conditions: VSD, MR, and TR.

    (c) Late systolic murmur of Perloff is the hallmark of MVP (see Fig. 4-7).

(2) Location. In addition to the type of murmur (ejection vs. regurgitant), the location of maximal intensity of the murmur is of great importance in determining the origin (Tables 1-4 through 1-7 and Fig. 1-7).

(3) Transmission. A systolic ejection murmur at the base that transmits well to the neck is likely to be aortic, and one that transmits well to the sides of the chest and the back is likely to arise in the pulmonary valve or pulmonary artery.

(4) Quality. Ejection systolic murmurs of AS or PS have a rough, grating quality. A common innocent murmur in children (Still murmur) has a characteristic vibratory or humming quality.

(5) Differential diagnosis by location. Figure 1-7 illustrates systolic murmurs that are audible at the various locations. Tables 1-4 through 1-7 summarize other clinical findings (e.g., physical

TABLE 1-4

DIFFERENTIAL DIAGNOSIS OF SYSTOLIC MURMURS AT THE ULSB
(PULMONARY AREA)

CONDITION	IMPORTANT PHYSICAL FINDINGS	CHEST X-RAY FINDINGS	ECG FINDINGS
PS	SEM grade 2-5/6 *Thrill (±) S2 may be split widely when mild *Ejection click (±) at 2LICS Transmit to back	*Prominent MPA segment (poststenotic dilation) Normal PVM	Normal if mild, RAD *RVH RAH if severe
ASD	SEM grade 2-3/6 *Widely split and fixed S2	*Increased PVM *RAE and RVE	RAD RVH *RBBB (rsR′ in V1)
Pulmonary Flow Murmur of Newborn	SEM grade 1-2/6 No thrill *Good transmission to back and axillae	Normal	Normal
Pulmonary Flow Murmur of Older Children	SEM grade 2-3/6 No thrill Poor transmission	Normal Occasional pectus excavatum or straight back	Normal
Pulmonary Artery Stenosis	SEM grade 2-3/6 Occasional continuous murmur in the back, if severe P2 may be loud *Transmits well to back and both axillae	Prominent hilar vessels (±)	RVH or normal
AS	SEM grade 2-5/6 *Also audible in 2RICS *Thrill (±) at 2RICS and SSN *Ejection click at apex, 3LICS, or 2RICS (±) Paradoxically split S2 if severe	Dilated aorta	Normal or LVH
TOF	*Long SEM, grade 2-4/6 Louder at MLSB *RVH or BVH Loud, single S2 Cyanosis, clubbing(±)	*Decreased PVM *Normal heart size Boot-shaped heart Right aortic arch (25%)	RAD *RVH or BVH RAH (±)

cont'd

TABLE 1-4—cont'd

DIFFERENTIAL DIAGNOSIS OF SYSTOLIC MURMURS AT THE ULSB
(PULMONARY AREA)

CONDITION	IMPORTANT PHYSICAL FINDINGS	CHEST X-RAY FINDINGS	ECG FINDINGS
COA	SEM grade 1-3/6 Loudest at left inter-scapular area (back) *Weak or absent femorals Hypertension in arms Frequently associated with AS, bicuspid aortic valve, or MR	*Classic 3 sign on plain film or E sign on barium esophagogram Rib notching (±)	LVH in children RBBB or RVH in newborns
PDA	*Continuous murmur, grade 2-4/6, at left infraclavicular area Occasional crescendo systolic only Thrill (±) Bounding pulses	*Increased PVM *LAE, LVE	Normal, LVH, or BVH
TAPVR	SEM grade 2-3/6 Widely split and fixed S2 (±) *Quadruple or quintuple rhythm Diastolic rumble at LLSB *Mild cyanosis and clubbing (±)	*Increased PVM RAE and RVE Prominent MPA Snowman sign	RAD RAH *RVH
PAPVR	Physical findings similar to those of ASD *S2 may not be fixed unless associated with ASD	Increased PVM *RAE and RVE Scimitar sign (±)	Same as in ASD

*Finding is particularly characteristic of the condition.

BVH, biventricular hypertrophy; 2LICS, second left intercostal space; LVE, left ventricular enlargement; SSN, suprasternal notch; (±), may be present. Other abbreviations are listed on pp. ix-xi.

examination, CXR, ECG) that may aid diagnosis according to the location of a systolic murmur.

d. Diastolic murmurs. Diastolic murmurs occur between S2 and S1. Three types exist.

(1) Early diastolic (protodiastolic) decrescendo murmurs are caused by AR or PR (Fig. 1-8). AR murmurs are high pitched, are best heard at the 3LICS, and radiate to the apex. PR murmurs are usually medium pitched but may be high if pulmonary hypertension is present, best heard at the 2LICS, and they radiate along the left sternal border.

TABLE 1-5

DIFFERENTIAL DIAGNOSIS OF SYSTOLIC MURMURS AT THE URSB (AORTIC AREA)

CONDITION	IMPORTANT PHYSICAL FINDINGS	CHEST X-RAY FINDINGS	ECG FINDINGS
Aortic Valve Stenosis	SEM grade 2-5/6 at 2RICS; may be loudest at 3LICS *Thrill (±), URSB, SSN, and carotid arteries *Ejection click *Transmits well to neck S2 may be single	Mild LVE (±) Prominent ascending aorta or aortic knob	Normal or LVH with or without strain
Subaortic Stenosis	SEM grade 2-4/6 *AR murmur may be present No ejection click	Usually normal	Normal or LVH
Supravalvular Aortic Stenosis	SEM grade 2-3/6 Thrill (±) No ejection click *Pulse and BP may be greater in right than left arm *Peculiar facies, mental retardation (±) Murmur may transmit well to back (PA stenosis)	Unremarkable	Normal, LVH, or BVH

*Finding is particularly characteristic of the condition.

BVH, biventricular hypertrophy; 3LICS, third left intercostal space; 2RICS, second right intercostal space; SSN, suprasternal notch; (±), may be present. Other abbreviations are listed on pp. ix-xi.

   (2) Middiastolic murmurs are low pitched, starting with a loud S3 (Fig. 1-8). Best heard with the bell of the stethoscope, these murmurs are caused by anatomic or relative stenosis of the mitral or tricuspid valve. MS murmurs are best heard at the apex (apical rumble), and TS murmurs are heard along the LLSB.
   (3) Presystolic, or late diastolic, murmurs are low pitched and occur late in diastole or just before the onset of systole (Fig. 1-8). They are found with anatomic stenosis of the mitral or tricuspid valve.
 e. Continuous murmurs. Continuous murmurs begin in systole and continue without interruption through the S2 into all or part of diastole (Fig. 1-8). A combined systolic and diastolic murmur, such as from AS and AR or PS

TABLE 1-6			
DIFFERENTIAL DIAGNOSIS OF SYSTOLIC MURMURS AT THE LLSB			
CONDITION	**IMPORTANT PHYSICAL FINDINGS**	**CHEST X-RAY FINDINGS**	**ECG FINDINGS**
VSD	*Regurgitant systolic, grade 2-5/6 May not be holosystolic Well localized at LLSB *Thrill often present P2 may be loud	*Increased PVM *LAE and LVE (cardiomegaly)	Normal, LVH, or BVH
Complete ECD	Similar to findings of VSD *Diastolic rumble at LLSB *Gallop rhythm common in infants (CHF)	Similar to large VSD	*Superior QRS axis, LVH or BVH
Vibratory Innocent Murmur (Still Syndrome)	SEM grade 2-3/6 *Musical or vibratory with midsystolic accentuation *Maximum between LLSB and apex	Normal	Normal
HOCM or IHSS	SEM grade 2-4/6, medium pitch Maximum LLSB or apex Thrill (±) *Sharp upstroke of brachial pulses May have MR murmur	Normal or globular LVE	LVH Abnormally deep Q waves in V5 and V6
Tricuspid Regurgitation (TR)	*Regurgitant systolic, grade 2-3/6 *Triple or quadruple rhythm (in Ebstein anomaly) Mild cyanosis (±) Hepatomegaly with pulsatile liver and neck vein distention when severe	Normal PVM RAE if severe	RBBB, RAH, and first-degree AV block in Ebstein anomaly
Tetralogy of Fallot (TOF)	Murmurs can be louder at ULSB (see Table 1-4)	See Table 1-4	See Table 1-4

*Finding is characteristic of the condition.
BVH, biventricular hypertrophy; ECD, endocardial cushion defect; HOCM, hypertrophic obstructive cardiomyopathy; IHSS, idiopathic hypertrophic subaortic stenosis; LVE, left ventricular enlargement; (±), may be present. Other abbreviations are listed on pp. ix-xi.

TABLE 1-7

DIFFERENTIAL DIAGNOSIS OF SYSTOLIC MURMURS AT THE APEX

CONDITION	IMPORTANT PHYSICAL FINDINGS	CHEST X-RAY FINDINGS	ECG FINDINGS
MR	*Regurgitant systolic murmur at apex, grade 2-3/6 Transmits to left axilla (less obvious in children) May be loudest in the midprecordium	LAE and LVE	LAH or LVH
MVP	*Midsystolic click with or without late systolic murmur *High incidence (85%) of thoracic skeletal anomalies (e.g., pectus excavatum, straight back)	Normal	Inverted T in aVF (±)
AS	Murmur and ejection click may be best heard at apex rather than at 2RICS	See Table 1-5	
HOCM or IHSS	Murmur of IHSS may be maximal at apex (may represent MR) (see Table 1-6)		
Vibratory Innocent Murmur	This innocent murmur may be loudest at apex (see Table 1-8)		

*Finding is characteristic of the condition.

(±), may be present. Other abbreviations are listed on pp. ix-xi.

and PR, is called a to-and-fro murmur to distinguish it from a machinery-like continuous murmur. Continuous murmurs are caused by the following:

(1) Aortopulmonary or arteriovenous connection (e.g., PDA, arteriovenous [AV] fistula, after S-P shunt surgery, or, rarely, persistent truncus arteriosus)

(2) Disturbances of flow patterns in veins (venous hum)

(3) Disturbances of flow patterns in arteries (COA, peripheral PA stenosis)

f. Innocent murmurs.

(1) Over 80% of children have innocent murmurs of one type or the other sometime during childhood, most commonly beginning about 3 or 4 years of age. All innocent heart murmurs are accentuated or brought out in high-output states, most importantly with fever. Clinical characteristics of these murmurs are summarized in Table 1-8.

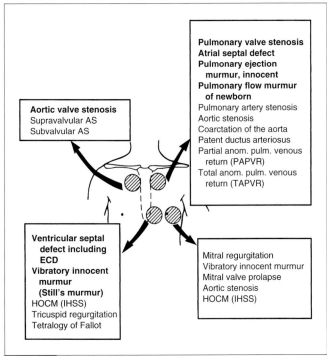

Aortic valve stenosis
Supravalvular AS
Subvalvular AS

Pulmonary valve stenosis
Atrial septal defect
Pulmonary ejection
  murmur, innocent
Pulmonary flow murmur
  of newborn
Pulmonary artery stenosis
Aortic stenosis
Coarctation of the aorta
Patent ductus arteriosus
Partial anom. pulm. venous
  return (PAPVR)
Total anom. pulm. venous
  return (TAPVR)

Ventricular septal
  defect including
  ECD
Vibratory innocent
  murmur
  (Still's murmur)
HOCM (IHSS)
Tricuspid regurgitation
Tetralogy of Fallot

Mitral regurgitation
Vibratory innocent murmur
Mitral valve prolapse
Aortic stenosis
HOCM (IHSS)

FIG. 1-7

Systolic murmurs audible at various locations. More common conditions are shown in boldface type (see also Tables 1-4 through 1-7). *(From Park MK: Pediatric cardiology for practitioners, ed 5, Philadelphia, 2008, Mosby.)*

(2) When one or more of the following are present, the murmur is likely to be pathologic and require cardiac consultation: (1) symptoms, (2) cyanosis, (3) abnormal CXR (heart size and/or silhouette and pulmonary vascularity), (4) abnormal ECG, (5) a systolic murmur that is loud (grade 3/6 or with a thrill) and long in duration, (6) a diastolic murmur, (7) abnormal heart sounds, and (8) abnormally strong or weak pulses.

III. ELECTROCARDIOGRAPHY

One normal cardiac cycle is represented by successive waveforms on an ECG tracing: the P wave, the QRS complex, and the T wave (Fig. 1-9, A). These waves produce two important intervals, PR and QT, and two segments, PQ and ST.

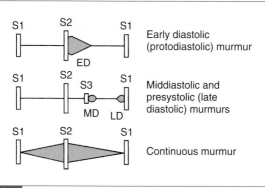

Diastolic murmurs and the continuous murmur. *(From Park MK:* Pediatric cardiology for practitioners, *ed 5, Philadelphia, 2008, Mosby.)*

TABLE 1-8

COMMON INNOCENT HEART MURMURS

TYPE (TIMING)	DESCRIPTION OF MURMUR	AGE GROUP
Classic Vibratory Murmur (Still Murmur) (Systolic)	Maximal at MLSB or between LLSB and apex Grade 2-3/6 Low-frequency vibratory, twanging string, groaning, squeaking, or musical	3-6 yr Occasionally in infancy
Pulmonary Ejection Murmur (Systolic)	Maximal at ULSB Early to midsystolic Grade 1-3/6 in intensity Blowing in quality	8-14 yr
Pulmonary Flow Murmur of New-born (Systolic)	Maximal at ULSB Transmits well to left and right chest, axillae, and back Grade 1-2/6 in intensity	Premature and full-term newborns Usually disappears by 3-6 mo of age
Venous Hum (Continuous)	Maximal at right (or left) supraclavicular and infraclavicular areas Grade 1-3/6 in intensity Inaudible in supine position Intensity changes with rotation of head and compression of jugular vein	3-6 yr
Carotid Bruit (Systolic)	Right supraclavicular area and over carotids Grade 2-3/6 in intensity Occasional thrill over carotid	Any age

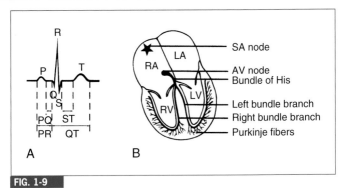

A, Definition of ECG configuration and **B,** diagrammatic representation of the conduction system of the heart. *(From Park MK, Guntheroth WG: How to read pediatric ECGs, ed 4, Philadelphia, 2006, Mosby.)*

In normal sinus rhythm the sinoatrial (SA) node is the pacemaker for the entire heart; the SA node impulse depolarizes the right and left atria by a contiguous spread, producing the P wave (Fig. 1-9, *A, B*). When the atrial impulse arrives at the atrioventricular (AV) node, it passes through the node much more slowly than in any other part of the heart, producing the PQ interval. Once the electrical impulse reaches the bundle of His, conduction becomes very fast and spreads simultaneously down the left and right bundle branches to the ventricular muscle through the Purkinje fibers, producing the QRS complex. The repolarization of the ventricle produces the T wave, but the repolarization of the atria is not usually visible on the ECG tracing.

A. VECTORIAL APPROACH TO THE ELECTROCARDIOGRAM

A scalar ECG, which is routinely obtained in clinical practice, shows only the magnitude of the forces against time. The vectorial approach views the standard scalar ECG as three-dimensional vector forces that vary with time. When leads, which represent the frontal projection and the horizontal projection, are combined, one can derive the direction of the force from scalar ECG. The limb leads (i.e., leads I, II, III, aVR, aVL, and aVF) provide information about the frontal projection, while the precordial leads (V4R, and V1 through V6) provide information about the horizontal plane (Fig. 1-10). The vectorial approach clarifies the meaning of the ECG waves and the concept of axes, such as the P axis, QRS axis, and T axis. It is important for the readers to become familiar with the orientation of each scalar ECG lead.

The *hexaxial reference system,* which is composed of six limb leads (leads I, II, III, aVR, aVL, and aVF), gives information about the left-right and superior-inferior relationships (Fig. 1-10, *A*). The positive pole of each lead is indicated by the lead labels. The positive deflection (i.e., the R wave) is the

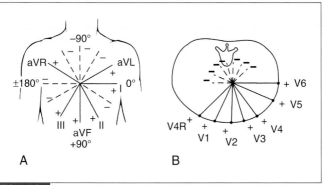

FIG. 1-10

A, Hexaxial reference system. **B,** Horizontal reference system. *(Adapted from Park MK, Guntheroth WG: How to read pediatric ECGs, ed 4, Philadelphia, 2006, Mosby.)*

force directed to the positive pole, and the negative deflection (i.e., the S wave) is the force directed toward the negative pole. Therefore, the R wave in lead I represents the leftward force and the S wave in lead I the rightward force. The R wave in aVF is the inferior force, and the S wave in the same lead represents the superior force. The R wave in lead II is the left and inferior force, and the R wave in lead III is the right and inferior force.

An easy way to memorize the hexaxial reference system is shown in Figure 1-11 by a superimposition of a body with stretched arms and legs on the X and Y axes. The hands and feet are the positive poles of certain leads. The left and right hands are the positive poles of leads aVL and aVR, respectively. The left and right feet are the positive poles of leads II and III, respectively. The bipolar limb leads I, II, and III are clockwise in sequence for the positive poles.

On the other hand, the *horizontal reference system* gives information about the anteroposterior and left-right relationships. The horizontal reference system uses precordial leads (e.g., V4R, V1, V2, V5, and V6) (Fig. 1-10, *B*). The positive poles of the precordial leads are marked by the lead labels. The R wave in V2 represents the anterior force, and the S wave in the same lead represents the posterior force. The R wave in V6 is the leftward force, and the S wave in the same lead is the rightward force. The R wave in V1 is the right and anterior force, and the S wave in this lead is the posterior and leftward force. The V4R lead is very useful in pediatrics. Its electrode position is in the right chest at the mirror image position of the V4 lead.

B.   NORMAL PEDIATRIC ELECTROCARDIOGRAMS

ECGs of normal infants and children are different from those of normal adults. The RV dominance seen in the ECG of neonates and infants is the result of the fetal circulation. The RV dominance is most marked in the neonate and is

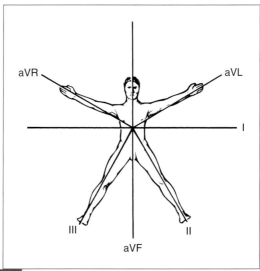

Easy way to memorize the hexaxial reference system.

gradually replaced by the LV dominance of later childhood and adulthood. By the time a child is age 3 to 4 years, pediatric ECGs resemble those of the adult. Figures 1-12 and 1-13 are ECGs from a newborn and an adult, respectively. The pediatric ECG has the following characteristics.

1. The heart rate is faster than in the adult.
2. All the durations and intervals (PR interval, QRS duration, and QT interval) are shorter than in the adult.
3. The RV dominance of the neonate and infant is expressed in the ECG by the following:
a. RAD is usually present.
b. Large rightward forces (tall R waves in aVR and the right precordial leads [RPLs, i.e., V4R, V1, and V2] and deep S waves in lead I and the left precordial leads [LPLs, i.e., V5 and V6]) are typically seen.
c. The R/S ratios in the RPLs are large and those in the LPLs are small. The R/S ratio is the ratio of the R amplitude and the S amplitude in a given lead.
d. The T wave is inverted in V1 in infants and small children, with the exception of the first 3 days when the T waves may be normally upright.

C. ROUTINE INTERPRETATION

The following sequence is one of many approaches that can be used in routine interpretation of an ECG.

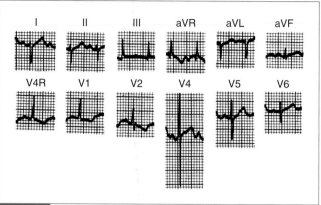

FIG. 1-12

ECG of a normal newborn infant.

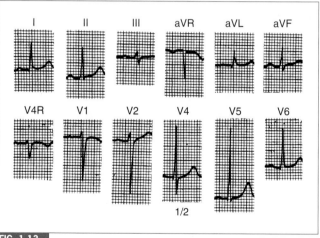

FIG. 1-13

ECG of a normal young adult.

- Rhythm (sinus or nonsinus), considering the P axis
- Heart rate (atrial and ventricular rates, if different)
- The QRS axis, the T axis, and the QRS-T angle
- Intervals and duration: PR, QRS, and QT
- The P wave amplitude and duration

- The QRS amplitude and R/S ratio; also note abnormal Q waves
- ST segment and T wave abnormalities

1. Rhythm. Sinus rhythm, the normal rhythm at any age, must meet the following two characteristics (Fig. 1-14).

a. A P wave preceding each QRS complex with a regular PR interval. (The PR interval may be prolonged as in first-degree AV block.)

b. The P axis between 0 and +90 degrees (with upright P waves in leads I and aVF).

Because the sinoatrial (SA) node is located in the right upper part of the atrial mass, the direction of atrial depolarization is from the right upper part toward the left lower part, with the resulting P axis in the left lower quadrant (0 to +90 degrees) (Fig. 1-15). For the P axis to be between 0 and +90 degrees, P waves must be upright in leads I and aVF. P waves may be flat, but they should not be inverted in these two leads.

2. Heart rate. At the usual paper speed of 25 mm/sec, 1 mm = 0.04 seconds and 5 mm = 0.2 seconds. The heart rate may be calculated by dividing 60 (seconds) by the RR interval in seconds. For quick estimation, inspect the RR interval in millimeters and use the following relationship: 5 mm, 300/sec; 10 mm, 150/sec; 15 mm, 100/sec; 20 mm, 75/sec; 25 mm, 60/sec (Fig. 1–16). Normal resting heart rates per minute according to age are shown in Table 1-9. Tachycardia is a heart

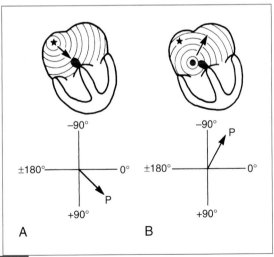

FIG. 1-14

A, Comparison of P axis in sinus rhythm and **B,** nonsinus rhythm (low atrial rhythm). In sinus rhythm the P axis is between 0 and +90 degrees, and in nonsinus rhythm the P axis is out of the 0- to +90-degree quadrant.

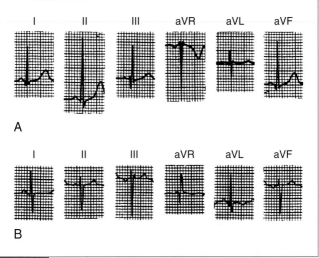

FIG. 1-15

Sinus or nonsinus rhythm determined by the P axis. **A,** Sinus rhythm with the P axis between 0 and +90 degrees. **B,** A nonsinus rhythm with the P axis in the 0- to −90-degree quadrant. The presence of a P wave in front of each QRS complex does not necessarily mean the rhythm is sinus rhythm; the P axis should be in the normal quadrant, as in **A.**

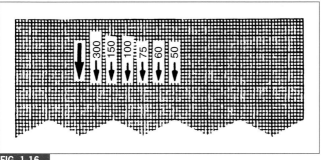

FIG. 1-16

Quick method of estimating heart rate.

rate faster than the upper range of normal, and bradycardia is a heart rate slower than the low range of normal for that age.

3. The QRS axis, the T axis, and the QRS-T angle

a. **Successive approximation method.** A convenient way of determining the QRS axis is by the use of the hexaxial reference system (Fig. 1-10, *A*).

TABLE 1-9

NORMAL RANGES OF RESTING
HEART RATE

AGE	BEATS/MIN
Neonates	110-150
2 yr	85-125
4 yr	75-115
Over 6 yr	60-100

(1) Step 1. Locate a quadrant using leads I and aVF (Fig. 1-17).
(2) Step 2. Find a lead with equiphasic QRS complex (in which the height of the R wave and the depth of the S wave are equal). The QRS axis is perpendicular to the lead with equiphasic QRS complex in the predetermined quadrant.
(3) **Example 1.** Determine the QRS axis in Figure 1-18, *A*.
   (a) Step 1. The axis is in the left lower quadrant (0 to +90 degrees) because the R waves are upright in both leads I and aVF.
   (b) Step 2. The QRS complex is equiphasic in aVL. Therefore, the QRS axis is +60 degrees, which is perpendicular to aVL (Fig. 1-18, *B*).
(4) **Example 2.** Determine the QRS axis in Figure 1-19, *A*.
   (a) Step 1. The QRS complexes are negative in lead I and negative in aVF, placing the axis in the right upper quadrant (−90 to −180 degrees) (Fig. 1-17, bottom panel).
   (b) Step 2a. It is almost equiphasic in aVL. Therefore, the axis is close to −120 degrees.
   (c) Step 2b. Lead II has the deepest negative deflection. The negative limb of lead II is −120 degrees. The QRS axis is *indeterminate,* that is, neither right nor left.
b. The normal QRS axis varies with age (Table 1-10). The abnormal QRS axis has the following significance.
   (1) LAD (with the QRS axis less than the lower limits of normal) is seen in LVH, LBBB, and left anterior hemiblock (or superior QRS axis, characteristically seen with endocardial cushion defect [ECD] and tricuspid atresia).
   (2) RAD (with the QRS axis greater than the upper limits of normal) is seen in RVH and RBBB.
   (3) Superior QRS axis is present when the S wave is greater than the R wave in aVF. It includes the left anterior hemiblock (in the range of −30 degrees to −90 degrees) and extreme RAD.
c. The T axis can be determined by the same method as that used to determine the QRS axis.
   (1) **Example.** Determine the T axis in Figure 1-19, *A*.
      (a) In Figure 1-19, *A*, the positive T wave in lead T and the positive T wave in aVF place the T axis in the left lower quadrant (0 to

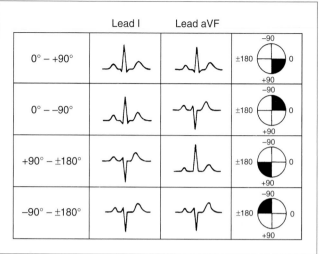

	Lead I	Lead aVF	
0° − +90°			
0° − −90°			
+90° − ±180°			
−90° − ±180°			

FIG. 1-17

Locating quadrants of the QRS axis using leads I and aVF. This figure is also used in determining the P and T axes. In the top panel the QRS complexes are upright in both leads I and aVF and thus the axis is in the 0- to +90-degree quadrant. The P and T waves are also upright in leads I and aVF, and thus the P and T axes are in the left lower quadrant (0 to +90 degrees) as well. The P axis in this quadrant indicates a sinus rhythm, which is the normal rhythm at any age. The normal T axis is always in the left lower quadrant (0 to +90 degrees) at any age. Using the similar approaches, the QRS axis can be located for other panels. *(From Park MK, Guntheroth WG: How to read pediatric ECGs, ed 4, Philadelphia, 2006, Mosby.)*

+90 degrees). The T wave is nearly flat in aVL, and therefore the T axis is perpendicular to this lead, close to +60 degrees (or the positive pole of lead II, which shows the tallest T wave).
(b) The normal T axis is 0 to +90 degrees.
(c) The abnormal T axis (outside the 0- to +90-degree quadrant) is present when the T wave is inverted in lead I or aVF, usually resulting in a wide QRS-T angle. An abnormal QRS axis suggests conditions with abnormal myocardial repolarization (myocarditis, myocardial ischemia), ventricular hypertrophy with strain, or RBBB.
d. The QRS-T angle is the angle formed by the QRS axis and the T axis. In Figure 1-19 the QRS-T angle is about 180 degrees (because the QRS axis is −120 degrees and the T axis is about +60 degrees).
(1) The normal QRS-T angle is less than 60 degrees except in the newborn period, when it may be more than 60 degrees.

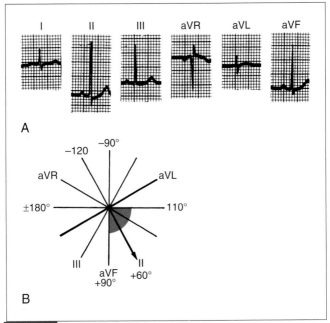

FIG. 1-18

An example of a QRS axis determination using the successive approximation method. The six limb leads shown at the top **(A)** are from a 6-year-old child. The QRS axis is plotted in a hexaxial reference system **(B)** (see text).

   (2) The QRS-T angle of more than 60 degrees is unusual and that of more than 90 degrees is certainly abnormal. The abnormal QRS-T angle (above 90 degrees) is seen in severe ventricular hypertrophy with strain, ventricular conduction disturbances, ventricular arrhythmias, and myocardial dysfunction of a metabolic or ischemic nature.
4. Intervals
a. The PR interval is measured from the onset of the P wave to the beginning of the QRS complex. The normal PR interval varies with age and heart rate (Table 1-11). The older the person and the slower the heart rate, the longer the PR interval.
   (1) A prolonged PR interval (first-degree AV block) may be seen in myocarditis (viral, rheumatic, or diphtheric), digitalis or quinidine toxicity, certain CHDs (ECD, ASD, Ebstein anomaly), hyperkalemia, other myocardial dysfunction, and in an otherwise normal heart.
   (2) A short PR interval is present in Wolff-Parkinson-White (WPW) pre-excitation, Lown-Ganong-Levine syndrome, Duchenne muscular

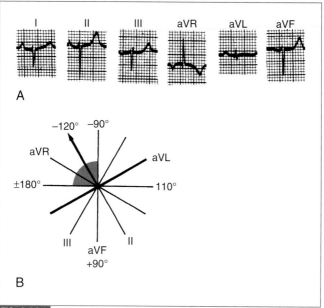

FIG. 1-19

An example of a QRS axis determination using the successive approximation method. The six limb leads shown at the top **(A)** are from a 2-year-old child with Down syndrome. The QRS axis is plotted in a hexaxial reference system **(B)** (see text).

TABLE 1-10

MEAN AND RANGE OR NORMAL QRS AXES

AGE	MEAN (RANGE)
1 wk-1 mo	+110 degrees (+30 to +180)
1-3 mo	+70 degrees (+10 to +125)
3 mo-3 yr	+60 degrees (+10 to +110)
>3 yr	+60 degrees (+20 to +120)
Adult	+50 degrees (−30 to +105)

dystrophy (or relative of these patients), Friedreich ataxia, pheochromocytoma, glycogen storage disease, and otherwise normal children.

(3) Variable PR intervals are seen in wandering atrial pacemaker and Wenckebach (Mobitz type I) second-degree AV block.

b. Normal QRS duration varies with age (Table 1-12). A prolonged QRS is characteristic of ventricular conduction disturbances, which include bundle branch blocks (BBBs), preexcitation (WPW type), and intraventricular block (see later section: "Ventricular Conduction Disturbances,"

TABLE 1-11

PR INTERVAL WITH RATE AND AGE (UPPER LIMITS OF NORMAL)

RATE (BEATS/MIN)	0-1 MO	1-6 MO	6 MO-1 YR	1-3 YR	3-8 YR	8-12 YR	12-16 YR	ADULT
<60						0.16 (0.18)	0.16 (0.19)	0.17 (0.21)
60-80	0.10 (0.12)				0.15 (0.17)	0.15 (0.17)	0.15 (0.18)	0.16 (0.21)
80-100	0.10 (0.12)				0.14 (0.16)	0.15 (0.16)	0.15 (0.17)	0.15 (0.20)
100-120	0.10 (0.11)			(0.15)	0.13 (0.16)	0.14 (0.15)	0.15 (0.16)	0.15 (0.19)
120-140	0.10 (0.11)	0.11 (0.14)	0.11 (0.14)	0.12 (0.14)	0.13 (0.15)	0.14 (0.15)		0.15 (0.18)
140-160	0.09 (0.11)	0.10 (0.13)	0.11 (0.13)	0.11 (0.14)	0.12 (0.14)			(0.17)
160-180	0.10 (0.11)	0.10 (0.12)	0.10 (0.12)	0.10 (0.12)				
>180	0.09	0.09 (0.11)	0.10 (0.11)					

From Park MK, Guntheroth WG: *How to read pediatric ECGs*, ed 4, Philadelphia, 2006, Mosby.

TABLE 1-12

QRS DURATION ACCORDING TO AGE: MEAN (UPPER LIMITS OF NORMAL*) (IN SEC)

	0-1 MO	1-6 MO	6-12 MO	1-3 YR	3-8 YR	8-12 YR	12-16 YR	ADULT
Seconds	0.05 (0.07)	0.055 (0.075)	0.055 (0.075)	0.055 (0.075)	0.06 (0.075)	0.06 (0.085)	0.07 (0.085)	0.08 (0.10)

Derived from percentile charts in Davignon A, Rautaharju P, Boisselle E et al: Normal ECG standards for infants and children, *Pediatr Cardiol* 1:123-131, 1979/80.

*Upper limit of normal refers to the 98th percentile.

Fig. 1-25). A slight prolongation of the QRS duration may also be seen in ventricular hypertrophy.

c. The QT interval normally varies primarily with heart rate. The heart rate–corrected QT interval (QTc) can be calculated with Bazett's formula:

$$QTc = QT / \sqrt{RR \text{ interval}}.$$

(1) According to Bazett's formula, the normal QTc interval (mean $\pm$ SD) is 0.40 ($\pm$0.014) seconds with the upper limit of normal 0.44 seconds in children 6 months and older. The QTc interval is slightly longer in the newborn and small infants with the upper limit of normal QTc 0.47 seconds in the first week of life and 0.45 seconds in the first 6 months of life.

(2) Prolonged QT intervals predispose to serious ventricular arrhythmias. Long QT intervals may be seen in long QT syndrome (e.g., Jervell and Lange-Nielsen syndrome, Romano-Ward syndrome), hypocalcemia, myocarditis, diffuse myocardial diseases (including hypertrophic and dilated cardiomyopathies), head injury, severe malnutrition, and so on. A number of drugs are also known to prolong the QT interval. Among these are antiarrhythmic agents (especially class IA, IC, and III), antipsychotic phenothiazines (e.g., thioridazine, chlorpromazine), tricyclic antidepressants (e.g., imipramine, amitriptyline), CNS stimulants used in ADHD (methylphenidate, dexmethylphenidate, atomoxetine, amphetamine), arsenics, organophosphates, antibiotics (e.g., azithromycin, erythromycin, trimethoprim-sulfa, amantadine), and antihistamines (e.g., terfenadine) (see Box 5-1, Acquired causes of QT prolongation).

(3) A short QT interval is a sign of a digitalis effect or of hypercalcemia. It is also seen with hyperthermia. Short QT syndrome is a familial cause of sudden death in which the QTc $\leq$ 300 ms.

(4) **The JT interval** is measured from the J point (the junction between the S wave and the ST segment) to the end of the T wave. Prolonged JT interval has the same significance as the prolonged QT interval. The JT interval is useful when the QT interval is prolonged secondary to a prolonged QRS duration, as seen with BBBs. The JT interval is also expressed as a rate-corrected interval (called JTc) using Bazett's formula. Normal JTc (mean $\pm$ SD) is 0.32 $\pm$ 0.02 seconds, with the upper limit of normal 0.34 seconds.

5. P wave duration and amplitude. Normally the P wave amplitude is less than 3 mm. The duration of the P waves is shorter than 0.09 seconds in children and shorter than 0.07 seconds in infants. Tall P waves indicate RAH. Long P wave durations are seen in LAH.

6. QRS amplitude, R/S ratio, and abnormal Q waves

a. QRS amplitude varies with age (Tables 1-13 and 1-14).

(1) Large QRS amplitudes are found in ventricular hypertrophy and ventricular conduction disturbances (e.g., BBBs, WPW preexcitation).

TABLE 1-13

R VOLTAGES ACCORDING TO LEAD AND AGE: MEAN (AND UPPER LIMIT*) (IN MM)

	0-1 MO	1-6 MO	6-12 MO	1-3 YR	3-8 YR	8-12 YR	12-16 YR	ADULT
I	4 (8)	7 (13)	8 (16)	8 (16)	7 (15)	7 (15)	6 (13)	6 (13)
II	6 (14)	13 (24)	13 (27)	12 (23)	13 (22)	14 (24)	14 (24)	5 (25)
III	8 (16)	9 (20)	9 (20)	9 (20)	9 (20)	9 (24)	9 (24)	6 (22)
aVR	3 (8)	2 (6)	2 (6)	2 (5)	2 (4)	1 (4)	1 (4)	1 (4)
aVL	2 (7)	4 (8)	5 (10)	5 (10)	3 (10)	3 (10)	3 (12)	3 (9)
aVF	7 (14)	10 (20)	10 (16)	8 (20)	10 (19)	10 (20)	11 (21)	5 (23)
V3R	10 (19)	6 (13)	6 (11)	6 (11)	5 (10)	3 (9)	3 (7)	
V4R	6 (12)	5 (10)	4 (8)	4 (8)	3 (8)	3 (7)	3 (7)	
V1	13 (24)	10 (19)	10 (20)	9 (18)	8 (16)	5 (12)	4 (10)	3 (14)
V2	18 (30)	20 (31)	22 (32)	19 (28)	15 (25)	12 (20)	10 (19)	6 (21)
V5	12 (23)	20 (33)	20 (31)	20 (32)	23 (38)	26 (39)	21 (35)	12 (33)
V6	5 (15)	13 (22)	13 (23)	13 (23)	15 (26)	17 (26)	14 (23)	10 (21)

Data are from percentile charts in Davignon A, Rautaharju P, Boisselle E et al: Normal ECG standards for infants and children, *Pediatr Cardiol* 1:123-131, 1979/80; data for leads I, II, III, aVL, and aVF are from Guntheroth WG: *Pediatric electrocardiography*, Philadelphia, 1965, WB Saunders; data for V4R and adults are from Park MK, Guntheroth WG: *How to read pediatric ECGs*, ed 3, St. Louis, 1992, Mosby-Year Book.

*Upper limit of normal refers to the 98th percentile.

Voltages measured in millimeters, when 1 mV = 10 mm paper.

TABLE 1-14

S VOLTAGES ACCORDING TO LEAD AND AGE: MEAN (AND UPPER LIMIT*) (IN MM)

	0-1 MO	1-6 MO	6-12 MO	1-3 YR	3-8 YR	8-12 YR	12-16 YR	ADULT
I	5 (10)	4 (9)	4 (9)	3 (8)	2 (8)	2 (8)	2 (8)	1 (6)
V3R	3 (12)	3 (10)	4 (10)	5 (12)	7 (15)	8 (18)	7 (16)	
V4R	4 (9)	4 (12)	5 (12)	5 (12)	5 (14)	6 (20)	6 (20)	
V1	7 (18)	5 (15)	7 (18)	8 (21)	11 (23)	12 (25)	11 (22)	10 (23)
V2	18 (33)	15 (26)	16 (29)	18 (30)	20 (33)	21 (36)	18 (33)	14 (36)
V5	9 (17)	7 (16)	6 (15)	5 (12)	4 (10)	3 (8)	3 (8)	
V6	3 (10)	3 (9)	2 (7)	2 (7)	2 (5)	1 (4)	1 (4)	1 (13)

Data are from percentile charts in Davignon A, Rautaharju P, Boisselle E et al: Normal ECG standards for infants and children, *Pediatr Cardiol* 1:123-131, 1979/80; data for lead are from Guntheroth WG: *Pediatric electrocardiography,* Philadelphia, 1965, WB Saunders; data for V4R and adults are from Park MK, Guntheroth WG: *How to read pediatric ECGs,* ed 3, St. Louis, 1992, Mosby-Year Book.

*Upper limit of normal refers to the 98th percentile.

Voltages measured in millimeters, when 1 mV = 10 mm paper.

   (2) Low QRS voltages are seen in pericarditis, myocarditis, hypothyroidism, and normal neonates.
b. In normal infants and small children the R/S ratio is large in the right
precordial leads (RPLs) and small in the left precordial leads (LPLs)
because of the presence of tall R waves in the RPLs and deep
S waves in the LPLs (Table 1-15). Abnormal R/S ratios are seen in
ventricular hypertrophy and ventricular conduction disturbances.
c. Normal Q waves are narrow (0.02 seconds) and are usually less than
5 mm in LPLs and aVF (Table 1-16). They may be as deep as 8 mm
in lead III in children younger than 3 years old.
   (1) Deep Q waves may be present in the LPLs in ventricular hypertrophy of the volume overload type.
   (2) Deep and wide Q waves are seen in myocardial infarction and
myocardial fibrosis.
d. Q waves are normally absent in RPLs.
   (1) Q waves in V1 may be seen in severe RVH, ventricular inversion
(L-TGA), single ventricle, and occasionally in neonates.
   (2) Absent Q waves in V6 may be seen in LBBB and ventricular
inversion.
7. ST segment and T waves
a. The normal ST segment is isoelectric. However, in infants and children, elevation or depression of the ST segment up to 1 mm in the
limb leads and up to 2 mm in the left precordial leads is not necessarily abnormal.
   (1) J depression is a nonpathologic ST segment shift in which the
junction between the QRS and the ST segment (i.e., J point) is
depressed without sustained ST segment shift (Fig. 1-20, A).
   (2) In early repolarization all leads with upright T waves have
elevated ST segments, and leads with inverted T waves have
depressed ST segments. This condition is seen in healthy adolescents and young adults.
b. Pathologic shift of the ST segment assumes either a downward slope
of the ST segment followed by a diphasic inverted T wave or a sustained horizontal segment 0.08 seconds or longer (Fig. 1-20, B, C). A
pathologic ST segment shift occurs in pericarditis, myocardial ischemia or infarction, severe ventricular hypertrophy (with strain), and
digitalis effect. Associated T wave changes are commonly present.
c. Tall peaked T waves may be seen in hyperkalemia, LVH (volume overload), and cerebrovascular accident. Flat or low T waves may occur in
normal neonates or with such conditions as hypothyroidism, hypokalemia, pericarditis, myocarditis, myocardial ischemia, hyperglycemia, or
hypoglycemia.

D. ATRIAL HYPERTROPHY

Abnormalities in the P wave amplitude and/or duration characterize atrial
hypertrophy (Fig. 1-21).

TABLE 1-15

R/S RATIO ACCORDING TO AGE: MEAN, LOWER, AND UPPER LIMITS OF NORMAL

	LEAD	0-1 MO	1-6 MO	6 MO-1 YR	1-3 YR	3-8 YR	8-12 YR	12-16 YR	ADULT
V1	LLN	0.5	0.3	0.3	0.5	0.1	0.15	0.1	0.0
	Mean	1.5	1.5	1.2	0.8	0.65	0.5	0.3	0.3
	ULN	19	S ≡ 0	6	2	2	1	1	1
V2	LLN	0.3	0.3	0.3	0.3	0.05	0.1	0.1	0.1
	Mean	1	1.2	1	0.8	0.5	0.5	0.5	0.2
	ULN	3	4	4	1.5	1.5	1.2	1.2	2.5
V6	LLN	0.1	1.5	2	3	2.5	4	2.5	2.5
	Mean	2	4	6	20	20	20	10	9
	ULN	S ≡ 0	S ≡ 0	S ≡ 0	S ≡ 0	S ≡ 0	S ≡ 0	S ≡ 0	S ≡ 0

From Guntheroth WG: *Pediatric electrocardiography,* Philadelphia, 1965, WB Saunders.
LLN, lower limit of normal; ULN, upper limit of normal.

TABLE 1-16

Q VOLTAGES ACCORDING TO LEAD AND AGE: MEAN (AND UPPER LIMIT*) (IN MM)

	0-1 MO	1-6 MO	6-12 MO	1-3 YR	3-8 YR	8-12 YR	12-16 YR	ADULT
III	1.5 (5.5)	1.5 (6.0)	2.1 (6.0)	1.5 (5.0)	1.0 (3.5)	0.6 (3.0)	1.0 (3.0)	0.5 (4)
aVF	1.0 (3.5)	1.0 (3.5)	1.0 (3.5)	1.0 (3.0)	0.5 (3.0)	0.5 (2.5)	0.5 (2.0)	0.5 (2)
V5	0.1 (3.5)	0.1 (3.0)	0.1 (3.0)	0.5 (4.5)	1.0 (5.5)	1.0 (3.0)	0.5 (3.0)	0.5 (3.5)
V6	0.5 (3.0)	0.5 (3.0)	0.5 (3.0)	0.5 (3.0)	1.0 (3.5)	0.5 (3.0)	0.5 (3.0)	0.5 (3)

Data are from percentile charts in Davignon A, Rautaharju P, Boisselle E et al: Normal ECG standards for infants and children, *Pediatr Cardiol* 1:123-131, 1979/80.
*Upper limit of normal refers to the 98th percentile.
Voltages measured in millimeters, when 1 mV = 10 mm paper.

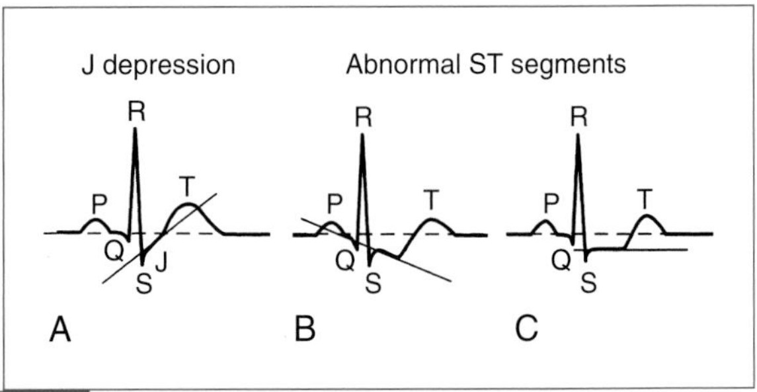

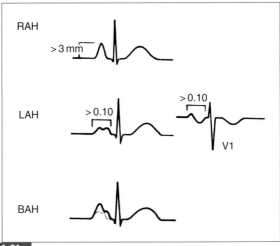

FIG. 1-20

Nonpathologic (nonischemic) and pathologic (ischemic) ST and T changes. **A,** Characteristic nonischemic ST segment alteration called J depression; note that the ST slope is upward. **B, C,** Ischemic or pathologic ST segment alterations. **B,** Downward slope of the ST segment. **C,** Horizontal segment is sustained.

FIG. 1-21

Criteria for atrial hypertrophy. *(From Park MK, Guntheroth WG: How to read pediatric ECGs, ed 4, Philadelphia, 2006, Mosby.)*

1. Right atrial hypertrophy (RAH) accompanies tall P waves (at least 3 mm).
2. Left atrial hypertrophy (LAH) accompanies wide P wave duration (at least 0.1 seconds in children and >0.08 seconds in infants).
3. Biatrial hypertrophy (BAH) accompanies a combination of tall and wide P waves.

E. VENTRICULAR HYPERTROPHY

Ventricular hypertrophy produces abnormalities in one or more of the following: the QRS axis, the QRS voltages, the R/S ratio, the T axis, and miscellaneous changes.

1. The QRS axis is usually directed toward the hypertrophied ventricle (see Table 1-10 for normal QRS axis); RAD seen with RVH; LAD with LVH. However, LAD is relatively rare with LVH due to pressure overload; in this situation, the QRS axis is more often directed inferiorly. RAD is almost always present with RVH.

2. Changes in QRS voltages. Anatomically, the RV occupies the right and anterior aspect, and the LV occupies the left, inferior, and posterior aspect of the ventricular mass. With ventricular hypertrophy the voltage of the QRS complex increases in the direction of the respective ventricle.

a. In the frontal plane (Fig. 1-22, A), LVH shows increased R voltages in leads I, II, aVL, aVF, and sometimes III, especially in small infants. RVH shows increased R voltages in aVR and III and increased S voltages in lead I (see Tables 1-13 and 1-14 for normal R and S voltages).

b. In the horizontal plane (Fig. 1-22, B), tall R waves in V4R, V1, and V2 or deep S waves in V5 and V6 are seen with RVH. With LVH, tall R waves in V5 and V6 and/or deep S waves in V4R, V1, and V2 are present (see Tables 1-13 and 1-14 for normal R and S voltages).

3. Changes in R/S ratio. An increase in the R/S ratio in the RPLs suggests RVH, and a decrease in the ratio in these leads suggests LVH. An increase in the R/S ratio in the LPLs suggests LVH, and a decrease in the ratio suggests RVH (Table 1-15).

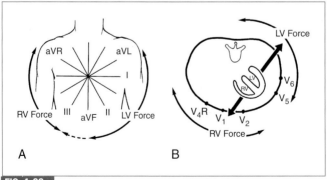

FIG. 1-22

Left and right ventricular forces on the frontal **(A)** and horizontal **(B)** projections. **A,** Hexaxial reference system. **B,** Horizontal plane. *(From Park MK, Guntheroth WG: How to read pediatric ECGs, ed 4, Philadelphia, 2006, Mosby.)*

4. Changes in the T axis. In severe ventricular hypertrophy with relative ischemia of the hypertrophied myocardium, the T axis changes. In the presence of criteria of ventricular hypertrophy, a wide QRS-T angle (≥90 degrees) with the T axis outside the normal range indicates a strain pattern. When the T axis remains in the normal quadrant (0 to +90 degrees), a wide QRS-T angle indicates a possible strain pattern.

5. Miscellaneous nonspecific changes

a. RVH: (1) A q wave in V1 (either qR or qRs) suggests RVH, although it may be present in ventricular inversion. (2) An upright T wave in V1 after 3 days of age is a sign of probable RVH.

b. LVH: Deep Q waves (≥5 mm) and/or tall T waves in V5 and V6 are signs of LVH of the volume overload type (often seen with a large-shunt VSD). Deep Q seen in the inferior leads (II, III, and aVF) may also be a sign of LVH (dilated or hypertrophied LV). Normally, the Q wave in lead III may be as deep as 8 mm in small children.

Criteria for Right Ventricular Hypertrophy

1. RAD for the patient's age (Table 1-10).

2. Increased rightward and anterior QRS voltages in the presence of normal QRS duration. Increased QRS voltages in the presence of a prolonged QRS duration indicate a ventricular conduction disturbance, such as BBB or WPW preexcitation.

a. R in V1, V2, or aVR greater than the upper limits of normal for the patient's age (Table 1-13)

b. S in I and V6 greater than the upper limits of normal for the patient's age (Table 1-14)

3. Abnormal R/S ratio (Table 1-15).

a. R/S ratio in V1 and V2 greater than the upper limits of normal for age

b. R/S ratio in V6 less than 1 after 1 month of age

4. Upright T in V1 in patients older than 3 days, provided that the T is upright in the LPLs (V5, V6). Upright T in V1 is not abnormal in patients 6 years or older.

5. A q wave in V1 (qR or qRs pattern) suggests RVH.

6. In the presence of RVH, a wide QRS-T angle (≥90 degrees) with T axis outside the normal range (usually in the 0- to −90-degree quadrant) indicates a strain pattern.

7. The more independent criteria for RVH that are satisfied, the more probable RVH is. An abnormal force both rightward and anterior is stronger evidence than one that is anterior only or rightward only. For example, large S waves seen in two leads, I and V6 (rightward forces), are not as strong as a large S wave seen in lead I and a large R wave seen in V2 (reflecting both rightward and anterior forces). An example of RVH with "strain" is shown in Figure 1-23.

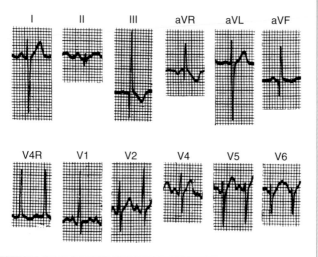

FIG. 1-23

Tracing from a 10-month-old infant with severe TOF. The tracing shows RVH with strain. There is RAD (+150 degrees). The R waves in III (22 mm) and aVR (9 mm) and the S waves in I (19 mm) and V6 (8 mm) are abnormally large, indicating RVH. The R/S ratios in V1 and V2 are abnormally large, and the ratio in V6 is smaller than the LLN (Table 1-15), also indicating RVH. The S wave is inverted in aVF, with a T axis of −10 degrees and a wide QRS-T angle (160 degrees).

Right Ventricular Hypertrophy in the Newborn

The diagnosis of RVH in the neonate is particularly difficult because of the normal dominance of the RV during that period of life. The following clues, however, are helpful.

1. S waves in lead I ≥ 12 mm.
2. R waves in aVR ≥ 8 mm.
3. The following abnormalities in V1 also suggest RVH.
a. Pure R wave (with no S wave) in V1 greater than 10 mm
b. R in V1 ≥ 25 mm
c. A qR pattern in V1 (also seen in 10% of healthy newborn infants)
d. Upright T waves in V1 in neonates older than 3 days of age (with upright T in V6)
4. RAD greater than +180 degrees.

Criteria for Left Ventricular Hypertrophy

1. LAD for the patient's age (Table 1-10).
2. QRS voltages in favor of the LV in the presence of normal QRS duration.

a. R in I, II, III, aVL, aVF, V5, or V6 greater than the upper limits of normal for age (Table 1-13)

b. S in V1 or V2 greater than the upper limits of normal for age (Table 1-14)

3. Abnormal R/S ratio: an R/S ratio in V1 and V2 less than the lower limits of normal for the patient's age (Table 1-15).

4. Q in V5 and V6, 5 mm or more, coupled with tall symmetric T waves in the same leads (volume overload type).

5. In the presence of LVH, a wide QRS-T angle ($\geq$90 degrees) with the T axis outside the normal range indicates a strain pattern. This is manifested by inverted T waves in lead I or aVF.

6. The more of the preceding independent criteria satisfied, the more probable LVH is. For example, abnormal leftward forces seen in three leads (I, V5, and V6) are not as strong as the situation in which abnormal leftward force (e.g., tall R in I) is combined with abnormal posterior forces (deep S in V2) or abnormal inferior force (tall R in aVF or tall R in II). With obstructive lesions (e.g., AS), the abnormal force is more likely inferior *(not showing LAD)*. With a volume overload (e.g., VSD), the abnormal force is more likely to the left. An example of LVH is shown in Figure 1-24.

Criteria for Biventricular Hypertrophy

Diagnosis of BVH is often difficult because the abnormal LV and RV forces are opposite in direction and therefore tend to cancel out, resulting in relatively small (or even normal) QRS forces.

1. Positive voltage criteria for RVH and LVH in the absence of ventricular conduction disturbances, such as BBB or WPW preexcitation. Many cases of large QRS voltages suggestive of BVH are seen in ventricular conduction disturbances with increased QRS duration.

2. Positive voltage criteria for RVH or LVH and large (but within normal limits) voltages for the other ventricle, again in the presence of normal QRS duration.

3. Large equiphasic QRS complexes in two or more of the limb leads and in the midprecordial leads (V2 through V5), called Katz-Wachtel phenomenon.

F. VENTRICULAR CONDUCTION DISTURBANCES

Conditions that are grouped together as ventricular conduction disturbances have in common abnormal prolongation of QRS duration (Fig. 1-25). Types of ventricular conduction disturbances and their characteristic findings include the following:

• Right and left bundle branch blocks, in which the prolongation of the QRS duration is in the terminal portion of the QRS complex (i.e., "terminal slurring") (Fig. 1-25, *B*).

• Wolff-Parkinson-White (WPW) preexcitation shows the prolongation in the initial portion of the QRS complex (i.e., initial slurring or delta wave) (Fig. 1-25, *C*).

• Intraventricular block in which the prolongation is throughout the QRS complex (see Fig. 1-25, *D*).

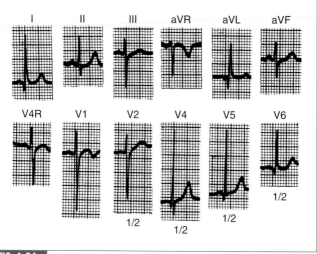

FIG. 1-24

Tracing from a 4-year-old boy with moderate VSD. The tracing shows LVH without strain pattern. The QRS axis is 0 degrees (LAD for age). The R waves in I (17 mm), aVL (12 mm), V5 (44 mm), and V6 (27 mm) are beyond the upper limits of normal, indicating abnormal LV force. The T axis (+50 degrees) is in the normal range. Note one-half standardization for some precordial leads.

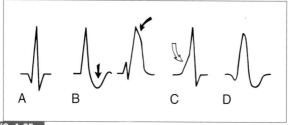

FIG. 1-25

Schematic diagram of three types of ventricular conduction disturbances. **A,** Normal QRS complex. **B,** QRS complexes in RBBB with terminal slurring *(black arrows).* **C,** Preexcitation with delta wave *(initial slurring, open arrow).* **D,** Intraventricular block in which the prolongation of the QRS complex is throughout the duration of the QRS complex. *(From Park MK: Pediatric cardiology for practitioners, ed 5, Philadelphia, 2008, Mosby.)*

The normal QRS duration varies with age (Table 1-12): In infants, QRS duration of 0.08 seconds (not 0.1, as in adults) meets the requirement for RBBB. Therefore, accurate determination of the QRS duration is necessary to diagnose ventricular conduction disturbances.

1. Right bundle branch block (RBBB). RBBB is the most common form of ventricular conduction disturbance in children. The RV depolarization is delayed with the terminal slurring of the QRS complex directed toward the RV (e.g., rightward and anteriorly). The RV depolarization is unopposed by the LV depolarization due to asynchronous depolarization of the opposing forces, and therefore the manifest QRS potentials are abnormally large, often a source of misinterpretation of the condition as ventricular hypertrophy. The same is the case with LBBB. Thus, larger QRS voltages for both the RV and the LV are seen in RBBB or LBBB.

a. Criteria for RBBB (Fig. 1-26)

    (1) RAD at least for the terminal portion of the QRS complex. The initial QRS vector is normal.

    (2) QRS duration longer than the upper limits of normal for the patient's age (Table 1-12).

    (3) Terminal slurring of the QRS complex directed to the right and usually, but not always, anteriorly.

        (a) Wide and slurred S in I, V5, and V6

        (b) Terminal, slurred R′ in aVR and the RPLs (i.e., V4R, V1, and V2), with an rsR′ pattern

    (4) ST segment shift and T wave inversion are common in adults but not in children.

    (5) It is unsafe to make a diagnosis of ventricular hypertrophy in the presence of RBBB because a greater manifest potential for both ventricles is expected to occur without actual ventricular hypertrophy as a result of asynchronous unopposed forces of the RV and LV (as explained earlier).

b. The two most common pediatric disorders that present with RBBB are ASD and conduction disturbances following open heart surgery involving a right ventriculotomy. Other conditions often associated with RBBB include Ebstein anomaly, COA in infants younger than 6 months of age, ECD, partial anomalous pulmonary venous return (PAPVR), and occasionally in normal children.

c. The significance of RBBB in children is different from that in adults. In many pediatric examples of RBBB, the right bundle is intact, unlike in adult patients with RBBB, who have abnormalities in the bundle. Although the rsR′ pattern in V1 is unusual in adults, it is normal in infants and small children, provided that:

    (1) The QRS duration is not prolonged.

    (2) The voltage of the primary or secondary R waves is not abnormally large.

2. Intraventricular block. In intraventricular block, the prolongation is throughout the duration of the QRS complex and does not resemble either

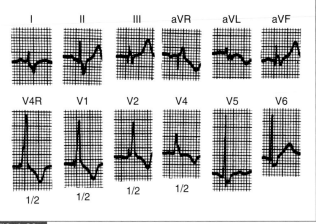

FIG. 1-26

Tracing from a 6-year-old boy who had corrective surgery for TOF that involved right ventriculotomy for repair of VSD and resection of infundibular narrowing. The QRS axis is only minimally rightward (about +115 degrees), but the terminal (slurred) portion of the QRS is clearly rightward. The QRS duration is prolonged (0.13 seconds). The T vector remains normal (+10 degrees). Although there are abnormally large R voltages in V4R, V1, and V2, with abnormal R/S ratios, one cannot make the diagnosis of an additional RVH; it may all be due to RBBB.

RBBB or LBBB (Fig. 1-25, *D*). It is associated with metabolic disorders (hyperkalemia), myocardial ischemia (e.g., during or after cardiopulmonary resuscitation), drugs (e.g., quinidine, procainamide, tricyclic antidepressants), and diffuse myocardial diseases (myocardial fibrosis and systemic diseases with myocardial involvement). Conditions seen with the intraventricular block are often more serious than those seen with BBB or WPW preexcitation.

3. Wolff-Parkinson-White preexcitation. In WPW preexcitation the initial portion of the QRS complex is slurred, with a "delta" wave (Fig. 1-25, *C*). WPW preexcitation results from an anomalous conduction pathway (i.e., bundle of Kent) between the atrium and the ventricle, bypassing the normal delay of conduction in the AV node. In the presence of this syndrome, diagnosis of ventricular hypertrophy cannot be made safely for the same reason as with BBB. Patients with WPW preexcitation are prone to attacks of paroxysmal SVT. When there is a history of supraventricular tachycardia (SVT), the diagnosis of WPW syndrome is justified.

a. Criteria for WPW syndrome.

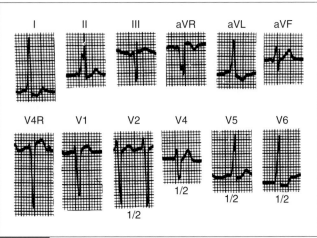

Tracing from a 6-month-old infant with possible glycogen storage disease. The QRS duration is increased to 0.1 seconds (ULN is 0.06 for age). There are delta waves in the initial portion of the QRS complex, which are best seen in I, aVL, and V5. The QRS axis is 0 degrees (LAD for age), and the large leftward and posterior QRS voltages are abnormal, but with preexcitation the diagnosis of LVH cannot be made.

(1) Short PR interval, less than the lower limits of normal for the patient's age. The lower limits of normal PR interval are as follows:

    (a) <3 years, 0.08 seconds

    (b) 3 to 16 years, 0.1 seconds

    (c) >16 years, 0.12 seconds

  (2) Delta wave (initial slurring of the QRS complex).

  (3) Wide QRS duration (beyond the ULN).

Figure 1-27 is an example of WPW preexcitation.

b. There are two other forms of preexcitation.

  (1) Lown-Ganong-Levine preexcitation is characterized by a short PR interval and normal QRS duration (without a delta wave).

  (2) Mahaim-type preexcitation is characterized by a normal PR interval and long QRS duration with a delta wave.

Ventricular Hypertrophy vs. Ventricular Conduction Disturbances

Two common pediatric ECG abnormalities, ventricular hypertrophy and ventricular conduction disturbances, often manifest with increased QRS voltages and thus are not always easy to differentiate from each other. An accurate measurement of the QRS duration is essential. The following approach may aid in separating these two conditions (Fig. 1-28).

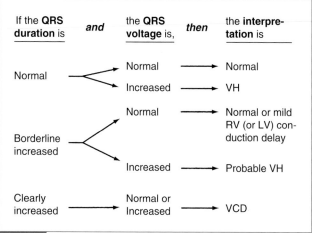

If the **QRS** duration is	*and*	the **QRS** voltage is,	*then*	the **interpre- tation** is
Normal		Normal		Normal
		Increased		VH
Borderline increased		Normal		Normal or mild RV (or LV) con- duction delay
		Increased		Probable VH
Clearly increased		Normal or Increased		VCD

FIG. 1-28

Algorithm for differentiating between ventricular hypertrophy and ventricular conduction disturbances. VCD, ventricular conductive disturbance; VH, ventricular hypertrophy.

1. When the QRS duration is normal, normal QRS voltages indicate a nor-mal ECG, and increased QRS voltages may indicate ventricular hypertrophy.
2. When the QRS duration is clearly prolonged, normal as well as in-creased QRS voltages indicate ventricular conduction disturbance. An increased QRS voltage does not indicate the presence of an additional ventricular hypertrophy.
3. When the QRS duration is only borderline increased, the separation of ventricular hypertrophy and ventricular conduction disturbances is not easy. In general, a borderline increase in the QRS voltage, especially without the terminal or initial slurring, indicates probable ventricular hypertrophy rather than conduction disturbances. The slight prolongation of the QRS duration may result from a hypertrophied ventricular myocardium, which takes lon-ger for depolarization. When the QRS voltage is normal, the ECG may be interpreted either as normal or as a mild RV or LV conduction delay.

G. PATHOLOGIC ST SEGMENT AND T WAVE CHANGES

Not all ST segment shifts are abnormal. Elevation or depression of up to 1 mm in the limb leads and up to 2 mm in the precordial leads is within normal limits.
1. **Nonpathologic ST segment shift.** Two common types of nonpathologic ST segment shifts are J depression and early repolarization. The T vector remains normal in these conditions.
a. **J depression.** J depression is a shift of the junction between the QRS complex and the ST segment (J point) without sustained ST segment depression (Fig. 1-20, *A*).

b. **Early repolarization.** In early repolarization all leads with upright T waves have elevated ST segments, and leads with inverted T waves have depressed ST segments. This condition, seen in healthy adolescents and young adults, resembles the ST segment shift seen in acute pericarditis; in the former, the ST segment is stable, and in the latter, the ST segment returns to the isoelectric line.

2. **Pathologic ST segment shift.** Abnormal shifts of the ST segment often are accompanied by T wave inversion. A pathologic ST segment shift assumes one of the following forms.

a. Downward slant followed by a diphasic or inverted T wave (Fig. 1-20, *B*).

b. Horizontal elevation or depression sustained for >0.08 seconds (Fig. 1-20, *C*).

c. Examples of pathologic ST segment shifts and T wave changes include LVH or RVH with strain, digitalis effects, pericarditis, myocarditis, and myocardial infarction.

    (1) Pericarditis. The ECG changes seen in pericarditis consist of the following:

        (a) Pericardial effusion may produce low QRS voltages (with <5 mm in every one of the limb leads).

        (b) Subepicardial myocardial damage produces the following time-dependent changes in the ST segment and T wave (Fig. 1-29).

            (i) ST segment elevation in the leads represents the LV.

            (ii) ST segment shift returns to normal within 2 or 3 days.

            (iii) T wave inversion (with isoelectric ST segment) occurs 2 to 4 weeks after the onset of pericarditis.

    (2) Myocarditis. ECG findings of rheumatic or viral myocarditis are relatively nonspecific and may involve all phases of the cardiac cycle: first- or second-degree AV block, low QRS voltages (≤5 mm in all six limb leads), decreased amplitude of the T wave, QT prolongation, and arrhythmias.

    (3) Myocardial infarction (MI). The ECG findings of myocardial infarction, which are time dependent, are illustrated in Figure 1-30. Leads that show these abnormalities vary with the location of the infarction. They are summarized in Table 1-17.

In adult patients with acute MI, the more common ECG findings are those of the early evolving phase, which consists of pathologic Q waves (abnormally wide and deep), ST segment elevation, and T wave inversion. The duration of the pathologic Q wave is ≥0.04 seconds in adults; it should be at least 0.03 seconds in children. Frequent ECG findings in children with acute MI include wide Q waves, ST segment elevation (>2 mm), and QTc prolongation (>0.44 seconds) with accompanying abnormal Q waves.

H. ELECTROLYTE DISTURBANCES

1. Calcium: Hypocalcemia produces the prolongation of the ST segment, with resulting prolongation of the QTc interval. The T wave duration remains normal. Hypercalcemia shortens the ST segment without affecting the T wave, with resultant shortening of the QTc interval (Fig. 1-31).

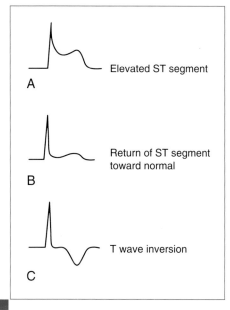

FIG. 1-29

Time-dependent changes of the ST segment and T wave in pericarditis. **A,** Acute phase with elevated ST-segment. **B,** Return of ST-segment toward the isoelectric line seen in 2 to 3 days. **C,** The T-wave inversion seen 2 to 4 weeks after the onset of pericarditis. *(From Park MK, Guntheroth WG: How to read pediatric ECGs, ed 4, Philadelphia, 2006, Mosby.)*

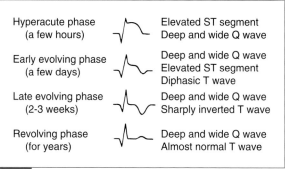

FIG. 1-30

Sequential changes in the ST segment and T wave in myocardial infarction. *(From Park MK, Guntheroth WG: How to read pediatric ECGs, ed 4, Philadelphia, 2006, Mosby.)*

TABLE 1-17

LEADS SHOWING ABNORMAL ECG FINDINGS IN MYOCARDIAL INFARCTION

	LIMB LEADS	PRECORDIAL LEADS
Lateral	I, aVL	V5, V6
Anterior		V1, V2, V3
Anterolateral	I, aVL	V2-V6
Diaphragmatic	II, III, aVF	

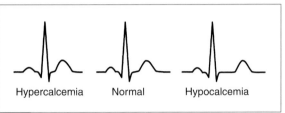

Hypercalcemia   Normal   Hypocalcemia

FIG. 1-31

ECG findings of hypercalcemia and hypocalcemia. *(From Park MK, Guntheroth WG: How to read pediatric ECGs, ed 4, Philadelphia, 2006, Mosby.)*

2. Potassium
a. Hypokalemia produces one of the least specific ECG changes. When the serum potassium K level is below 2.5 mEq/L, ECG changes consist of a prominent U wave with apparent prolongation of the QTc interval, flat or diphasic T waves, and ST segment depression (Fig. 1-32). With further lowering of serum K, the PR interval becomes prolonged, and sinoatrial block may occur.
b. A progressive hyperkalemia produces the following sequential changes in the ECG (Fig. 1-32): (1) tall, tented T waves, best seen in the precordial leads; (2) prolongation of QRS duration; (3) prolongation of PR interval; (4) disappearance of P waves; (5) wide, bizarre diphasic QRS complexes (sine wave); and (6) eventual asystole. These ECG changes are usually seen best in leads II and III and the left precordial leads.

IV. CHEST ROENTGENOGRAPHY

Information to be gained from CXR includes (1) heart size and silhouette, (2) enlargement of specific cardiac chambers, (3) pulmonary blood flow (PBF) or pulmonary vascular marking (PVM), and (4) other information regarding lung parenchyma, spine, bony thorax, abdominal situs, and so on.

A. HEART SIZE AND SILHOUETTE

1. Heart size: The cardiothoracic (CT) ratio is obtained by dividing the largest transverse diameter of the heart with the widest internal diameter of the chest (Fig. 1-33). A CT ratio of more than 0.5 is considered to indicate cardiomegaly. However, the CT ratio cannot be used with any

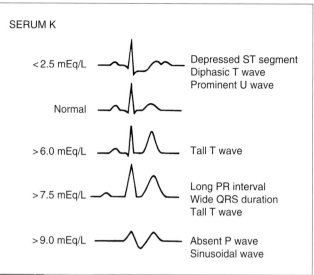

FIG. 1-32

ECG findings of hypokalemia and hyperkalemia. *(From Park MK, Guntheroth WG: How to read pediatric ECGs, ed 4, Philadelphia, 2006, Mosby.)*

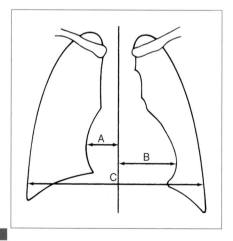

FIG. 1-33

Measurement of the cardiothoracic (CT) ratio from the posteroanterior view of a CXR. The CT ratio is obtained by dividing the largest horizontal diameter of the heart *(A + B)* by the longest internal diameter of the chest *(C)*.

accuracy in neonates and small infants, in whom a good inspiratory chest film is rarely obtained.

2. Normal cardiac silhouette: The structures that form the cardiac borders in the posteroanterior and lateral projections of a CXR are shown in Figure 1-34. In the neonate, however, a typical normal cardiac silhouette, as shown in Figure 1-34, is rarely seen because of the presence of a large thymus.

3. Abnormal cardiac silhouette: The overall shape of the heart sometimes provides important clues to the type of defect (Fig. 1-35).

a. Boot-shaped heart with decreased PVM is seen in infants with cyanotic TOF and in some infants with tricuspid atresia (Fig. 1-35, A).

b. Narrow waist and egg-shaped heart with increased PVM in a cyanotic infant strongly suggest TGA (Fig. 1-35, B).

c. Snowman sign with increased PVM is seen in infants with the supracardiac type of total anomalous pulmonary venous return (TAPVR) (Fig. 1-35, C).

B. CARDIAC CHAMBERS AND GREAT ARTERIES

1. Individual chamber enlargement

a. Left atrial enlargement (LAE): Mild LAE is best recognized in the lateral projection by posterior protrusion of the LA border (Fig. 1-36). An enlargement of the LA may produce a double density on the posteroanterior view. With further enlargement the left atrial appendage becomes prominent on the left cardiac border, and the left main-stem bronchus is elevated.

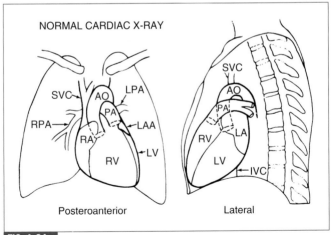

FIG. 1-34

Posteroanterior and lateral projections of normal cardiac silhouette. *(From Park MK: Pediatric cardiology for practitioners, ed 5, Philadelphia, 2008, Mosby.)*

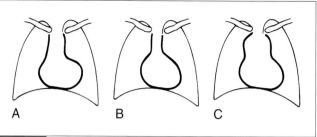

FIG. 1-35

Abnormal cardiac silhouette. **A,** Boot-shaped heart. **B,** Egg-shaped heart. **C,** Snowman sign. *(From Park MK: Pediatric cardiology for practitioners, ed 5, Philadelphia, 2008, Mosby.)*

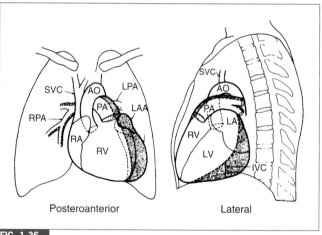

Posteroanterior   Lateral

FIG. 1-36

Posteroanterior and lateral view diagrams of CXR demonstrating an enlargement of the LA and LV, as seen in a patient with a moderate VSD. The enlargement of the LA, LV, and main PA and increased pulmonary vascular markings are present.

b. Left ventricular enlargement (LVE): In the posteroanterior view the apex of the heart is displaced to the left and inferiorly. In the lateral view the lower posterior cardiac border is displaced further posteriorly (Fig. 1-36).
c. Right atrial enlargement (RAE): In the posteroanterior projection an enlargement of the RA results in an increased prominence of the right lower cardiac border (Fig. 1-37).
d. Right ventricular enlargement (RVE): RVE is best recognized in the lateral view by the filling of the retrosternal space (Fig. 1-37).

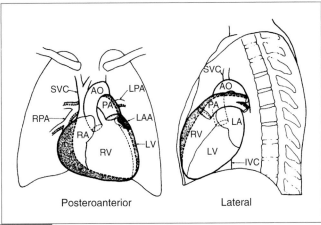

FIG. 1-37

Posteroanterior and lateral view diagrams of CXR demonstrating an enlargement of the RA and RV, as seen in a patient with a large ASD. The pulmonary vascular markings are also increased. The RV enlargement is best seen in the lateral view. AO, aorta; LAA, left atrial appendage. Other abbreviations are found on pp. ix-xi.

2. The size of the great arteries
a. Prominent main pulmonary artery (MPA) segment in the posteroanterior view is due to one of the following (Fig. 1-38, *A*):
   (1) Poststenotic dilation (e.g., pulmonary valve stenosis)
   (2) Increased blood flow through the PA (e.g., ASD, VSD)
   (3) Increased pressure in the PA (i.e., pulmonary hypertension)
   (4) Occasional normal adolescence, especially in girls
b. A concave MPA segment with resulting boot-shaped heart is seen in TOF and tricuspid atresia (Fig. 1-38, *B*).
c. Dilation of the aorta. An enlarged ascending aorta (AA) is seen in AS (poststenotic dilation) and TOF and less often in PDA, COA, or systemic hypertension. When the ascending aorta and aortic arch are enlarged, the aortic knob (AK) may become prominent on the posteroanterior view (Fig. 1-38, *C*).

C. PULMONARY VASCULAR MARKINGS

One of the major goals of radiologic examination is the assessment of the pulmonary vasculature.
1. Increased pulmonary vascular marking (PVM) is present when the pulmonary arteries appear enlarged and extend into the lateral third of the lung field, where they are not usually present, and there is an increased vascularity to the lung apices where the vessels are normally collapsed. Increased PVM in an acyanotic child suggests ASD, VSD, PDA,

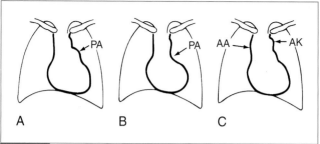

FIG. 1-38

Abnormalities of the great arteries. **A**, Prominent main PA segment. **B**, Concave PA segment. **C**, Dilation of the ascending aorta (AA) and prominence of the aortic knob (AK). *(From Park MK: Pediatric cardiology for practitioners, ed 5, Philadelphia, 2008, Mosby.)*

ECD, PAPVR, or any combination of these. In a cyanotic infant an increased PVM may indicate TGA, TAPVR, HLHS, persistent truncus arteriosus, or single ventricle.

2. A decreased PVM is suspected when the hilum appears small, the remaining lung fields appear black, and the vessels appear small and thin. Ischemic lung fields in cyanotic patients suggest critical stenosis or atresia of the pulmonary or tricuspid valves or TOF.

3. Pulmonary venous congestion, which is characterized by a hazy and indistinct margin of the pulmonary vasculature, is seen with HLHS, MS, TAPVR, cor triatriatum, and so on.

4. Normal pulmonary vasculature is present in patients with mild to moderate PS and in patients with small L-R shunt lesions.

D.   SYSTEMATIC APPROACH

The interpretation of CXRs should include a systematic routine to avoid overlooking important anatomic changes relevant to cardiac diagnosis.

1. Location of the liver and stomach gas bubble: The cardiac apex should be on the same side as the stomach or opposite the hepatic shadow. When there is heterotaxia, with the apex on the right and the stomach on the left, or vice versa, the likelihood of a serious heart defect is great. A midline liver is associated with asplenia (Ivemark) syndrome or polysplenia syndrome.

2. Skeletal aspect of CXR: Pectus excavatum may create the false impression of cardiomegaly in the posteroanterior projection. Thoracic scoliosis and vertebral abnormalities are frequent findings in cardiac patients. Rib notching is a specific finding of COA in a child usually older than 5 years, generally seen between the fourth and eighth ribs.

3. Identification of the aorta: When the descending aorta is seen on the left of the vertebral column, a left aortic arch is present. When the

descending aorta is seen on the right of the vertebral column, a right arch is present. A right aortic arch is frequently associated with TOF or persistent truncus arteriosus. A figure 3 in a heavily exposed film or an E-shaped indentation in a barium esophagogram is seen with COA.

4. Upper mediastinum: The thymus is prominent in healthy infants and may give a false impression of cardiomegaly. A narrow mediastinal shadow is seen in TGA or DiGeorge syndrome. A snowman figure (figure 8 configuration) is seen in infants (usually older than 4 months) with supracardiac TAPVR.

5. Pulmonary parenchyma: A long-standing density, particularly in the right lower lung field, suggests bronchopulmonary sequestration. A vertical vascular shadow along the right lower cardiac border may suggest PAPVR from the lower lobe (the scimitar syndrome).

V. FLOWCHART

A flowchart that often helps in arriving at a diagnosis of CHD is shown in Box 1-2. It is based on the presence or absence of cyanosis and the status of pulmonary blood flow (PBF). Ventricular hypertrophy on the ECG further narrows the possibilities. Only common entities are listed in the flowchart.

Using the flowchart often requires certain adjustments. For example, in some instances when the PVM on CXR films may be interpreted as normal or the upper limits of normal, the list of defects in the flowchart may need

---

BOX 1-2

FLOWCHART FOR THE DIAGNOSIS OF CONGENITAL HEART DEFECTS

ACYANOTIC DEFECTS

INCREASED PBF
    LVH or BVH: VSD, PDA, ECD
    RVH: ASD (often RBBB), PAPVR, Eisenmenger physiology (secondary to VSD, PDA, and so on)

NORMAL PBF
    LVH: AS or AR, COA, endocardial fibroelastosis, MR
    RVH: PS, COA in infants, MS

CYANOTIC DEFECTS

INCREASED PBF
    LVH or BVH: Persistent truncus arteriosus, single ventricle, TGA + VSD
    RVH: TGA, TAPVR, HLHS

DECREASED PBF
    BVH: TGA + PS, truncus with hypoplastic PA, single ventricle + PS
    LVH: Tricuspid atresia, pulmonary atresia with hypoplastic RV
    RVH: TOF, Eisenmenger physiology (secondary to ASD, VSD, PDA), Ebstein anomaly (RBBB)

BVH, biventricular hypertrophy; ECD, endocardial cushion defect. Other abbreviations are listed on pp. ix-xi.

to be checked under both normal and increased PBF. Likewise, an ECG may show RV dominance yet not meet strict criteria for RVH. Such a case may need to be treated as RVH. It should also be remembered that normal ECG and normal PVM on CXR do not rule out CHD. In fact, many mild acyanotic heart defects do not show abnormalities on the ECG or CXR films. Diagnosis of these defects rests primarily on the physical examination, particularly auscultation, and other special tools of cardiac evaluation.

Special Tools in Cardiac Evaluation

A number of special tools are available to the cardiologist in the evaluation of cardiac patients. Noncardiologists have access to some noninvasive tools, such as echocardiography, exercise stress test, and ambulatory ECG (e.g., Holter monitor). Magnetic resonance imaging (MRI) and computed tomography (CT) are other noninvasive tools that have become popular in recent years. Cardiac catheterization and angiocardiography are invasive tests. Although catheter intervention procedures are not diagnostic, they are included here because they are usually performed with cardiac catheterization.

I. ECHOCARDIOGRAPHY

Echocardiography (echo) is an extremely useful, safe, and noninvasive test used in the diagnosis and management of heart disease. Echo studies, which use ultrasound, provide anatomic diagnosis as well as functional information, especially with the incorporation of Doppler echo and color flow mapping.

A. M-MODE ECHOCARDIOGRAPHY

The M-mode echo provides an "ice-pick" view of the heart. It has limited capability in demonstrating the spatial relationship of structures but remains an important tool in the evaluation of certain cardiac conditions and functions, particularly by measurements of dimensions and timing. It is usually performed as part of two-dimensional echo studies.

Figure 2-1 shows three important structures of the left side of the heart that are imaged using the M-mode echo. The following are some applications of the M-mode echo.

- Measurement of the dimensions of cardiac chambers and vessels, thickness of the ventricular septum and free walls
- LV systolic function (e.g., fractional shortening, ejection fraction)
- Study of the motion of the cardiac valves (e.g., MVP, MS) and the interventricular septum
- Detection of pericardial fluid

1. **Normal M-mode echo values.** The dimensions of the cardiac chambers and the aorta are measured during diastole, coincident with the onset of the QRS complex; the LA dimension and LV systolic dimension are exceptions (see Fig. 2-1). Table 2-1 shows normal M-mode values of cardiac chamber size, wall thickness, and aortic size, according to the patient's weight. More detailed normal values of chamber

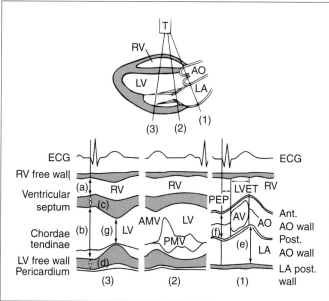

FIG. 2-1

Cross-sectional view of the left side of the heart along the long axis *(top)* through which ice-pick views of the M-mode echo recordings are made *(bottom)*. *(a)*, RV dimension. *(b)*, LV diastolic dimension (Dd). *(c)*, Thickness of ventricular septum. *(d)*, Thickness of posterior free wall. *(e)*, LA dimension. *(f)*, Aortic dimension. *(g)*, LV systolic dimension (Ds). AMV, Anterior mitral valve; PMV, posterior mitral valve; LVET, LV ejection time; PEP, preejection period. *(From Park MK: Pediatric cardiology for practitioners, ed 5, Philadelphia, 2008, Mosby.)*

dimensions and LV wall thickness by stand-alone M-mode echo are shown according to body surface area in Appendix D (Table D-1). M-mode echo measurement of the aortic annulus, LA, and LV dimensions as part of a two-dimensional study are shown by age in Table D-2. Table D-3 shows M-mode echo measurements of the LA and LV dimensions by height.

2. **Left ventricular systolic function**

a. Fractional shortening

   (1) Fractional shortening (or shortening fraction) is derived by the following:

$$FS(\%) \equiv Dd - Ds/Dd \times 100,$$

   where *FS* is fractional shortening, *Dd* is end-diastolic dimension of the LV, and *Ds* is end-systolic dimension of the LV. This is a reliable

TABLE 2-1
NORMAL M-MODE ECHO VALUES (MM) BY WEIGHT (LB): MEAN (RANGES)

	0-25 LB	26-50 LB	51-75 LB	76-100 LB	101-125 LB	126-200 LB
RV Dimension	9 (3-15)	10 (4-15)	11 (7-18)	12 (7-16)	13 (8-17)	13 (12-17)
LV Dimension	24 (13-32)	34 (24-38)	38 (33-45)	41 (35-47)	43 (37-49)	49 (44-52)
LV Free Wall (or Septum)	5 (4-6)	6 (5-7)	7 (6-7)	7 (7-8)	7 (7-8)	8 (7-8)
LA Dimension	17 (7-23)	22 (17-27)	23 (19-28)	24 (20-30)	27 (21-30)	28 (21-37)
Aortic Root	13 (7-17)	17 (13-22)	20 (17-23)	22 (19-27)	23 (17-27)	24 (22-28)

Modified from Feigenbaum H: *Echocardiography*, ed 5, Philadelphia, 1995, Lea & Febiger.

LA, left atrium; LV, left ventricle; RV, right ventricle.

and reproducible index of LV systolic function, provided there is no regional wall-motion abnormality or abnormal motion of the interventricular septum.

(2) Normal FS is 36% (range 28% to 44%). Fractional shortening is decreased in a poorly compensated LV regardless of cause (e.g., pressure overload, volume overload, primary myocardial disorders, doxorubicin cardiotoxicity, and so on). It is increased in volume-overloaded ventricle (e.g., VSD, PDA, AR, MR) and pressure overload lesions (e.g., moderately severe AS, HOCM).

b. Ejection fraction. Ejection fraction relates to the change in volume of the LV with cardiac contraction. It is obtained by the following formula:

$$EF(\%) \equiv (Dd)^3 - (Ds)^3/(Dd)^3 \times 100,$$

where *EF* is ejection fraction and *Dd* and *Ds* are end-diastolic and end-systolic dimensions, respectively, of the LV. In the preceding formula the minor axis is assumed to be half of the major axis of the LV; this assumption is incorrect in children. Normal mean ejection fraction is 66% (range 56% to 78%).

c. Systolic time intervals

(1) The method of measuring left preejection period (LPEP) and left ventricular ejection time (LVET) is shown in the lower right panel of Figure 2-1. The preejection period usually reflects the rate of pressure rise in the ventricle during isovolumic systole (i.e., dp/dt). The ratio of preejection period to ventricular ejection time for both right and left sides is little affected by changes in the heart rate.

(2) Normal values (and ranges) for the RV and LV are as follows:
   (a) RPEP/RVET, 0.24 (0.16 to 0.3)
   (b) LPEP/LVET, 0.35 (0.3 to 0.39)

B. TWO-DIMENSIONAL ECHOCARDIOGRAPHY

The two-dimensional (2D) echo has an enhanced ability to demonstrate the spatial relationship of cardiovascular structures. The Doppler and color mapping study has added the ability to easily detect valve regurgitation and cardiac shunts during the echo examination. It also provides some quantitative information such as pressure gradients across cardiac valves and estimation of pressures in the great arteries and ventricles.

Routine 2D echo is obtained from four transducer locations: parasternal, apical, subcostal, and suprasternal notch positions. Sometimes, abdominal and subclavicular views are also obtained. Figures 2-2 through 2-10 illustrate selected standard images of the heart and great vessels. Selected normal dimensions of cardiac chambers and the great arteries are presented in Appendix D. Table D-4 shows the dimensions of the aorta and pulmonary arteries. Table D-5 shows the aortic root dimensions. Table D-6 shows the mitral and tricuspid valve annulus dimensions, and Table D-7 shows the valve annulus in the neonate.

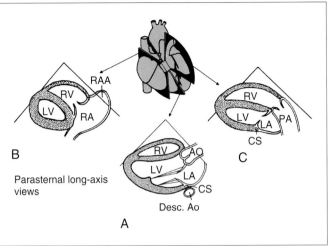

FIG. 2-2

Diagram of 2D echo views obtained from the parasternal long-axis transducer position. Standard long-axis view **(A)**, RV inflow view **(B)**, and RV outflow view **(C)**. AO, aorta; CS, coronary sinus; Desc. Ao, descending aorta; LA, left atrium; LV, left ventricle; PA, pulmonary artery; RA, right atrium; RAA, right atrial appendage; RV, right ventricle. *(From Park MK:* Pediatric cardiology for practitioners, *ed 5, Philadelphia, 2008, Mosby.)*

C. COLOR FLOW MAPPING

A color-coded Doppler provides images of the direction and disturbances of blood flow superimposed on the echo structural image. In general, red is used to indicate flow toward the transducer and blue is used to indicate flow away from the transducer. A turbulent flow appears as light green. This is useful in the detection of shunt or valvular lesions. Color may not appear when the direction of flow is perpendicular to the ultrasound beam.

D. DOPPLER ECHOCARDIOGRAPHY

A Doppler echo combines the study of cardiac structure and blood flow profiles. Doppler ultrasound equipment detects frequency shifts and thus determines the direction and velocity of blood flow with respect to the ultrasound beam. By convention, velocities of red blood cells moving toward the transducer are displayed above a zero baseline; those moving away from the transducer are displayed below the baseline. The Doppler echo is usually used with color flow mapping (see following) to enhance the technique's usefulness.

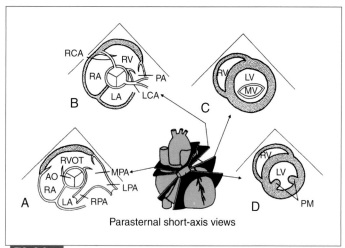

Parasternal short-axis views

FIG. 2-3

Diagram of a family of parasternal short-axis views. Semilunar valves and great artery level **(A)**, coronary arteries **(B)**, mitral valve level **(C)**, and papillary muscle level **(D)**. AO, aorta; LA, left atrium; LCA, left coronary artery; LPA, left pulmonary artery; LV, left ventricle; MPA, main pulmonary artery; MV, mitral valve; PM, papillary muscle; RA, right atrium; RCA, right coronary artery; RPA, right pulmonary artery; RV, right ventricle; RVOT, right ventricular outflow tract. *(From Park MK:* Pediatric cardiology for practitioners, *ed 5, Philadelphia, 2008, Mosby.)*

The two commonly used Doppler techniques are continuous wave and pulsed wave. The pulsed wave (PW) emits a short burst of ultrasound, and the Doppler echo receiver "listens" for returning information. The continuous wave (CW) emits a constant ultrasound beam with one crystal, and another crystal continuously receives returning information. The pulsed-wave Doppler can control the site at which the Doppler signals are sampled, but the maximal detectable velocity is limited, making it unusable for quantification of severe obstruction. In contrast, continuous-wave Doppler can measure extremely high velocities (e.g., for the estimation of severe stenosis), but it cannot localize the site of the sampling; rather, it picks up the signal anywhere along the Doppler beam. When these two techniques are used in combination, clinical application expands.

Normal Doppler velocities in children and adults are shown in Table 2-2. Normal Doppler velocity is less than 1 m/sec for the pulmonary valves, but it may be up to 1.8 m/sec for the ascending and descending aortas. With stenosis of the atrioventricular valves, the flow velocity of the E and A waves increases (Fig. 2-11). Normally, the E wave is taller than the A wave, except for the first 3 weeks of life, during which the A

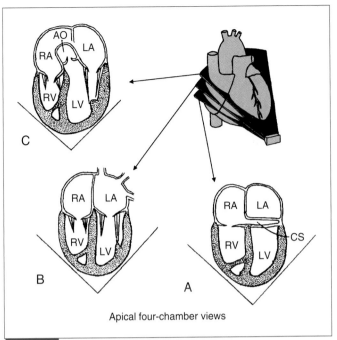

Apical four-chamber views

FIG. 2-4

Diagram of 2D echo views obtained with the transducer at the apical position.
A, A posterior plane view showing the coronary sinus. **B,** The standard apical four-chamber view. **C,** The apical "five-chamber" view is obtained with further anterior angulation of the transducer. AO, aorta; CS, coronary sinus; LA, left atrium; LV, left ventricle; RA, right atrium; RV, right ventricle. *(From Park MK: Pediatric cardiology for practitioners, ed 5, Philadelphia, 2008, Mosby.)*

wave may be taller than the E wave. In normal subjects 11 to 40 years of age, mitral Doppler indexes are as follows (mean ± SD). The average peak E velocity is 0.73 ± 0.09 m/sec, the average peak A velocity is 0.38 ± 0.089 m/sec, and the average E:A velocity ratio is 2.0 ± 0.5.

1. Measurement of pressure gradients
a. The simplified Bernoulli equation can be used to estimate the pressure gradient across a stenotic lesion, regurgitant lesion, or shunt lesion. One may use one of the following equations:

$$P_1 - P_2 \text{ (mm Hg)} \equiv 4(V_2^2 - V_1^2),$$

$$P_1 - P_2 \text{ (mm Hg)} = 4(V \, max)^2,$$

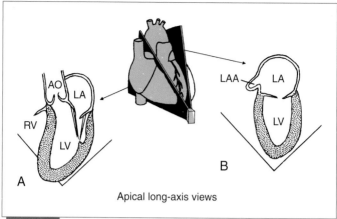

FIG. 2-5

Apical long-axis views. **A,** Apical "three-chamber" view. **B,** Apical "two-chamber" view. AO, aorta; LA, left atrium; LAA, left atrial appendage; LV, left ventricle; RV, right ventricle. *(From Park MK:* Pediatric cardiology for practitioners, *ed 5, Philadelphia, 2008, Mosby.)*

where $(P_1 - P_2)$ is the pressure difference across an obstruction, V_1 is the velocity (m/sec) proximal to the obstruction, and V_2 is the velocity (m/sec) distal to the obstruction in the first equation. When V_1 is less than 1 m/sec, it can be ignored, as in the second equation. However, when V_1 is more than 1.5 m/sec, it should be incorporated in the equation to obtain a more accurate estimation of pressure gradients. This is important in the study of the ascending and descending aortas where flow velocities are often more than 1.5 m/sec. Ignoring V_1 may significantly overestimate pressure gradient in patients with aortic stenosis or coarctation of the aorta.

b. The pressure gradient calculated from the Bernoulli equation is the peak instantaneous pressure gradient, *not* the peak-to-peak pressure gradient measured during cardiac catheterization. The peak instantaneous pressure gradient is in general larger than the peak-to-peak pressure gradient. The difference between the two is more noticeable in patients with mild to moderate obstruction and less apparent in patients with severe obstruction.

2. **Prediction of intracardiac or intravascular pressures.** The Doppler echo allows estimation of pressures in the RV, PA, and LV using the flow velocity of valvular or shunt jets. The following are some examples of such applications.

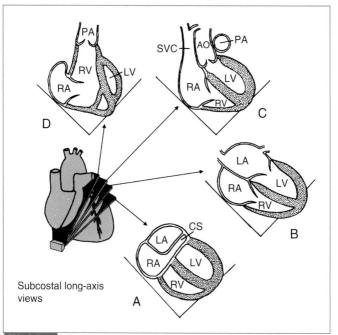

FIG. 2-6

Diagram of subcostal long-axis views. **A,** Coronary sinus view posteriorly. **B,** Standard subcostal four-chamber view. **C,** View showing the left ventricular outflow tract and the proximal aorta. **D,** View showing the right ventricular outflow tract and the proximal main pulmonary artery. AO, aorta; CS, coronary sinus; LA, left atrium; LV, left ventricle; PA, pulmonary artery; RA, right atrium; RV, right ventricle; SVS, superior vena cava. *(From Park MK: Pediatric cardiology for practitioners, ed 5, Philadelphia, 2008, Mosby.)*

a. RV (or PA) systolic pressure (SP) can be estimated from the velocity of the tricuspid regurgitation (TR) jet, if present, by the following equation:

$$RVSP \text{ (or } PASP) \equiv 4(V)^2 + RA \text{ pressure,}$$

where V is the TR jet velocity. For example, if the TR velocity is 2.0 m/sec, the instantaneous pressure gradient is $4 \times (2.0)2 \equiv 4 \times 4.0 \equiv 16$ mm Hg. Using an assumed RA pressure of 10 mm Hg, the RV systolic pressure (or PA systolic pressure in the absence of PS) is 26 mm Hg. The upper limit of normal Doppler-estimated PA systolic pressure is about 37 mm Hg.

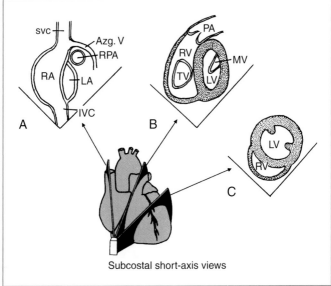

Subcostal short-axis views

FIG. 2-7

Subcostal short-axis (sagittal) views. **A,** Entry of venae cavae with drainage of the azy-gous vein. **B,** View showing the RV, RVOT, and pulmonary artery. **C,** Short-axis view of the ventricles. Azg. V, azygous vein; LA, left atrium; LV, left ventricle; MV, mitral valve; PA, pulmonary artery; RA, right atrium; RPA, right pulmonary vein; RV, right ventricle; SVC, superior vena cava; TV, tricuspid valve. *(From Park MK: Pediatric car-diology for practitioners, ed 5, Philadelphia, 2008, Mosby.)*

b. RV (or PA) systolic pressure can also be estimated from the velocity of the VSD jet by the following equation:

$$RVSP \text{ (or } PASP) \equiv \text{Systemic } SP \text{ (or arm } SP) - 4(V)^2$$

where V is the VSD jet. For example, if the VSD jet flow velocity is 3 m/sec, the instantaneous pressure drop between the LV and RV is $4 \times 3^2 = 36$ mm Hg. That is, the RV systolic pressure is 36 mm Hg lower than the LV systolic pressure. If the arm systolic blood pressure is 90 mm Hg (which is close to but usually higher than the LV systolic pressure), the RV pressure is estimated to be $90 - 36 = 54$ mm Hg. In the absence of PS, the PA systolic pressure will be approximately 54 mm Hg.

3. **Diastolic function.** Signs of diastolic dysfunction may precede those of systolic dysfunction. Using mitral inflow velocities obtained in the apical four-chamber view, LV diastolic function can be evaluated. LV diastolic

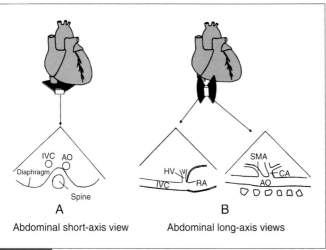

A
Abdominal short-axis view

B
Abdominal long-axis views

FIG. 2-8

Abdominal views. **A,** Abdominal short-axis view. **B,** Abdominal long-axis views. AO, aorta; CA, celiac axis; HV, hepatic vein; IVC, inferior vena cava; RA, right atrium; SMA, superior mesenteric artery. *(From Park MK:* Pediatric cardiology for practitioners, *ed 5, Philadelphia, 2008, Mosby.)*

dysfunction is easy to find but is usually nonspecific and does not provide independent diagnostic information. Two well-known patterns of abnormal diastolic function are a decreased relaxation pattern and a "restrictive" pattern (see Fig. 4-2).

II. MAGNETIC RESONANCE IMAGING AND COMPUTED TOMOGRAPHY

Rapid evolution in technology has brought other imaging methods to the arsenal of pediatric cardiologists. Complementary imaging modalities to echocardiography, magnetic resonance imaging (MRI), and computed tomography (CT) have gained momentum because they prevail over the limitations of the former technique. Both systems produce images not only of the cardiac anatomy but also of the adjacent structures. Furthermore, cardiac MRI and magnetic resonance angiography (MRA) provide information about flow dynamics and ventricular function and dimensions. As with any other technique, full knowledge of their indications and limitations is mandatory. Both of these methods are superior to echocardiography in patients with poor acoustic windows (e.g., postsurgical patients) and allow three-dimensional reconstruction. Sedation is usually not required in older children; however, younger children or uncooperative patients may require conscious sedation or general anesthesia.

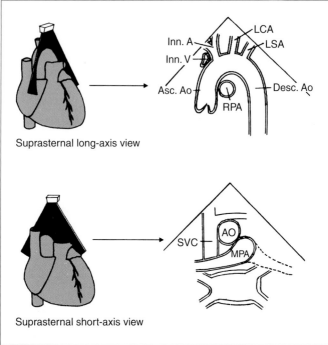

Suprasternal long-axis view

Suprasternal short-axis view

FIG. 2-9

Diagram of suprasternal notch views. *Top panel*, Long-axis view. *Bottom panel*, Short-axis view. AO, aorta; Asc. Ao, ascending aorta; Desc. Ao, descending aorta; Inn. A, innominate artery; Inn. V, innominate vein; LA, left atrium; LCA, left carotid artery; LSA, left subclavian artery; MPA, main pulmonary artery; PA, pulmonary artery; RPA, right pulmonary artery; SVC, superior vena cava. *(From Park MK:* Pediatric cardiology for practitioners, *ed 5, Philadelphia, 2008, Mosby.)*

A. MAGNETIC RESONANCE IMAGING AND MAGNETIC RESONANCE ANGIOGRAPHY

These are noninvasive alternatives to cardiac catheterization and angiography, eliminate the exposure to ionizing radiation, and reduce the procedural risks (e.g., perforation, arrhythmia, and stroke).

1. Indications
a. Evaluation of extracardiac vascular structures (e.g., systemic and pulmonary veins, pulmonary arteries, aortic arch) and their relationship to adjacent structures (e.g., vascular ring, pulmonary artery sling)
b. Evaluation of intracardiac anatomy
c. Evaluation of origin and course of coronary arteries

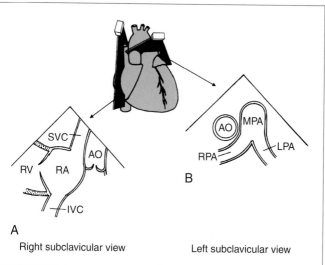

FIG. 2-10

Diagram of subclavicular views. **A,** Right subclavicular view. **B,** Left subclavicular view. AO, aorta; IVC, inferior vena cava; LPA, left pulmonary artery; MPA, main pulmonary artery; RA, right atrium; RPA, right pulmonary artery; RV, right ventricle; SVC, superior vena cava. *(From Park MK: Pediatric cardiology for practitioners, ed 5, Philadelphia, 2008, Mosby.)*

TABLE 2-2

NORMAL DOPPLER VELOCITIES IN CHILDREN AND ADULTS: MEAN (RANGES) (IN M/SEC)

	CHILDREN	**ADULTS**
Mitral Flow	1.0 (0.8-1.3)	0.9 (0.6-1.3)
Tricuspid Flow	0.6 (0.5-0.8)	0.6 (0.3-0.7)
Pulmonary Artery	0.9 (0.7-1.1)	0.75 (0.6-0.9)
Left Ventricle	1.0 (0.7-1.2)	0.9 (0.7-1.1)
Aorta	1.5 (1.2-1.8)	1.35 (1.0-1.7)

From Hatle L, Angelsen B: *Doppler ultrasound in cardiology,* ed 2, Philadelphia, 1985, Lea & Febiger.

d. Evaluation of surgically created vascular connections (e.g., S-P shunts, Glenn shunt)

e. Evaluation of ventricular dimensions and function

f. Evaluation of flow dynamics

g. Evaluation of myocardial abnormalities (e.g., ischemic myocardium, RV arrhythmogenic cardiomyopathy, LV noncompaction)

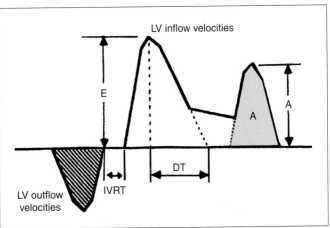

FIG. 2-11

Selected parameters of diastolic function. A, second peak velocity; DT, deceleration time; E, early peak velocity; IVRT, isovolumic relaxation time; LV, left ventricle. *(From Park MK: Pediatric cardiology for practitioners, ed 5, Philadelphia, 2008, Mosby.)*

h. Evaluation of pericardium (e.g., pericardial effusion, constrictive pericarditis)

2. Contraindications and limitations

a. Contraindicated in patients with implanted pacemaker and automated implantable cardioverter-defibrillator (may cause pacer malfunction, arrhythmia, or heat generation at the tip of the electrode).

b. Contraindicated in patients with intracranial, intraocular, or intracochlear metallic object.

c. Implanted intracardiac or intravascular devices (e.g., stents, coils) may produce significant artifacts but are usually not contraindicated (some authorities recommend that MRI should be delayed for 6 weeks after deployment of the device).

d. ECG gating is required for cardiac imaging; tachycardia and some arrhythmias limit optimal image acquisition.

e. Claustrophobic patients may require sedation.

f. Procedure is lengthy.

B. COMPUTED TOMOGRAPHY AND COMPUTED TOMOGRAPHY ANGIOGRAPHY

The introduction of ultrafast 64-multidetector spiral CT scanners (commercial availability of 256-slice scanners is on the horizon), with their superior temporal and spatial resolution, has provided physicians with an accurate and noninvasive tool to visualize the minute cardiovascular structures of children. This has resulted in short study time, obviating the need for sedation even in some neonates. Unlike MRI, CT and CT angiography are not contraindicated in patients with implanted pacemakers or ferromagnetic devices.

1. Indications
a. Evaluation of extracardiac vascular structures (e.g., systemic and pulmonary veins, pulmonary arteries, aortic arch) and their relationship to adjacent structures (e.g., vascular ring, pulmonary artery sling). This modality is superior to MRI for evaluation of patients with vascular stents (fewer artifacts).
b. Evaluation of origin and course of the coronary arteries.
c. Evaluation of surgically created vascular connections (e.g., S-P shunts, Glenn shunt).
d. Evaluation of ventricular dimensions and function.
e. Evaluation of pericardium (e.g., pericardial effusion, constrictive pericarditis).
f. Rapid assessment of the lungs and airways in conjunction with cardiac evaluation.
g. Less iodinated contrast (2 mL/kg) is necessary compared with the quantity required for cardiac catheterization ($\approx$ 4 to 5 mL/kg).
h. Short study time.

2. Contraindications and limitations
a. Angiography is relatively contraindicated in patients with renal insufficiency. Patients may need to be hydrated with IV normal saline or isotonic sodium bicarbonate. Adjunctive medications such as antioxidant N-acetylcysteine or ascorbic acid (vitamin C) may have beneficial effect. One such regimen is continuous IV infusion of 154 mEq/L sodium bicarbonate in D_5W (at 3 mL/kg/hr IV for 1 hour immediately before, and at 1 mL/kg/hr during and for 6 hours after contrast exposure), plus N-acetylcysteine (1200 mg PO every 12 hours on the day before and on the day of the study). Of note is that these recommendations to prevent contrast-induced nephropathy are from studies performed in adults.
b. Contraindicated in patients with allergy to iodinated contrast material.
c. Contraindicated in pregnancy.
d. Exposure to ionizing radiation.
e. Need of withholding potentially nephrotoxic medications (e.g., nonsteroidal anti-inflammatory drugs, cyclosporine, vancomycin, amphotericin, metformin-containing medications [e.g., Glucophage®]).
f. For optimal imaging, ECG gating is required; some arrhythmias limit optimal image acquisition. ECG gating will be suboptimal if heart rate is higher than 110 beats per minute (may require β-receptor blockade to decrease heart rate).
g. Respiratory artifacts.

III. EXERCISE STRESS TESTING

Exercise stress testing plays an important role in the evaluation of cardiac symptoms by quantifying the severity of the cardiac abnormality and assessing the effectiveness of management. Although some exercise laboratories have developed bicycle ergometer protocols, the treadmill protocols, such as Bruce protocol, are well standardized and widely used because most hospitals have treadmills.

During upright dynamic exercise in normal subjects, the heart rate, cardiac index, and mean arterial pressure increase. The systemic vascular resistance drops, and blood flow to the exercising leg muscles greatly increases. Heart rate increase is the major determinant of increased cardiac output seen during exercise. During *dynamic exercise,* systolic blood pressure increases but diastolic and mean arterial pressures remain nearly identical. On the contrary, with *isometric exercise,* both systolic and diastolic pressures increase.

A. MONITORING DURING EXERCISE STRESS TESTING

During exercise stress testing, the patient is continually monitored for symptoms such as chest pain or faintness, ischemic changes or arrhythmias on the ECG, oxygen saturation, and responses in heart rate and blood pressure.

1. **Endurance time.** There is a high correlation between maximal Vo_2 and endurance time and thus endurance time is the best predictor of exercise capacity in children. Endurance data from a recently published U.S. study are presented in Table 2-3.

TABLE 2-3

PERCENTILES OF ENDURANCE TIME (MIN) BY BRUCE TREADMILL PROTOCOL

AGE GROUP (YR)	PERCENTILES					MEAN ± SD
	10	25	50	75	90	
Boys						
4-5	6.8	7.0	8.2	10.0	12.7	8.9 ± 2.4
6-7	6.6	7.7	9.6	10.4	13.1	9.6 ± 2.3
8-9	7.0	9.1	9.9	11.1	15.0	10.2 ± 2.5
10-12	8.1	9.2	10.7	12.3	13.2	10.7 ± 2.1
13-15	9.6	10.3	12.0	13.5	15.0	12.0 ± 2.0
16-18	9.6	11.1	12.5	13.5	14.6	12.2 ± 2.2
Girls						
4-5	6.8	7.2	7.4	9.1	10.0	8.0 ± 1.1
6-7	6.5	7.3	9.0	9.2	12.4	8.7 ± 2.0
8-9	8.0	9.2	9.8	10.6	10.8	9.8 ± 1.6
10-12	7.3	9.3	10.4	10.8	12.7	10.2 ± 1.9
13-15	6.9	8.1	9.6	10.6	12.4	9.6 ± 2.1
16-18	7.4	8.5	9.5	10.1	12.0	9.5 ± 2.0

From Chatrath R, Shenoy R, Serratto M et al: Physical fitness of urban American children, *Pediatric Cardiol* 23:608-612, 2002.

2. **Heart rate.** Heart rate is measured from the electrocardiographic (ECG) signal. The maximal heart rate ranges between 188 and 210. Heart rate declines abruptly during the first minute of recovery to 140s to 150s. Inadequate increments in heart rate may be seen with sinus node dysfunction, in congenital heart block, and after cardiac surgery. An extremely high heart rate at low levels of work may indicate physical decondition or marginal circulatory compensation.

3. **Blood pressure.** Blood pressure (BP) is measured in the arm with an auscultatory method or oscillometric devices. Accuracy of BP measurement is doubtful during exercise. Systolic pressure usually rises to as high as 180 mm Hg, and rarely in excess of 200 mm Hg, with little change in diastolic pressure. During recovery, BPs return to baseline in about 10 minutes.

a. Systolic pressure in the arm may rise very high, to the level that is considered hypertensive emergency, but the arm systolic pressure probably does not reflect the central aortic pressure. The high systolic pressure in the arm may be caused by the peripheral amplification of systolic pressure due to vasoconstriction in the nonexercising arm. The central aortic pressure is likely to be much lower than the arm systolic pressure in most cases. Thus, the usefulness of arm BP in assessing CV function during upright exercise is questionable. It has been shown that when the radial artery systolic pressure is over 230 mm Hg, the aortic pressure is only 160 mm Hg in healthy young adults.

b. However, failure of BP to rise to the expected level may be significant, which may reflect an inadequate increase in cardiac output, such as that seen with cardiomyopathy, LVOT obstruction, coronary artery diseases, or ventricular or atrial arrhythmias.

4. **ECG monitoring.** The major reasons for ECG monitoring are to detect exercise-induced arrhythmias and ischemic changes.

a. Exercise-induced arrhythmias: Arrhythmias that increase in frequency or begin with exercise are usually significant. Occurrence of serious ventricular arrhythmias may be an indication to terminate the test.

b. ST segment depression is the most common manifestation of exercise-induced myocardial ischemia. For children, down-sloping or sustained horizontal depression of the ST segment of 2 mm or greater when measured at 80 ms after the J point is considered abnormal (see Fig. 1-20).

c. If the ST segment is depressed at rest, an additional depression of 1 mm or greater should be present to be significant. Specificity of the exercise ECG is poor in the presence of ST-T abnormalities on a resting ECG or with digoxin use. When there is an abnormal depolarization (such as BBB, ventricular pacemaker, or WPW preexcitation), interpretation of ST segment displacement is impossible.

5. **Oximetry.** Normal children maintain oxygen saturation greater than 90% during maximal exercise when monitored by pulse oximetry. Desaturation (<90%) is considered an abnormal response and may reflect pulmonary,

cardiac, or circulatory compromise. Children who received lateral tunnel Fontan operation with fenestration may desaturate during exercise due to R-L shunt through the fenestration.

B. INDICATIONS FOR EXERCISE STRESS TESTING IN CHILDREN

1. To evaluate specific signs or symptoms that are induced or aggravated by exercise
2. To assess or identify abnormal responses to exercise in children with cardiac, pulmonary, or other organ disorders, including the presence of myocardial ischemia and arrhythmias
3. To assess efficacy of specific medical or surgical treatments
4. To assess functional capacity for recreational, athletic, and vocational activities
5. To evaluate prognosis, including both baseline and serial testing measurements
6. To establish baseline data for institution of cardiac, pulmonary, or musculoskeletal rehabilitation

C. CONTRAINDICATIONS

Absolute contraindications include patients with acute myocardial or pericardial inflammatory diseases or patients with severe obstructive lesions in whom surgical intervention is clearly indicated. Patients with pulmonary hypertension, documented long QT syndrome, uncontrolled hypertension, unstable arrhythmias, Marfan syndrome, and those who have undergone heart transplantation are at high risk (and they may be relative contraindications).

D. TERMINATION OF EXERCISE TESTING

Three general indications to terminate an exercise test are (1) when diagnostic findings have been established and further testing would not yield any additional information, (2) when monitoring equipment fails, and (3) when signs or symptoms indicate that further testing may compromise the patient's well-being. The following are some indications for termination of exercise testing in the pediatric age group.

1. Failure of heart rate to increase or a decrease in ventricular rate with increasing workload associated with symptoms (such as extreme fatigue, dizziness)
2. Progressive fall in systolic pressure with increasing workload
3. Severe hypertension, >250 mm Hg systolic or 125 mm Hg diastolic, or BP higher than can be measured by the laboratory equipment
4. Dyspnea that the patient finds intolerable
5. Symptomatic tachycardia that the patient finds intolerable
6. Progressive fall in oxygen saturation to <90% or a 10-point drop from resting saturation in a patient who is symptomatic
7. Presence of ≥3 mm flat or downward-sloping ST segment depression
8. Increasing ventricular ectopy with increasing workload
9. Request by patient to terminate the study

E. ALTERNATIVE STRESS TESTING PROTOCOLS

1. Exercise-induced bronchospasm provocation

a. Exercise in cold or dry air typically induces airway obstruction in asthmatic patients. Bronchial reactivity is measured while a subject exercises for 5 to 8 minutes on a treadmill. The exercise protocol used should increase the heart rate to 80% of predicted maximum within 2 minutes; the usual incremental workload used in many exercise tests is not appropriate because, if the intensity of exercise is raised slowly, the patient may develop refractoriness to bronchospasm. Starting with stage 4, Bruce protocol may be appropriate.

b. Exercise is preceded by baseline spirometry. Spirometry is repeated immediately after exercise and again at minutes 5, 10, and 15 of recovery. Most pulmonary function test nadirs occur within 5 to 10 minutes after exercise. Declines of 12% to 15% in FEV_1 are typically diagnostic.

2. **Six-minute walk test.** This test may be used in children with moderate to severe exercise limitation to follow disease progression or when measuring the effectiveness of medical interventions. The patient is encouraged to try to cover as many laps on a measured course (often 30 m) as possible in 6 minutes. Oxygen saturation and heart rate are monitored before, during, and after the test. The total distance walked is the primary outcome. At least two practice tests performed on a separate day are advisable.

IV. LONG-TERM ELECTROCARDIOGRAM RECORDING

Long-term ECG recording is the most useful method to document and quantify the frequency of arrhythmias, correlate the arrhythmia with the patient's symptoms, and evaluate the effect of antiarrhythmic therapy.

Ambulatory ECG monitoring is obtained for the following reasons.

• To determine whether symptoms such as chest pain, palpitation, or syncope are caused by cardiac arrhythmias

• To evaluate the adequacy of medical therapy for an arrhythmia

• To screen high-risk cardiac patients (such as those with hypertrophic cardiomyopathy or those in postoperative status after operations known to predispose to arrhythmias (e.g., Fontan-type operation)

• To evaluate possible intermittent pacemaker failure in patients who have an implanted pacemaker

• To determine the effect of sleep on potentially life-threatening arrhythmias

There are several different types of long-term ECG recorders.

1. Holter recording: The Holter monitoring records the heart rhythm continuously for 24 hours, using ECG electrodes attached on the chest. This type of recording is useful when the child has symptoms almost daily.

2. Event recorders: Event monitors are devices used by patients for a longer period (weeks to months, typically 1 month). The monitor is used

when symptoms suggestive of an arrhythmia occur infrequently. Two general types of cardiac event monitors are available.

a. Looping memory (presymptom) event monitor. Two electrodes are attached on the chest. The monitor is always on but will store the patient's rhythm only when the patient or caregiver pushes the button. Most monitors will save the rhythm for 30 seconds before the device is activated.

b. Postsymptom event monitor. It does not have electrodes that are attached to the chest. One type is worn on the wrist like a watch. When symptoms occur, a button is pressed to start the recording. The other type is a small device that has small metal discs that function as the electrodes. When symptoms occur, the device is pressed against the chest to start the recording.

3. Implantable loop recorder: This device is indicated in patients with very infrequent symptoms, such as once every 6 months. Implantable loop recorders, about the size of a pack of chewing gum, are implanted beneath the skin in the upper left chest. The patient uses a handheld activator to record and permanently store the cardiac rhythm when symptoms occur. The device can be "interrogated" through the skin to determine what the heart was doing when the symptoms occurred.

V. AMBULATORY BLOOD PRESSURE MONITORING

Blood pressure is not a static variable; it changes not only from daytime to nighttime but also from minute to minute. In some patients there is a transient elevation of BP when BP is measured in a health care facility (i.e., "white coat hypertension"). This could lead to an overdiagnosis of hypertension and to unnecessarily aggressive and costly diagnostic studies and treatment. Some researchers advocate the use of ambulatory BP monitoring (ABPM) in all patients with casual BP elevation.

In ABPM, BP is measured multiple times during a predefined period in the patient's normal living environment during both awake and sleep periods, thus helping to identify those with "white coat hypertension." Typically, BP measurements are programmed to occur every 20 minutes during awake periods and every 30 to 60 minutes during expected sleep periods. Although the advantages of ABPM are clear, there are still some technical difficulties and problems with normative ambulatory BP levels in children.

There are three basic calculations of ABPM.

1. The *mean BP value* can be determined for the entire 24-hour period or for awake and sleep periods separately.

2. Alternatively, the *BP load* can be calculated. BP load is the percentage of BP readings for a given period that exceeds the 95th percentile of normal for the individual patient.

3. The *percent sleep decline* in BP (nocturnal dipping) is calculated by subtracting the mean sleep BP from the mean awake BP and dividing this value by the mean awake BP. Normal nocturnal dipping is at least 10% of mean awake BP. Nondipping (defined as a decline of <10%) has

been associated with hypertensive end-organ injury, end-stage renal disease, renal transplantation, or insulin-dependent diabetes mellitus. Black children have higher sleep BP levels and less significant decreases in BP during sleep compared with age-matched white counterparts.

VI. CARDIAC CATHETERIZATION AND ANGIOCARDIOGRAPHY

Cardiac catheterization and angiocardiography are the definitive invasive diagnostic tests for most cardiac patients. They are carried out under sedation. For neonates, cyanotic infants, and hemodynamically unstable children, general anesthesia with intubation may be employed.

A. INDICATIONS

Indications for these invasive studies vary from institution to institution and from cardiologist to cardiologist. With improved capability of noninvasive techniques (2D echo and color flow Doppler studies), many cardiac problems are adequately diagnosed and managed without the invasive studies. The following are considered indications by most but not all cardiologists.

1. Selected neonates with cyanotic CHD who may require palliative surgery or balloon atrial septostomy during the procedure
2. Selected children with CHD when the lesion is severe enough to require surgical intervention
3. Children who appear to have had unsatisfactory results from cardiac surgery
4. Infants and children with lesions amenable to balloon angioplasty or valvuloplasty

B. SEDATION

The following sedatives have been used singly or in combination by different institutions with equally good success rates. In general, smaller doses of sedatives are used in cyanotic infants.

1. General anesthesia is often used in the newborn and cyanotic infants.
2. For infants less than 10 kg, a combination of chloral hydrate, 75 mg/kg (maximum 2 g) PO, and diphenhydramine, 2 mg/kg (maximum 100 mg) PO, has been used with good results.
3. For older children, Demerol compound, a solution containing 25 mg/mL of meperidine (Demerol), 12.5 mg/mL of promethazine (Phenergan), and 12.5 mg/mL of chlorpromazine (Thorazine) is popular. The dose of the Demerol compound is 0.11 mL/kg IM. Some centers exclude chlorpromazine from the mixture. In cyanotic children the dose is reduced by one third. For children with severe CHF the dose is reduced by half.
4. A combination of meperidine 1 mg/kg and hydroxyzine (Vistaril) 1 mg/kg IM, or of fentanyl 1.25 μg/kg and droperidol 62.5 μg/kg IM, gives an equally good result.
5. Ketamine, 3 mg/kg IM or 1 to 2 mg/kg IV, may be used, but it can change the hemodynamic data because it increases the systemic vascular resistance and blood pressure.

6. Morphine 0.1 to 0.2 mg/kg administered subcutaneously has been used in cyanotic infants to prevent or treat hypoxic spells.

7. If more sedation is required during the study, intravenous diazepam (Valium), 0.1 mg/kg, or morphine, 0.1 mg/kg, is used.

C. NORMAL HEMODYNAMIC VALUES AND THEIR CALCULATIONS

Pressure and oxygen saturation values for normal children are shown in Figure 2-12. During cardiac catheterization, cardiac output, cardiac shunt, and vascular resistance are routinely calculated.

1. Flows (cardiac output) are calculated by the Fick formula:

$$\text{Pulmonary flow (Qp)} = \frac{Vo_2}{C_{PV} - C_{PA}},$$

$$\text{Systemic flow (Qs)} = \frac{Vo_2}{C_{AO} - C_{MV}},$$

where flows are in liters per minute, Vo_2 is oxygen consumption in milliliters per minute, C is oxygen content in milliliters per liter at the various positions; the pulmonary vein (PV), pulmonary artery (PA), aorta (AO), and mixed systemic venous blood (MV).

Oxygen consumption is either directly measured during the procedure or estimated from a table (see Appendix A, Table A-5). Oxygen content (milliliters per 100 mL of blood) is derived by multiplying oxygen capacity by percent saturation. Oxygen capacity (milliliters per 100 mL of blood) is the total

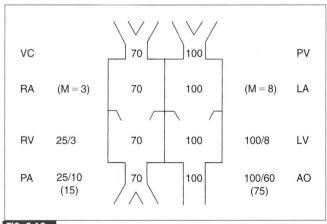

FIG. 2-12

Average pressure and oxygen saturation values in normal children. AO, aorta; LA, left atrium; LV, left ventricle; M, mean pressure; PA, pulmonary artery; PV, pulmonary vein; RA, right atrium; RV, right ventricle; VC, vena cava.

content of oxygen that hemoglobin contains when it is 100% saturated (1.36 × hemoglobin in grams per 100 mL). Normal systemic flow (or pulmonary flow in the absence of shunt) is 3.1 ± 0.4 L/min/m² (i.e., cardiac index).

2. The magnitude of the shunt is calculated as follows:

$$\text{L-R shunt} = Qp - Qs,$$

$$\text{R-L shunt} = Qs - Qp,$$

In pediatrics, the ratio of pulmonary to systemic flow (Qp/Qs), which does not require an oxygen consumption value, is often used. The ratio provides information on the magnitude of the shunt. Patients with an L-R shunt greater than 2:1 are usually candidates for surgery.

3. Vascular resistances are calculated by using formulas derived from Ohm's law ($R \equiv \Delta P/Q$):

$$\text{PVR} = \frac{\text{Mean PA pressure} - \text{Mean LA pressure}}{Qp},$$

$$\text{SVR} = \frac{\text{Mean arotic pressure} - \text{Mean RA pressure}}{Qs},$$

The normal systemic vascular resistance (SVR) varies between 15 and 30 units/m². The normal pulmonary vascular resistance (PVR) is high at birth but reaches near-adult values (1 to 3 units/m²) after 2 to 4 months. The normal ratio of PVR/SVR ranges from 1:20 to 1:10.

D.   SELECTIVE ANGIOCARDIOGRAPHY

A radiopaque dye is rapidly injected through a cardiac catheter into a certain site in the cardiovascular system, and angiograms are recorded on film, often on biplane views. Nonionizing contrast media with low osmolality (e.g., Isovue, Omnipaque) are widely used because of their low incidence of side effects. The dose of angiographic dyes for an angiogram ranges from 1 to 2 mL/kg of body weight, depending on the nature of the defect.

E.   RISKS

Cardiac catheterization and angiocardiography can lead to serious complications, including (rarely) death. Complications include serious arrhythmias, heart block, cardiac perforation, hypoxic spells, arterial obstruction, hemorrhage, infection, reactions to the contrast material, intramyocardial injection of the contrast, and renal complications (hematuria, proteinuria, oliguria, and anuria). Hypothermia, acidemia, hypoglycemia, convulsions, hypotension, and respiratory depression are more likely in the newborn infant.

In general, the risk of cardiac catheterization and angiocardiography varies with the age and illness of the patient, the type of lesion, and the experience of those doing the procedure. The reported rate of fatal complications varies from less than 1% to as high as 5% in neonates. About 3% to 5% of patients have significant nonfatal complications such as arrhythmias and arterial complications. However, careful preparation and monitoring and the use of prostaglandin infusion in selected neonates can keep the mortality and morbidity to a minimum.

F. PREPARATION AND MONITORING

Adequate preparation of the patient and careful monitoring during the procedure can minimize complications and fatality from the invasive studies. The following areas are particularly important.

1. Avoiding hypothermia when an infant is being studied, by increasing temperature in the cardiac catheterization laboratory, using a warming blanket, and monitoring rectal temperature

2. Monitoring oxygen saturation transcutaneously, checking arterial blood gases and pH, and correcting acidemia and hypoxemia; correcting hypoglycemia or hypocalcemia before the start of the procedure

3. Administering oxygen, if indicated, during the procedure

4. Intubating or readiness for intubating in infants with respiratory difficulties, and having emergency medications (e.g., atropine, epinephrine, bicarbonate) drawn up and ready

5. Initiating prostaglandin infusion in cyanotic infants who appear to have a ductus-dependent lesion

6. Whenever possible, having another physician or an anesthesiologist available to monitor noncardiac aspects of the patient

G. CATHETER INTERVENTION PROCEDURES

Catheter intervention procedures can save lives of critically ill neonates and may eliminate or delay the need for elective surgical procedures. Blood vessels and heart valves that are too small can be enlarged using balloon catheters and/or implantable devices known as stents. Too small an opening in the atrial septum can be enlarged by using a balloon or blade catheter. An opening can be created in an intact atrial septum for left-to-right or right-to-left shunt to occur. Abnormal connections within the heart (ASDs and VSDs) can be closed using innovative devices. Abnormal blood vessels (PDAs or collaterals) can also be closed using coils or plugging devices.

1. **Atrial septostomy.** In balloon atrial septostomy (Rashkind's procedure), an opening is created or enlarged in the atrial septum, using a special balloon-tipped catheter, to improve shunting at the atrial level (such as TGA, pulmonary atresia, tricuspid atresia, TAPVR, and so on). In infants older than 6 to 8 weeks of age, the atrial septum may be too thick to allow an effective balloon septostomy. In such cases, the atrial septum can be opened using a blade catheter (i.e., Park blade). The opening can then be torn further with a balloon catheter.

2. **Balloon valvuloplasty.** The balloons used in this interventional procedure are made of special plastic polymers and retain their predetermined diameters.

a. Pulmonary valve stenosis. Balloon pulmonary valvuloplasty is the treatment of choice for valvular pulmonary stenosis (PS) in children and, to a large extent, has replaced the surgical pulmonary valvotomy. Balloon valvuloplasty may be indicated in patients with Doppler peak gradient of 40 mm Hg or greater.

b. Aortic valve stenosis. This procedure is more difficult and carries a higher complication rate than does pulmonary valvuloplasty, especially for infants. The gradient reduction is less effective than for the pulmonary valve. Indications for balloon valvotomy include peak systolic pressure gradients >50 to 60 mm Hg without significant aortic regurgitation (AR). Complications include production or worsening of AR, iliofemoral artery injury and occlusion, ventricular arrhythmias, and even death in small infants.

c. Mitral stenosis. Balloon dilation valvuloplasty has been effective for rheumatic mitral stenosis (MS) but less effective for congenital MS.

d. Stenosis of prosthetic conduits and valves within conduits. The balloon dilation procedure may reduce the transconduit gradient across stenotic areas of prosthetic conduits and across valves contained within conduits.

3. **Balloon angioplasty.** Balloon catheters similar to those used in balloon valvuloplasties are used for the relief of stenosis of blood vessels. This procedure has been used for coarctation of the aorta, pulmonary artery branch stenosis, and stenosis of the systemic veins. Following the balloon procedure, some blood vessels recoil and do not maintain the dilated caliber of the vessel. Endovascular stents are sometimes used to maintain vessel patency after balloon angioplasty of any vascular structure. After stent placement, the vascular endothelium grows over the struts of the stent over several months, functionally incorporating the stent into the vessel wall. Occasionally, however, the endothelialization may go awry, resulting in a thick neointimal layer causing a functional stenosis.

a. Recoarctation of the aorta. Balloon angioplasty has become the procedure of choice for patients with postoperative residual obstruction of coarctation of the aorta. Some centers use a stent to prevent restenosis.

b. Native (or unoperated) coarctation of the aorta. Balloon angioplasty for native unoperated coarctation is controversial because the long-term effects of the procedure for native coarctation are unknown.

c. Branch pulmonary artery stenosis. The most frequent use of stent in the pediatric patient is to treat peripheral PA stenosis. Surgical treatment of peripheral PA stenosis is often impossible. Hypoplastic and stenotic branch PAs are seen with postoperative tetralogy of Fallot, pulmonary atresia, and hypoplastic left heart syndrome. When a stent is placed, an antiplatelet dose of aspirin is given for 6 months.

d. Systemic venous stenosis. The balloon procedure may be performed for obstructed venous baffles after the Senning operation for TGA.

4. **Closure techniques.** Various closure devices have been used for nonsurgical closure of ASD, PDA, and muscular VSD in the cardiac catheterization laboratory.

a. Atrial septal defect. Currently, there are several devices available; some are approved by the U.S. Food and Drug Administration (FDA) and others are in clinical trial stages. They include the Sideris buttoned device, Angel Wings ASD device, CardioSEAL device, ASDOS (Atrial Septal Defect Occluder System), Amplatzer ASD occlusion device, and modified clamshell double-umbrella device. The Amplatzer device is being used worldwide and is most popular. After the procedure an antiplatelet dose of aspirin is given for 6 months.

b. Ventricular septal defect. Successful closure of a muscular VSD, which is remote from cardiac valves, has been reported by using the double-umbrella clamshell device and others.

c. Patent ductus arteriosus. Most transcatheter PDA closures are now performed using Gianturco vascular occlusion coils. They are small, coiled wires coated with thrombogenic Dacron strands that open like a small "pigtail" when placed in the vessel. Good candidates for the coil occlusion are those children weighing 6 kg and larger with the ductus 4 mm and smaller. For a larger ductus the Amplatzer PDA occluder may be used.

d. Occlusion of collaterals and other vessels. This technique closes aorto-pulmonary collaterals (often seen with TOF), systemic arteriovenous fistulas, pulmonary arteriovenous fistulas, or surgically placed shunts that are no longer necessary. The Gianturco coil and the White balloon are examples. Peripheral embolization of the coil or balloon into the PAs or the aorta is a major risk.

Congenital Heart Defects

3

I. LEFT-TO-RIGHT SHUNT LESIONS

A. ATRIAL SEPTAL DEFECT (OSTIUM SECUNDUM ASD)

PREVALENCE. 5% to 10% of all congenital heart diseases (CHDs). Female preponderance (male-to-female ratio of 1:2).

PATHOLOGY AND PATHOPHYSIOLOGY

1. Three types of atrial septal defects (ASDs) occur in the atrial septum (Fig. 3-1). Secundum ASD is in the central portion of the septum and is the most common type (50% to 70% of ASDs). Primum ASD (or partial endocardial cushion defect [ECD]) is in the lower part of the septum (30% of ASDs). Sinus venosus defect is near the entrance of the superior vena cava (SVC) or inferior vena cava (IVC) to the right atrium (RA) (about 10% of all ASDs). Partial anomalous pulmonary venous return (PAPVR) is common with a sinus venous defect.

2. A left-to-right shunt (L-R shunt) is present through the defect, with a volume overload to the RA and right ventricle (RV) and an increase in pulmonary blood flow.

CLINICAL MANIFESTATIONS

1. The patients are usually asymptomatic.

2. A widely split and fixed S2 and a grade 2 to 3/6 systolic ejection murmur at the upper left sternal border (ULSB) are characteristic of moderate-size ASD (Fig. 3-2). With a large L-R shunt a middiastolic rumble (resulting from relative tricuspid stenosis [TS]) may be audible at the lower left sternal border (LLSB). The typical auscultatory findings are usually absent in infants and toddlers, even in those with a large defect, because the RV is poorly compliant.

3. The ECG shows right axis deviation (RAD) (+90 to +180 degrees) and mild right ventricular hypertrophy (RVH) or right bundle branch block (RBBB) with an rsR′ pattern in V1.

4. Chest x-ray (CXR) films show cardiomegaly (with right atrial enlargement [RAE] and right ventricular enlargement [RVE]), increased pulmonary vascular markings (PVMs), and a prominent main pulmonary artery (MPA) segment.

5. Two-dimensional echo shows the position and the size of the defect. Cardiac catheterization is usually not necessary.

6. Spontaneous closure of the defect occurs more than 80% of the time in patients with defects 3 to 8 mm (diagnosed by echo) before 1½ years of age. An ASD with a diameter greater than 8 mm rarely closes spontaneously. The defect may reduce in size in some patients. If the defect is

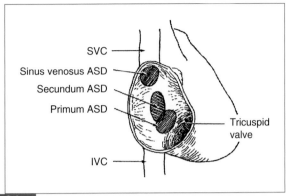

Anatomic types of atrial septal defect (ASD) viewed with the right atrial wall removed. IVC, inferior vena cava; SVC, superior vena cava. *(From Park MK: Pediatric cardiology for practitioners, ed 5, Philadelphia, 2008, Mosby.)*

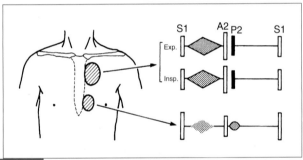

Cardiac findings of ASD. Throughout this book, heart murmurs with solid borders are the primary murmurs, and those without solid borders are transmitted murmurs or those occurring occasionally. Abnormalities in heart sounds are shown in black. Exp., expiration; Insp., inspiration.

large and left untreated, pulmonary hypertension develops in the third and fourth decades of life. Cerebrovascular accident due to paradoxical embolization through an ASD is possible.

MANAGEMENT
MEDICAL

1. Exercise restriction is not required.
2. Nonsurgical closure of the defect using a catheter-delivered closure device has become a preferred method, provided the indications are met.

These devices are applicable only to secundum ASD. The use of the closure device may be indicated for a defect measuring ≥5 mm in diameter (but <32 mm) with an adequate septal rim (4 mm), and evidence of RA and RV volume overload. Among several devices available, the Amplatzer Septal Occluder appears to be most popular. Following the device closure, the patients are placed on aspirin 81 mg per day for 6 months. Advantages of nonsurgical closure would include a hospital stay of less than 24 hours, rapid recovery, and no residual thoracotomy scar.

SURGICAL. For patients with primum ASD and sinus venosus defect, and some patients with secundum ASD for which the device closure is considered inappropriate, surgical closure is indicated when there is a significant L-R shunt with Qp/Qs of 1.5:1 or greater. Surgery is usually delayed until 2 to 4 years of age, unless congestive heart failure (CHF) develops. Open repair with a midsternal incision or minimally invasive cardiac surgical technique (with a smaller skin incision) is used. Surgical mortality rate is less than 1%. High pulmonary vascular resistance (PVR) ($10 units/m^2) is a contraindication to surgery.

POSTSURGICAL FOLLOW-UP. Atrial or nodal arrhythmias occur in 7% to 20% of patients. Occasional sick sinus syndrome requires pacemaker therapy.

B. VENTRICULAR SEPTAL DEFECT

PREVALENCE. Ventricular septal defect (VSD) is the most common form of CHD, accounting for 15% to 20% of all CHDs, not including those occurring as part of cyanotic CHD.

PATHOLOGY AND PATHOPHYSIOLOGY

1. The ventricular septum consists of a small membranous septum and a larger muscular septum. The muscular septum has three components: the inlet, infundibular, and trabecular (or simply muscular) septa (Fig. 3-3). A membranous VSD often involves a varying amount of muscular septum adjacent to it (i.e., perimembranous VSD). The perimembranous defect is more common (70%) than the trabecular (5% to 20%), infundibular (5% to 7%), or inlet defects (5% to 8%). In Far Eastern countries the infundibular defects account for about 30%.

2. The perimembranous VSD is frequently associated with patent ductus arteriosus (PDA) and coarctation of aorta (COA). The VSD seen with tetralogy of Fallot (TOF) is a large nonrestrictive perimembranous defect with extension into the subpulmonary region. The inlet VSD is typically seen with endocardial cushion defects.

3. In subarterial infundibular or supracristal VSD the aortic valve may prolapse through the VSD, with resulting aortic regurgitation (AR) and reduction of the VSD shunt. The prolapse may occasionally occur with the perimembranous VSD.

4. In VSDs with small to moderate L-R shunts, volume overload is placed on the left atrium (LA) and left ventricle (LV) (but not on the RV). With larger defects the RV is also under volume and pressure overload, in addition to a greater volume overload on the LA and LV. Pulmonary

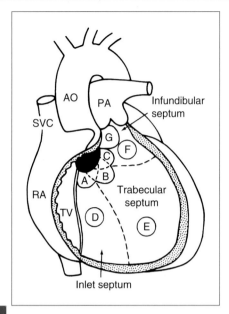

Anatomic locations of various types of VSDs, viewed with the RV free wall removed. Black area is the membranous ventricular septum. **A,** Perimembranous inlet ("AV canal-type") VSD; **B,** perimembranous trabecular (typical membranous) VSD; **C,** perimembranous infundibular ("tetralogy-type") VSD; **D,** inlet muscular VSD; **E,** trabecular muscular VSD; **F,** infundibular or outlet muscular VSD; **G,** subarterial infundibular (supracristal) VSD. AO, aorta; PA, pulmonary artery; RA, right atrium; SVC, superior vena cava; TV, tricuspid valve.

blood flow (PBF) is increased to a varying degree depending on the size of the defect and the pulmonary vascular resistance. With a large VSD, pulmonary hypertension results. With a long-standing large VSD, pulmonary vascular obstructive disease (PVOD) develops, with severe pulmonary hypertension and cyanosis resulting from a right-to-left shunt (R-L shunt). At this stage, surgical correction is nearly impossible.

CLINICAL MANIFESTATIONS

1. Patients with small VSDs are asymptomatic, with normal growth and development. With large VSDs, delayed growth and development, repeated pulmonary infections, CHF, and decreased exercise tolerance are relatively common. With PVOD, cyanosis and a decreased level of activity may result.

2. With a small VSD, a grade 2 to 5/6 regurgitant systolic murmur (holosystolic or less than holosystolic) maximally audible at the LLSB is characteristic (Fig. 3-4). A systolic thrill may be present at the LLSB. With

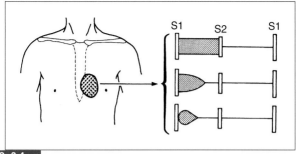

FIG. 3-4
Cardiac findings of a small VSD. A regurgitant systolic murmur is best audible at the LLSB; it may be holosystolic or less than holosystolic. Occasionally the heart murmur is in early systole. A systolic thrill may be palpable at the LLSB (*dots*). The S2 splits normally, and the P2 is of normal intensity.

a large defect, an apical diastolic rumble is audible, which represents a relative stenosis of the mitral valve due to large pulmonary venous return to the LA (Fig. 3-5). The S2 may split narrowly, and the intensity of the P2 increases if pulmonary hypertension is present (Fig. 3-5).
3. ECG findings: Small VSD, normal; moderate VSD, left ventricular hypertrophy (LVH) and left atrial hypertrophy (LAH) (±); large VSD, biventricular hypertrophy (BVH) and LAH (±); PVOD, pure RVH.

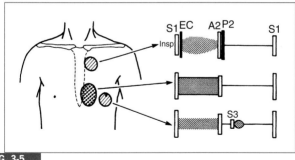

FIG. 3-5
Cardiac findings of a large VSD. A classic holosystolic regurgitant murmur is audible at the LLSB. A systolic thrill is also palpable at the same area *(dots)*. There is usually a middiastolic rumble, resulting from relative MS, at the apex. The S2 is narrowly split, and the P2 is accentuated in intensity. Occasionally an ejection click (EC) may be audible in the ULSB when associated with pulmonary hypertension. The heart murmurs shown without solid borders are transmitted from other areas and are not characteristic of the defect. Abnormal sounds are shown in black.

4. CXR films reveal cardiomegaly of varying degrees with enlargement of the LA, LV, and possibly the RV. PVMs are increased. The degree of cardiomegaly and the increase in PVMs are directly related to the magnitude of the L-R shunt. In PVOD the heart size is no longer enlarged and the MPA and the hilar pulmonary arteries are notably enlarged, but the peripheral lung fields are ischemic.

5. Two-dimensional echo studies provide accurate diagnosis of the position and size of the VSD. LA and LV dimensions provide indirect assessment of the magnitude of the shunt. Figure 3-6 shows selected 2D echo views of the ventricular septum, which helps locate the VSD position. The Doppler studies of the pulmonary artery (PA), tricuspid regurgitation (TR) (if present), and the VSD itself are useful in indirect assessment of RV and PA pressures (see Doppler Echocardiography, Chapter 2).

6. Spontaneous closure occurs in 30% to 40% of all VSDs, most often in small trabecular VSDs, more frequently in small defects than in large defects, and more often in the first year of life than thereafter. Large defects tend to become smaller with age. Inlet and infundibular VSDs do not become smaller or close spontaneously. CHF develops in infants with a large VSD but usually not until 6 or 8 weeks of age, when the PVR drops below a critical level. PVOD may begin to develop as early as 6 to 12 months of age in patients with a large VSD.

MANAGEMENT

MEDICAL. Treatment of CHF with digitalis and diuretics (see Chapter 6). No exercise restriction is required in the absence of pulmonary hypertension.

SURGICAL
1. Procedure
a. PA banding is rarely performed unless additional lesions make the complete repair difficult.
b. Direct closure of the defect is performed under cardiopulmonary bypass and/or deep hypothermia, preferably through an atrial approach rather than through a right ventriculotomy.
2. Indications and timing
a. A significant L-R shunt with Qp/Qs of greater than 2:1 is an indication for surgical closure. Surgery is not indicated for a small VSD with Qp/Qs less than 1.5:1.
b. Infants with CHF and growth retardation unresponsive to medical therapy should be operated on at any age, including early infancy. Infants with a large VSD and evidence of increasing PVR should be operated on as soon as possible. Infants who respond to medical therapy may be operated on by the age of 12 to 18 months. Asymptomatic children may be operated on between 2 and 4 years of age.
c. Contraindications: PVR/SVR ratio 0.5 or greater or PVOD with a predominant R-L shunt.
3. Surgical approaches for special situations

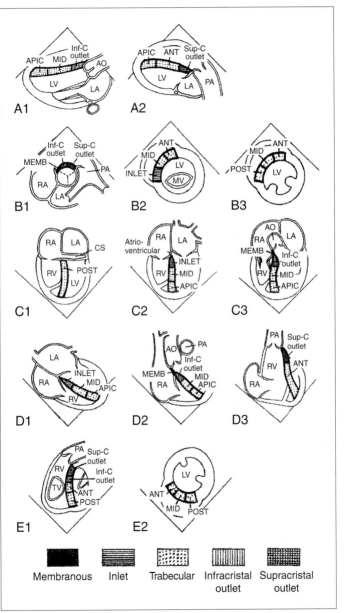

For figure legend see next page.

Selected 2D echo views of the ventricular septum. These schematic drawings are helpful in determining the site of a VSD. Different shading has been used for easy recognition of different parts of the ventricular septum. Row A, parasternal long-axis views; row B, parasternal short-axis views; row C, apical four-chamber and "five-chamber" views; row D, subcostal long-axis views; and row E, subcostal short-axis views. ANT, anterior muscular; AO, aorta; APIC, apical; CS, coronary sinus; Inf-C outlet, infracristal outlet; INLET, inlet; LA, left atrium; LV, left ventricle; MEMB, membranous; MID, midmuscular; PA, pulmonary artery; POST, posterior muscular; RA, right atrium; RV, right ventricle; Sup-C outlet, supracristal outlet. *(From Park MK: Pediatric cardiology for practitioners, ed 5, Philadelphia, 2008, Mosby.)*

a. VSD + large PDA: If PDA is large, the ductus alone may be closed in the first 6 to 8 weeks, and the VSD may be closed later. If the VSD is large and nonrestrictive, VSD should be closed early and the PDA ligated at the time of VSD repair.

b. VSD + COA: Controversies exist. One approach is the repair of COA alone initially and the VSD is closed later if indicated. Other options include COA repair and PA banding if the VSD appears large or repair of both defects at the same time using one or two incisions.

c. VSD + AR is usually associated with subarterial infundibular (or supracristal) VSD and occasionally with perimembranous VSD. When AR is present, a prompt closure of the VSD is recommended, even if the Qp/Qs is less than 2:1, to abort progression of or to abolish AR. Some centers close VSD if aortic prolapse is evident even in the absence of AR.

POSTSURGICAL FOLLOW-UP. An office follow-up should be done every 1 to 2 years. The ECG shows RBBB in 50% to 90% of the patients who had VSD repair through right ventriculotomy and in up to 40% of patients who had repair through right atrial approach.

C. PATENT DUCTUS ARTERIOSUS

PREVALENCE. 5% to 10% of all CHDs, excluding those in premature infants. PDA in premature infants is presented under a separate heading.

PATHOLOGY AND PATHOPHYSIOLOGY

1. There is a persistent postnatal patency of a normal fetal structure between the PA and the descending aorta.

2. The magnitude of the L-R shunt is determined by the diameter and length of the ductus and the level of PVR. With a long-standing large ductus, pulmonary hypertension and PVOD may develop with an eventual R-L shunt and cyanosis.

CLINICAL MANIFESTATIONS
1. Asymptomatic when the ductus is small. When the defect is large, signs of CHF may develop.
2. A grade 1 to 4/6 continuous (machinery) murmur best audible at the ULSB or left infraclavicular area is the hallmark of the condition (Fig. 3-7). An apical diastolic rumble is audible with a large-shunt PDA. Bounding peripheral pulses with wide pulse pressure are present with a large-shunt PDA.
3. ECG findings are similar to those of VSD: Normal or LVH in a small to moderate PDA; BVH in a large PDA; RVH if PVOD develops.
4. CXR findings are also similar to those of VSD: normal with a small-shunt PDA. With a large-shunt PDA, cardiomegaly (with LA and LV enlargement) and increased PVM are present. With PVOD the heart size is normal, with a marked prominence of the MPA and hilar vessels.
5. The PDA can be directly imaged and its hemodynamic significance determined by 2D echo and color flow Doppler examination. Cardiac catheterization is usually not indicated in isolated PDA.
6. CHF or recurrent pneumonia or both develop if the shunt is large. Spontaneous closure of PDA usually does not occur in term infants.

MANAGEMENT
MEDICAL
1. No exercise restriction is required in the absence of pulmonary hypertension.
2. Indomethacin is ineffective in term infants with PDA.
3. Catheter closure of the ductus may be employed. Small ductus <4 mm in diameter are closed by Gianturco stainless coils and larger ones by Amplatzer PDA device. An optimal candidate for the coil occlusion has the ductus 2.5 mm or less in size, but the use of multiple coils can close a ductus up to 5 mm. Amplatzer device may be used for PDAs ranging in size from 4 to 10 mm (with 100% closure rate). Complications may include residual

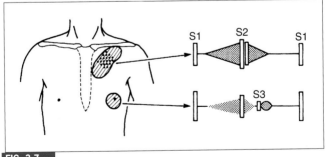

FIG. 3-7

Cardiac findings of PDA. A continuous murmur, maximally audible at the ULSB or left infraclavicular area, is a typical finding. When the shunt is large, a diastolic rumble is audible at the apex. A systolic thrill may be present in the area shown by dots.

leaks, pulmonary artery coil embolization, hemolysis, left PA stenosis, aortic occlusion with the Amplatzer device, and femoral vessel occlusion.

SURGICAL. Surgical closure is reserved for those patients in whom nonsurgical closure technique is not considered applicable. Ligation and division through left posterolateral thoracotomy without cardiopulmonary bypass is indicated for all significant PDAs. Surgical mortality is near 0%. PVOD is a contraindication to surgery. Repair through a smaller incision with video-assisted thoracoscopy is becoming popular.

POSTSURGICAL FOLLOW-UP. No restriction of activity is indicated unless pulmonary hypertension persists.

DIFFERENTIAL DIAGNOSIS. The following conditions require differentiation from PDA because they may present with a heart murmur similar to that of PDA and/or with bounding pulses.

1. Coronary atrioventricular (AV) fistula (the murmur is audible over the precordium, not at the ULSB)
2. Systemic AV fistula (a wide pulse pressure with bounding pulse, CHF, and a continuous murmur over the fistula [head or liver] are characteristic)
3. Pulmonary AV fistula (a continuous murmur over the back, cyanosis, and clubbing in the absence of cardiomegaly)
4. Venous hum (an innocent condition that disappears when the patient is supine)
5. Murmurs of collaterals in patients with COA or TOF (audible in the intercostal spaces)
6. VSD + AR (maximally audible at the mid-left sternal border [MLSB] or LLSB, it is actually a to-and-fro murmur, rather than a continuous murmur)
7. Absence of pulmonary valve (a to-and-fro murmur, or "sawing-wood sound," at the ULSB; large central pulmonary arteries on CXR films; RVH on ECG; and cyanosis)
8. Persistent truncus arteriosus (occasional continuous murmur, cyanosis, BVH on the ECG, cardiomegaly, and increased PVM on CXR films)
9. Aortopulmonary septal defect (AP window) (bounding peripheral pulses, a murmur resembling that of VSD, and signs of CHF)
10. Peripheral PA stenosis (a continuous murmur may be audible all over the thorax, unilateral or bilateral)
11. Ruptured sinus of Valsalva aneurysm (sudden onset of chest pain and severe heart failure, a continuous murmur or a to-and-fro murmur, and often Marfan features)
12. Total anomalous pulmonary venous return (TAPVR) draining into the RA (a murmur similar to venous hum along the right sternal border, mild cyanosis, RVH on ECG, and cardiomegaly with increased PVM on CXR)

D. PATENT DUCTUS ARTERIOSUS IN PRETERM NEONATES

PREVALENCE. Clinical evidence of PDA appears in 45% of infants less than 1750 g birth weight (with CHF occurring in 15%) and in about 80% of infants less than 1200 g birth weight (with CHF occurring in 40% to 50%).

PATHOPHYSIOLOGY

1. PDA is a special problem in premature infants with hyaline membrane disease. With improvement in oxygenation the PVR falls rapidly, but the ductus remains patent because its responsiveness to oxygen is immature in premature newborns. The resulting large L-R shunt makes the lung stiff, and weaning the infant from the ventilator and oxygen therapy becomes difficult.
2. If the ductus is not closed, the infant remains on ventilator therapy, with development of bronchopulmonary dysplasia and pulmonary hypertension (cor pulmonale) with right-sided heart failure.

CLINICAL MANIFESTATIONS

1. It is important to predict a significant PDA in a premature neonate in whom weaning from ventilator is delayed or fails. Episodes of apnea or bradycardia may be the initial sign of PDA in infants who are not on ventilators.
2. The physical examination reveals bounding peripheral pulses, a hyperactive precordium, and tachycardia with or without gallop rhythm. The classic continuous murmur at the left infraclavicular area or ULSB is diagnostic, but the murmur may be only systolic and is difficult to hear in infants who are on ventilators.
3. The ECG is usually normal but occasionally shows LVH.
4. CXR films show cardiomegaly and increased PVM in larger premature infants who are not intubated. In infants who are intubated and on high ventilator settings, CXR films may show the heart to be either of normal size or only mildly enlarged.
5. Two-dimensional echo and color flow Doppler studies provide accurate anatomic and functional information. Doppler studies of the ductus (with the sample volume placed at the pulmonary end of the ductus) provide important functional information, such as ductal shunt patterns (pure left-to-right, bidirectional, or predominant R-L shunt), pressures in the PA, and magnitude of the ductal shunt or pulmonary perfusion status.

MANAGEMENT. For symptomatic infants, either pharmacologic or surgical closure of the ductus is indicated. A small PDA that does not cause symptoms should be followed medically for 6 months because of the possibility of spontaneous closure.

MEDICAL

1. Fluid restriction to 120 mL/kg per day and a diuretic (e.g., furosemide, 1 mg/kg, 2 to 3 times a day) may be tried for 24 to 48 hours, but these regimens have a low success rate. Digoxin is not used because it has little hemodynamic benefit and a high incidence of digitalis toxicity.
2. Pharmacologic closure of the PDA can be achieved with intravenous administration of indomethacin, every 12 hours, a total of three doses. One example of the dosage regimens is as follows. The dose is given intravenously every 12 hours, a total of three doses. For patients younger than 48 hours old, 0.2 mg/kg is followed by 0.1 mg/kg times 2; for patients 2 to 7 days old, 0.2 mg/kg times 3; and for those older than 7 days old, 0.2 mg/kg followed by 0.25 mg/kg times 2. A second course

of indomethacin treatment is occasionally necessary to achieve adequate ductal closure. Contraindications to the use of indomethacin include high blood urea nitrogen (>25 mg/dL) or creatinine (>1.8 mg/dL) levels, low platelet count (<80,000/mm^3), bleeding tendency (including intracranial hemorrhage), necrotizing enterocolitis, and hyperbilirubinemia.

3. In Europe, intravenous ibuprofen (10 mg/kg, followed at 24-hour intervals by two doses of 5 mg/kg) is popular. Ibuprofen appears to have a significantly lower incidence of oliguria and a less deleterious effect on cerebral blood flow.

SURGICAL. If medical treatment is unsuccessful or if the use of indometha-cin is contraindicated, surgical ligation of the ductus is indicated. Many centers now perform PDA ligation in the neonatal intensive care unit at the bedside. The operative mortality is 0% to 3%. The use of minimally inva-sive video-assisted thoracoscopic surgery (VATS) is popular in the manage-ment of PDA in low-birth-weight infants.

E. COMPLETE ENDOCARDIAL CUSHION DEFECT (COMPLETE AV CANAL)

PREVALENCE. 2% of all CHDs. 30% of the defects occur in children with Down syndrome.

PATHOLOGY AND PATHOPHYSIOLOGY

1. Complete ECD consists of an ostium primum ASD, an inlet VSD, and clefts in the anterior mitral valve leaflet and in the septal leaflet of the tricuspid valve, forming common anterior and posterior cusps of the AV valve (Fig. 3-8). When the ventricular septum is intact, the defect is termed partial ECD or ostium primum ASD.

2. In complete ECD a single valve orifice connects the atrial and ventricular chambers, whereas in the partial form there are separate mitral and tricus-pid orifices. In the majority of complete ECDs the AV valve orifice is equally committed to the RV and LV. In some patients, however, the orifice is com-mitted primarily to one ventricle, with hypoplasia of the other ventricle (i.e., "unbalanced" AV canal with RV or LV dominance). Hypoplasia of one ven-tricle may necessitate one ventricular repair (Fontan-type operation).

3. Additional cardiac anomalies may include TOF (called "canal tet," occurring in 6% of patients with ECD), double-outlet right ventricle (DORV) with more than 50% overriding of the aorta (occurring in 6%), and transposition of the great arteries (TGA) (occurring in 3%). Associ-ated defects are rare in children with Down syndrome.

4. The combination of these defects may result in an interatrial and/or interventricular shunt, AV valve regurgitation, or LV-to-RA shunt. CHF with or without pulmonary hypertension usually develops early in infancy.

CLINICAL MANIFESTATIONS

1. Failure to thrive, repeated respiratory infections, and signs of CHF are common during early infancy.

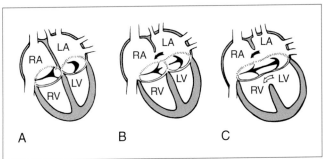

FIG. 3-8

AV valve and cardiac septa in partial and complete ECDs. **A,** Normal AV valve anatomy with no septal defects. **B,** Partial ECD with clefts in the mitral and tricuspid valves and an ostium primum ASD *(arrow).* **C,** Complete ECD. There is a common AV valve with large anterior and posterior bridging leaflets. An ostium primum ASD *(solid arrow)* and an inlet VSD *(open arrow)* are present. LA, left atrium; LV, left ventricle; RA, right atrium; RV, right ventricle.

2. Hyperactive precordium with a systolic thrill at the LLSB and a loud S2 are frequent findings. A grade 3 to 4/6 holosystolic regurgitant murmur is audible along the LLSB. The systolic murmur of mitral regurgitation (MR) may be audible at the apex. A middiastolic rumble at the LLSB or at the apex (from relative stenosis of the tricuspid and/or mitral valve) and gallop rhythm may be present.

3. The ECG finding of a "superior" QRS axis (with the axis between −40 and −150 degrees) is characteristic. RVH or RBBB is present in all, and many have LVH as well. Most patients have a prolonged PR interval (first-degree AV block).

4. CXR films always show cardiomegaly with increased PVMs.

5. Two-dimensional echo and color flow Doppler studies allow imaging of all components of ECD, as well as an assessment of the hemodynamic severity.

6. CHF occurs 1 to 2 months after birth, and recurrent pneumonia is commonly seen. Children with Down syndrome and ECD begin to develop PVOD in infancy. The survivors develop PVOD and die in late childhood or as young adults.

MANAGEMENT

MEDICAL. Medical management is recommended initially for small infants with CHF, as surgical mortality is relatively high in this age group.

SURGICAL

1. PA banding is no longer recommended unless other associated anomalies make complete repair a high-risk procedure. The mortality rate for PA banding is as high as 15%.

2. Closure of ASD and VSD and reconstruction of cleft AV valves under cardiopulmonary bypass and/or deep hypothermia are carried out between 2 and 4 months of age. Surgical mortality is 3% to 10%. Most of these infants have CHF that is unresponsive to medical therapy, and some have elevated PVR. Early surgical repair of the defect is especially important for infants with Down syndrome because of their known tendency to develop early PVOD.

3. Complications of the surgery include MR (which is persistent or has been worsened), sinus node dysfunction (with resulting bradyarrhythmias), and complete heart block (occurring in <5% of the patients).

4. Those patients with unbalanced AV canal (with hypoplasia of right or left ventricle) may be treated by an earlier PA banding and later by a modified Fontan operation.

5. In patients with "canal tet" who are severely cyanotic a systemic-to-PA shunt is carried out during infancy and a complete repair done between 2 and 4 years of age.

POSTSURGICAL FOLLOW-UP. For patients with a significant regurgitation of the AV valve or residual ventricular shunts, anticongestive medications (e.g., digoxin, diuretics, captopril, etc.) may be required. Some restriction of activities may be required if residual hemodynamic abnormalities are present.

F. PARTIAL ENDOCARDIAL CUSHION DEFECT (OSTIUM PRIMUM ASD)

PREVALENCE. 1% to 2% of all CHDs (much lower than secundum ASD).

PATHOLOGY AND PATHOPHYSIOLOGY

1. A defect is present in the lower part of the atrium septum near the AV valves, without an interventricular communication (Fig. 3-8). The anterior and posterior bridging leaflets are fused by a connecting tongue to form separate right and left AV orifices. Clefts of the mitral and occasionally of the tricuspid valve are present.

2. Less common forms of partial ECD include common atrium (which is a characteristic lesion seen in Ellis-van Creveld syndrome), VSD of the inlet septum (i.e., AV canal-type VSD), and isolated cleft of the mitral valve.

3. Pathophysiology of ostium primum ASD is similar to that of ostium secundum ASD.

CLINICAL MANIFESTATIONS

1. Usually asymptomatic during childhood.

2. Physical findings are identical to those of secundum ASD (Fig. 3-2), except for a regurgitant systolic murmur of MR, which may be present at the apex.

3. The ECG shows a "superior" QRS axis, as in complete ECD. First-degree AV block (50%) and RVH or RBBB (rsR′ pattern in V1) are common.

4. CXR findings are identical to those of secundum ASD except for the enlargement of the LA and LV when MR is significant.

5. Two-dimensional echo allows accurate diagnosis of primum ASD.

6. CHF may develop in childhood and pulmonary hypertension in adulthood. Spontaneous closure of the defect does not occur. Cardiac arrhythmias (20%) may complicate the defect.

MANAGEMENT

MEDICAL. No exercise restriction is required in asymptomatic children. Occasionally, anticongestive measures with digoxin and diuretic may be indicated.

SURGICAL. Closure of the primum ASD and reconstruction of the cleft mitral and tricuspid valves are performed electively between 2 and 4 years of age. Surgical mortality is approximately 3%.

POSTSURGICAL FOLLOW-UP. Sinus node dysfunction may develop and require pacemaker therapy.

G.   PARTIAL ANOMALOUS PULMONARY VENOUS RETURN

PREVALENCE. Less than 1% of all children with CHDs.

PATHOLOGY AND PATHOPHYSIOLOGY

1. One or more but not all pulmonary veins (PVs) drain into the RA or its venous tributaries such as the SVC, IVC, coronary sinus, or left innominate vein.

2. The right PVs are involved twice as often as the left PVs. The right PVs may drain into the SVC, often associated with sinus venous ASD, or drain into the IVC in association with an intact atrial septum and bronchopulmonary sequestration. The left PVs drain either into the left innominate vein or into the coronary sinus.

3. The hemodynamic alteration is similar to that seen with ASD. The magnitude of the pulmonary blood flow is determined by the number of anomalous PVs and the presence and size of the ASD.

CLINICAL MANIFESTATIONS

1. Children with PAPVR are usually asymptomatic.

2. Physical findings are similar to those of ASD (Fig. 3-2). When associated with ASD, the S2 is split widely and fixed. When the atrial septum is intact, the S2 is normal.

3. The ECG shows RVH or RBBB or is normal.

4. CXR films show RAE, RVE, and increased PVMs.

5. Echo diagnosis of PAPVR is less reliable.

6. If PAPVR is undetected, cyanosis and exertional dyspnea may develop during the third and fourth decades, resulting from pulmonary hypertension and PVOD.

MANAGEMENT

MEDICAL. Exercise restriction is not required.

SURGICAL

1. Surgical correction is carried out when the patient is 2 to 5 years of age. A significant L-R shunt with Qp/Qs greater than 1.5:1 or 2:1 is an indication for surgery. Isolated single lobe anomaly is not ordinarily corrected.

2. For the anomalous drainage into the SVC a tunnel is created between the anomalous vein and the ASD using a Teflon or pericardial patch and the SVC is widened to prevent obstruction of flow. For the anomalous drainage into the IVC an intraatrial tunnel drains the venous blood into the LA. When this is associated with the bronchopulmonary sequestration, the involved lobes(s) may be resected (without connecting the anomalous vein to the heart). When the left PVs drain into the coronary sinus, the sinus is unroofed and the orifice of the coronary sinus is closed.

II. OBSTRUCTIVE LESIONS

A. PULMONARY STENOSIS

PREVALENCE. 5% to 8% of children with CHDs.

PATHOLOGY AND PATHOPHYSIOLOGY

1. Pulmonary stenosis (PS) may be valvular (90%), subvalvular (infundibular), or supravalvular (i.e., stenosis of the PA). In valvular PS the pulmonary valve is thickened, with fused or absent commissures and a small orifice. A poststenotic dilation of the MPA usually develops in valvular PS. Dysplastic pulmonary valve (with thickened, irregular, immobile tissue) is frequently seen with Noonan syndrome. Infundibular PS is usually associated with a large VSD, as seen in TOF. The poststenotic dilation is not seen with subvalvular stenosis.
2. Abnormal muscular bands (running between the ventricular septum and the anterior wall) divide the RV cavity into a proximal high-pressure chamber and a distal low-pressure chamber (called "double-chambered" RV).
3. Depending on the severity of PS, a varying degree of RVH develops. The RV is usually normal in size but, with critical pulmonary stenosis, the RV is hypoplastic.
4. In general, three pathophysiologic changes occur in obstructive lesions such as PS or aortic stenosis (AS). They are (1) systolic ejection murmur on auscultation, (2) hypertrophy of the responsible ventricle, and (3) poststenotic dilation (Fig. 3-9).

CLINICAL MANIFESTATIONS

1. Usually asymptomatic with mild PS. Exertional dyspnea and easy fatigability may be seen in moderately severe cases and CHF occurs in severe cases. Neonates with critical PS are cyanotic and tachypneic.
2. An ejection click is present at the ULSB with valvular PS (Fig. 3-10). The S2 may split widely, and the P2 may be diminished in intensity. A systolic ejection murmur (grade 2 to 5/6) with or without systolic thrill is best audible at the ULSB and transmits fairly well to the back and the sides. The louder and longer the murmur, the more severe is the stenosis. Neonates with critical PS may have only a faint heart murmur, if any.
3. The ECG is normal in mild PS. RAD and RVH are present in moderate PS. RAH and RVH with "strain" pattern are present in severe PS. Neonates with critical PS may show LVH (due to hypoplastic RV and relatively large LV).

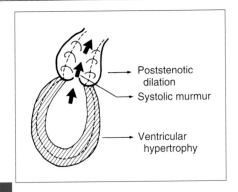

FIG. 3-9

Three secondary changes in ventricular outflow obstructive lesions that are typically seen in aortic valve stenosis and pulmonary valve stenosis.

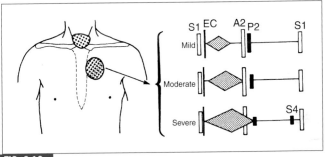

FIG. 3-10

Cardiac findings of pulmonary valve stenosis. Abnormal sounds are shown in black. Dots represent areas with systolic thrill. EC, ejection click.

4. CXR films show normal heart size and a prominent MPA segment (i.e., poststenotic dilation). PVMs are normal but may be decreased in severe PS.

5. Two-dimensional echo may show thick pulmonary valves with restricted systolic motion (doming) and a poststenotic dilation of the MPA. The Doppler study can estimate the pressure gradient across the stenotic valve.

6. The severity of the obstruction is usually not progressive in mild PS, but it tends to progress with age in moderate or severe PS. CHF may develop in patients with severe stenosis. Sudden death during heavy physical activities is possible in patients with severe stenosis.

MANAGEMENT

MEDICAL

1. For neonates with critical PS and cyanosis, prostaglandin E_1 (PGE_1) infusion to reopen the ductus should be started. Balloon valvuloplasty is the procedure of choice in critically ill neonates. Even dysplastic valves appear to mature after the procedure. Some patients require reintervention (either repeat valvuloplasty or surgery) at a later time.

2. Balloon valvuloplasty is the procedure of choice for significant pulmonary valve stenosis. Indications for the balloon procedure include (a) symptomatic patients (with angina, syncope or presyncope, and exertional dyspnea) with catheterization pressure gradient ≥ 30 mm Hg and (b) asymptomatic patients with cath gradient greater than 40 mm Hg. Cardiac catheterization is recommended in patients with a Doppler-estimated pressure gradient near 50 mm Hg. This procedure is useful even for dysplastic pulmonary valve.

3. Surgical treatment is not possible for PA branch stenosis that is within the lung parenchyma. In such cases the balloon angioplasty with balloon-expandable intravascular stent is effective (with effectiveness of 75% to 100%).

4. Restriction of activity is usually not indicated except for severe PS.

SURGICAL

1. Surgical valvotomy is occasionally indicated in patients with valvular PS in whom balloon valvuloplasty is unsuccessful.

2. Surgery is indicated in patients with dysplastic pulmonary valves that are resistant to dilation. Dysplastic valve may need to be completely excised because simple valvotomy may be ineffective.

3. Surgery is also indicated for infundibular stenosis and anomalous RV muscle bundle with significant pressure gradients.

4. If balloon valvuloplasty is unsuccessful, infants with critical PS require surgery on an urgent basis.

5. Stenosis at the main PA requires patch widening of the narrow portion.

POSTSURGICAL FOLLOW-UP. Periodic echo studies are indicated to detect recurrences of the stenosis.

B. AORTIC STENOSIS

PREVALENCE. A group of lesions that produce LV outflow tract obstruction accounts for 10% of all CHDs. Aortic valve stenosis occurs more often in males (male-to-female ratio of 4:1).

PATHOLOGY AND PATHOPHYSIOLOGY

1. Left ventricular outflow tract (LVOT) obstruction may occur at the valvular, subvalvular, or supravalvular levels (Fig. 3-11).

2. Valvular AS is caused most often by a bicuspid aortic valve (with a fused commissure) and less commonly by a unicuspid valve (with one lateral attachment) or stenosis of the tricuspid valve (Fig. 3-12). Many cases of bicuspid aortic valve are nonobstructive during childhood.

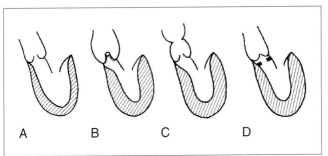

FIG. 3-11

Anatomic types of aortic stenosis. **A,** Normal. **B,** Valvular stenosis. **C,** Supravalvular stenosis. **D,** Discrete subaortic stenosis. *(Modified from Park MK: Pediatric cardiology for practitioners, ed 5, Philadelphia, 2008, Mosby.)*

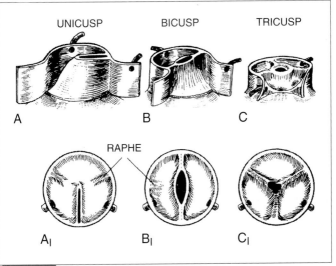

FIG. 3-12

Anatomic types of aortic valve stenosis. Top row is the side view, and bottom row is the view as seen in surgery during aortotomy. **A,** Unicuspid aortic valve. **B,** Bicuspid aortic valve. **C,** Stenosis of a tricuspid aortic valve. *(From Goor DA, Lillehei CW: Congenital malformations of the heart, New York, 1975, Grune & Stratton.)*

3. Symptomatic neonates with so-called critical neonatal aortic valve stenosis have primitive, myxomatous valve tissue, with a pinhole opening. The aortic valve ring and ascending aorta, the mitral valve, and the LV cavity are almost always hypoplastic (often requiring a Norwood operation followed by a Fontan operation).

4. Supravalvular AS occurs at the upper margin of the sinus of Valsalva. This is often associated with Williams syndrome.

5. Subvalvular (subaortic) stenosis may be in the form of simple diaphragm (discrete) or a long, tunnel-like fibromuscular narrowing (tunnel stenosis).

   a. Discrete subaortic stenosis is more common than tunnel stenosis and is often associated with other lesions such as VSD, PDA, or COA. Occasionally its development follows surgical interventions, such as closure of VSD or PA banding.

   b. Tunnel-like subaortic stenosis is often associated with hypoplasia of the valve ring and the ascending aorta. It may be a part of Shone complex (comprising supramitral ring, parachute mitral valve, subaortic stenosis, and COA).

6. Hypertrophy of the LV may develop if the stenosis is severe. A poststenotic dilation of the ascending aorta develops with valvular AS. AR usually develops in subaortic AS.

CLINICAL MANIFESTATIONS

1. Patients with mild to moderate AS are asymptomatic. Exertional chest pain or syncope may occur with severe AS. CHF develops within the first few months of life with critical AS.

2. In symptomatic infants with critical AS the heart murmur may be absent or faint, and the peripheral pulses are weak and thready.

3. Blood pressure is normal in most patients, but a narrow pulse pressure is present in severe AS. Patients with supravalvular AS may have a higher systolic pressure in the right arm than in the left (due to the jet of stenosis directed into the innominate artery, the so-called Coanda effect).

4. A systolic thrill may be present at the upper right sternal border (URSB), in the suprasternal notch, or over the carotid arteries. An ejection click may be audible with valvular AS. A harsh systolic ejection murmur (grade 2 to 4/6) is best audible at the second right intercostal space (2RICS) or third left intercostal space (3LICS) (Fig. 3-13), with good transmission to the neck and frequently to the apex. A high-pitched, early diastolic decrescendo murmur of AR may be audible in patients with bicuspid aortic valve and those with discrete subvalvular stenosis.

5. The ECG is normal in mild cases. LVH with or without a strain pattern is seen in more severe cases.

6. CXR films are usually normal in children, but a dilated ascending aorta may be seen occasionally in valvular AS. A significant cardiomegaly develops with CHF or substantial AR.

7. Echo studies are diagnostic. Two-dimensional echo may show the anatomy of the aortic valve (bicuspid, tricuspid, or unicuspid) and that of subvalvular and supravalvular AS. The Doppler-derived pressure gradient

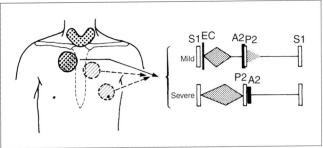

FIG. 3-13

Cardiac findings of aortic valve stenosis. Abnormal sounds are indicated in black. Systolic thrill may be present in areas with dots. EC, ejection click.

(instantaneous gradient) is approximately 20% higher than the peak-to-peak systolic pressure gradient obtained during cardiac catheterization. The degree of LV hypertrophy can be measured.

8. Mild stenosis becomes frequently more severe with time. The stenosis may worsen with aging as the result of calcification of the valve cusps (requiring valve replacement surgery in some adult patients). Progressive AR is possible in discrete subaortic stenosis.

MANAGEMENT

MEDICAL

1. In critically ill neonates and infants with CHF, anticongestive measures with fast-acting inotropic agents and diuretics, with or without PGE_1 infusion, are indicated, in preparation for either balloon valvuloplasty or surgery.

2. Serial echo-Doppler studies are needed every 1 to 2 years because AS of all severities tends to worsen with time. Exercise stress test (EST) may be indicated in asymptomatic children who want to participate in sports activities.

3. Percutaneous balloon valvuloplasty is now regarded as the first step in management of symptomatic neonates in many centers. It is also the first interventional method for children older than 1 year of age. Although the results are promising, they are not as good as those for PS. A survival rate of 50% has been reported in neonates. Serious complications (major hemorrhage, loss of femoral artery pulse, avulsion of part of the aortic valve leaflet, perforation of the mitral valve or LV) can occur. Indications for the balloon procedure are as follows:

a. Symptomatic patients (with angina, syncope, or dyspnea on exertion) with a catheterization pressure gradient ≥50 mm Hg

b. Asymptomatic patients with a catheterization pressure gradient greater than 60 mm Hg

c. Asymptomatic patients who develop ST or T wave changes on ECG at rest or during EST and who have a catheterization pressure gradient of greater than 50 mm Hg

d. Asymptomatic patients with a catheterization pressure gradient greater than 50 mm Hg when the patient wants to play competitive sports (balloon angioplasty is not indicated when the catheterization pressure gradient is <40 mm Hg)

4. Activity restrictions. No limitation in activity is required for mild AS (with peak Doppler gradient <40 mm Hg). Moderate AS (peak Doppler gradient 40 to 70 mm Hg) requires restriction from high dynamic or static competitive athletics (allowing only golf, baseball, doubles tennis, etc.). With severe AS (peak Doppler gradient >70 mm Hg), no competitive sports are allowed.

SURGICAL. Generally accepted indications for surgery and surgical procedures are as follows:

1. For valvular AS, failed balloon valvuloplasty or severe AR resulting from the procedure is an indication. A sick newborn with critical AS who has failed balloon valvuloplasty requires surgery. Surgery is indicated in children with symptoms (chest pain, syncope) with a strain pattern on the ECG or abnormal exercise test, even with a systolic pressure gradient slightly less than 50 mm Hg.

a. Either aortic valve commissurotomy, aortic valve replacement (using mechanical or biological valves), or the Ross procedure (see following) is performed. The advantage of the mechanical valve is durability, but it has the tendency of thrombus formation with a potential embolization, requiring anticoagulation (with warfarin) with its attendant risks of bleeding. Biologic valves have the advantage of a lower incidence of thromboembolism, but the deterioration occurs within a decade or two because of degeneration and calcification. For adolescent girls or women of childbearing age, homografts may be a good alternative because of the known teratogenic effects of warfarin.

b. In the Ross procedure (or pulmonary root autografts) the autologous pulmonary valve replaces the aortic valve, and an aortic or a pulmonary allograft replaces the pulmonary valve (Fig. 3-14). The pulmonary valve autograft has the advantage of documented long-term durability; it does not require anticoagulation and there is evidence of the autograft's growth. The patient's own aortic valve may be used for pulmonary position after aortic valvotomy ("double" Ross procedure).

2. For discrete subaortic stenosis, a systolic pressure gradient greater than 30 mm Hg or the onset of an AR is an indication for an elective operation. Some centers consider the mere presence of a significant membrane as an indication for surgery. Excision of the discrete membrane is performed. It is advisable to wait if possible until beyond 10 years of age because the recurrence rate of the subaortic membrane is higher before that age.

3. For tunnel-type subaortic stenosis, a pressure gradient ≥50 mm Hg is an indication. Valve replacement following aortic root enlargement (Kono procedure) may be performed.

4. For supravalvular AS, the peak pressure gradient greater than 50 to 60 mm Hg, severe LVH, or appearance of new AR is an indication for surgery.

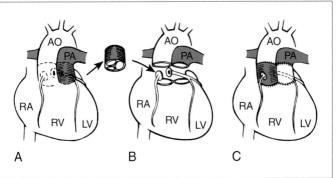

FIG. 3-14

Ross procedure (pulmonary root autograft). **A,** The two horizontal lines on the aorta (AO) and PA and two broken circles around the coronary artery ostia are lines of proposed incision. The pulmonary valve, with a small rim of right ventricle (RV) muscle, and the adjacent PA are removed. **B,** The aortic valve and the adjacent aorta have been removed, leaving buttons of aortic tissue around the coronary arteries. **C,** The pulmonary autograft is sutured to the aortic annulus and to the distal aorta, and the coronary arteries are sutured to openings made in the PA. The pulmonary valve is replaced with either an aortic or a pulmonary allograft. LV, left ventricle; RA, right atrium. *(From Park MK: Pediatric cardiology for practitioners, ed 5, Philadelphia, 2008, Mosby.)*

Widening of the stenotic area using a diamond-shaped fabric patch may be performed.

POSTSURGICAL OR POSTPROCEDURAL FOLLOW-UP
1. Annual follow-up is required for all patients who have had a balloon or surgical procedure done for the aortic valve because significant AR develops in 10% to 30% of the patients and the discrete subaortic membrane recurs in 25% to 30% after surgical resection.
2. Anticoagulation is needed after a prosthetic mechanical valve replacement. The INR should be maintained between 2.5 and 3.5 for the first 3 months and 2.0 to 3.0 beyond that time. Low-dose aspirin (81 mg per day) is also indicated in addition to warfarin.
3. After aortic valve replacement with bioprosthesis, aspirin (81 mg) is indicated (without warfarin).
4. Subacute bacterial endocarditis (SBE) prophylaxis is required after placement of prosthetic material or valve, when indications arise.
5. Restriction from competitive sports may be necessary for children with moderate residual AS and/or AR.

C.   COARCTATION OF THE AORTA

PREVALENCE. 8% to 10% of CHDs, with a male preponderance (2:1). Among patients with Turner syndrome, 30% have COA.

PATHOLOGY AND PATHOPHYSIOLOGY

1. In COA a narrowing of the upper thoracic aorta is present. There are two groups of patients with COA: one group of patients presenting symptoms early in life and the other group remaining asymptomatic.

a. In *symptomatic infants* with COA, other cardiac defects (such as aortic hypoplasia, VSD, PDA, and mitral valve anomalies) are often present. These abnormalities may have reduced antegrade flow through the aorta during fetal life and may have caused a poor development of collateral circulation around the COA.

b. In *asymptomatic children* with COA, associated anomalies are uncommon. The antegrade flow through the aorta has resulted in a pressure gradient and stimulated the development of the collateral circulation during the fetal life.

2. COA also occurs as part of other CHDs, such as TGA and DORV (e.g., Taussig-Bing abnormality).

3. As many as 85% of patients with COA have a bicuspid aortic valve.

Clinical manifestation and management of symptomatic neonates and asymptomatic children are quite different; therefore, they will be presented under separate headings.

Symptomatic Infants

CLINICAL MANIFESTATIONS

1. Signs of CHF (poor feeding, dyspnea) and renal failure (oliguria, anuria) with general circulatory shock may develop in the first 2 to 6 weeks of life.

2. A loud gallop is usually present, but heart murmur may be absent with weak and thready pulses in sick infants.

3. The ECG usually shows RVH or RBBB rather than LVH.

4. CXR films show a marked cardiomegaly and signs of pulmonary edema or pulmonary venous congestion.

5. Two-dimensional echo shows the site and extent of the COA and other associated cardiac defects. The Doppler examination reveals a disturbed flow distal to the COA and signs of delayed emptying in the proximal aorta.

6. In symptomatic infants with COA, early death from CHF and renal failure is possible.

MANAGEMENT

MEDICAL

1. Intensive anticongestive measures should be given with fast-acting inotropic agents (catechols), diuretics, and oxygen to stabilize the patient. PGE_1 infusion is indicated to reopen the ductus before any intervention takes place (see Appendix E for the dosage of PGE_1).

2. Balloon angioplasty is controversial, but it can be a useful procedure for sick infants. However, balloon angioplasty is associated with a higher rate of recoarctation (>50%) than surgical repair, and the rate of complications (including femoral artery injury) is high during infancy.

SURGICAL

1. If CHF develops, the need for surgery or nonsurgical intervention
is urgent. Surgical procedure of choice varies from institution to institution. Resection and end-to-end anastomosis (preferable when possible),
subclavian flap aortoplasty, or patch angioplasty is performed (Fig. 3-15).
The mortality rate for isolated COA is less than 5%. Postoperative renal
failure is the most common cause of death. Residual obstruction and/or
recoarctation occur in up to one third of all cases, but the recurrence rate
is lower than that following balloon angioplasty.

2. If it is associated with a VSD, one of the following procedures may be
performed.

a. If the VSD appears restrictive, COA repair only without PA banding.
   If CHF persists, VSD closure is indicated.
b. If the PA pressure remains high after completing the COA repair, PA
   banding is performed. Later VSD repair and removal of the PA band
   is performed when the patient is 6 to 24 months of age.
c. If the VSD appears nonrestrictive, repairing COA and VSD at the same
   operative setting is preferred by many centers.

POSTOPERATIVE

1. Reexamination every 6 to 12 months is indicated because recoarctation is possible, especially if surgery is performed in the first year of life.

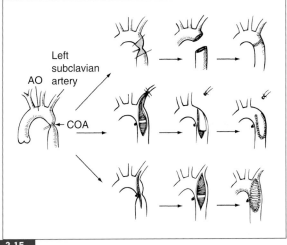

FIG. 3-15

Surgical techniques for repair of coarctation of the aorta (COA). *Top,* End-to-end anastomosis. *Middle,* Subclavian flap procedure. *Bottom,* Patch aortoplasty. AO, aorta. *(From
Park MK: Pediatric cardiology for practitioners, ed 5, Philadelphia, 2008, Mosby.)*

2. Balloon angioplasty may be performed if a significant recoarctation develops.

3. Surveillance for and treatment of systemic hypertension.

Asymptomatic Children
CLINICAL MANIFESTATIONS
1. These patients are usually asymptomatic except for rare complaints of leg pain.

2. The pulse in the leg is absent or weak and delayed. Hypertension in the arm or higher blood pressure (BP) readings in the arm than the thigh may be present. An ejection click resulting from the bicuspid aortic valve is frequently audible at the apex and/or base. A systolic ejection murmur, grade 2 to 3/6, is audible at the URSB and MLSB and in the left inter-scapular area in the back.

3. The ECG usually shows LVH, but it may be normal.

4. CXR films show a normal or slightly enlarged heart. An E sign on the barium-filled esophagus or 3 sign on overpenetrated films may be found. Rib notching may be seen in children after about 5 years of age.

5. Two-dimensional echo shows a discrete, shelflike membrane in the pos-terolateral aspect of the descending aorta. The Doppler examination reveals disturbed flow and increased flow velocity distal to the coarctation. The full Bernoulli equation (using the flow velocities proximal and distal to the coarctation site) provides more accurate assessment of the severity of the obstruction. The bicuspid aortic valve is frequently imaged.

6. The presence of PDA makes the diagnosis of COA less certain in neo-nates. In addition to the presence of a posterior shelf and BP discrepancies between the arms and the legs, the ratio of isthmus to descending aorta di-ameter (measured at the level of diaphragm) less than 0.64 strongly sug-gests COA in the presence of PDA (Lu et al. J Pediatr. 2006). Others suggest that the isthmic diameter ≤3 mm or the isthmic diameter 4 mm plus the continuous antegrade flow by Doppler is a probable sign of PDA + COA.

7. Bicuspid aortic valve may cause stenosis and/or regurgitation later in life. If a COA is left untreated, LV failure, intracranial hemorrhage, or hypertensive encephalopathy may develop in childhood or adult life.

MANAGEMENT
MEDICAL
1. Hypertension or hypertensive crisis should be detected and treated.

2. Balloon angioplasty for native (unoperated) COA is controversial. Some centers use the balloon procedure for native COA, while other cen-ters prefer a surgical approach. There appears to be a higher incidence of aortic aneurysm formation following the balloon procedure than surgery.

3. A balloon-expandable, stainless-steel stent implanted concurrently with balloon angioplasty is in the early stage of experience. An absorbable metal stent is also in the experimental stage.

SURGICAL
1. Indications for surgery

a. If severe hypertension, CHF, or cardiomegaly is present, surgery is indicated even during infancy.

b. Hypertension in the upper extremity or a large pressure gradient ≥20 mm Hg between the arms and legs is an indication for elective surgery at age of 1 to 2 years (optimal age about $1\frac{1}{2}$ years).

c. Even with a pressure gradient less than 20 mm Hg, surgery is indicated if imaging studies show the aortic diameter at the level of coarctation to be 50% or less.

2. Resection of the coarctation segment and end-to-end anastomosis constitute the procedure of choice. Other surgical options are illustrated in Figure 3-15.

POSTOPERATIVE

1. Annual examination should be performed with attention to (a) BP differences in the arms and leg (recoarctation), (b) persistence or resurgence of hypertension in the arms *and* legs, (c) status of associated abnormalities such as bicuspid aortic valve or mitral valve disease, and (d) possible development of subaortic AS.

2. Residual pressure gradient is common but usually less than 10 to 20 mm Hg.

3. If COA recurs following either surgery or angioplasty, balloon angioplasty is the procedure of choice.

D. INTERRUPTED AORTIC ARCH

PREVALENCE. 1% of critically ill infants with CHDs.

PATHOLOGY AND PATHOPHYSIOLOGY

1. This extreme form of COA is divided into three types according to the location of the interruption (Fig. 3-16).

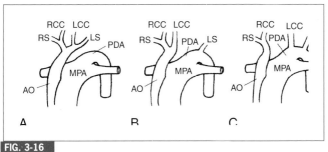

FIG. 3-16

Three types of aortic arch interruption. **A,** Type A. **B,** Type B. **C,** Type C (see text). AO, aorta; LCC, left common carotid; LS, left subclavian; MPA, main pulmonary artery; PDA, patent ductus arteriosus; RCC, right common carotid; RS, right subclavian. *(From Park MK: Pediatric cardiology for practitioners, ed 5, Philadelphia, 2008, Mosby.)*

a. In type A the interruption is distal to the left subclavian artery (occurring in 30% of patients).

b. In type B the interruption is between the left carotid and left subclavian arteries (occurs in 43% of cases). DiGeorge syndrome occurs in about 50% of patients with type B interruption.

c. In type C the interruption is between the innominate and left carotid arteries (occurs in 17% of cases).

2. PDA and VSD are almost always associated with this defect. A bicuspid aortic valve (60%), mitral valve deformity (10%), persistent truncus arteriosus (10%), or subaortic stenosis (20%) may be present.

3. DiGeorge syndrome occurs in at least 15% of these patients.

CLINICAL MANIFESTATIONS

1. Respiratory distress, cyanosis, poor peripheral pulse, or circulatory shock develops in the first few days of life.

2. Cardiac findings are nonspecific.

3. CXR films show cardiomegaly, increased PVMs, and pulmonary edema. The upper mediastinum may be narrow (due to the absence of thymus, i.e., DiGeorge syndrome).

4. The ECG may show RVH.

5. Echo studies are useful in the diagnosis of the condition. Angiocardiography is usually indicated for accurate diagnosis of the anatomy before surgery.

MANAGEMENT

1. Medical treatment consists of PGE_1 infusion (see Appendix E for dosage), intubation, and oxygen administration. Workup for DiGeorge syndrome (i.e., serum calcium) should be carried out. Citrated blood (that causes hypocalcemia by chelation) should not be transfused, and blood should be irradiated before transfusion in patients with DiGeorge syndrome.

2. Surgical repair of the interruption (primary anastomosis, Dacron vascular graft, or venous homograft) and closure of a simple VSD are recommended if possible. If the interruption is associated with complex defects, repair of the interruption and PA banding are performed, with complete repair later.

III. CYANOTIC CONGENITAL HEART DEFECTS

A. COMPLETE TRANSPOSITION OF THE GREAT ARTERIES

PREVALENCE. TGA constitutes 5% of all CHDs. It is more common in boys (3:1).

PATHOLOGY AND PATHOPHYSIOLOGY

1. The aorta (AO) and the pulmonary artery are transposed, with the AO arising anteriorly from the RV, and the PA arising posteriorly from the LV. The end result is complete separation of the two circuits, with hypoxemic blood circulating in the body and hyperoxemic blood circulating in the pulmonary circuit (Fig. 3-17). The classic complete TGA is called D-transposition, in which the aorta is located anteriorly and to the right of

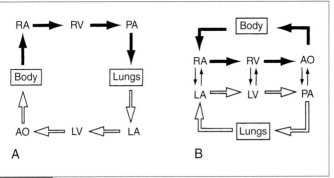

FIG. 3-17

Circulation pathways of normal serial circulation **(A)** and parallel circulation of TGA **(B).** Open arrows indicate oxygenated blood, and solid arrows, desaturated blood. AO, aorta; LA, left atrium; LV, left ventricle; PA, pulmonary artery; RA, right atrium; RV, right ventricle.

the PA, hence D-TGA. (When the transposed aorta lies to the left of the PA, it is called L-transposition.)

2. Defects that permit mixing of the two circulations, such as ASD, VSD, and PDA, are necessary for survival. A VSD is present in 40% of cases. In about 50% of the patients no associated defects are present other than patent foramen ovale (PFO), small ASD, or small PDA.

3. LVOT obstruction (subpulmonary stenosis) occurs in about 5% of the patients without VSD, either dynamic or fixed obstruction. PS occurs in 30% to 35% of patients with VSD.

4. In neonates with poor mixing of the two circulations, progressive hypoxia and acidosis result in early death, requiring an early intervention.

CLINICAL MANIFESTATIONS

1. Cyanosis and signs of CHF develop in the newborn period.

2. Severe arterial hypoxemia unresponsive to oxygen inhalation and acidosis are present in infants with poor mixing. Hypoglycemia and hypocalcemia are occasionally present.

3. Auscultatory findings are nonspecific. The S2 is single and loud. No heart murmur is audible in infants with an intact ventricular septum. When TGA is associated with VSD or PS, a systolic murmur of these defects may be audible.

4. The ECG shows RAD and RVH. An upright T wave in V1 after 3 days of age may be the only abnormality suggestive of RVH. BVH may be present in infants with large VSD, PDA, or PS.

5. CXR films show cardiomegaly with increased PVMs. An egg-shaped cardiac silhouette with a narrow superior mediastinum is characteristic.

6. Two-dimensional echo study is diagnostic. It fails to show a "circle-and-sausage" pattern of the normal great arteries in the parasternal short-axis view. Instead, it shows two circular structures. Other views reveal the PA arising from the LV and the aorta arising from the RV. Associated anomalies (VSD, LVOT obstruction, PS, ASD, and PDA) are imaged.

7. Natural history and prognosis depend on anatomy.

a. Infants with intact ventricular septum are the sickest group, but they demonstrate the most dramatic improvement following PGE_1 infusion or the Rashkind balloon atrial septostomy.

b. Infants with VSD or large PDA are the least cyanotic group but are most likely to develop CHF and PVOD (beginning as early as 3 or 4 months of age).

c. Combination of VSD and PS allows considerably longer survival without surgery, but repair surgery carries a high risk.

d. Cerebrovascular accident and progressive PVOD, particularly in infants with large VSD or PDA, are rare late complications.

MANAGEMENT

MEDICAL

1. Metabolic acidosis, hypoglycemia, and hypocalcemia should be treated if present.

2. PGE_1 infusion is started to raise arterial oxygen saturation by reopening the ductus.

3. Administration of oxygen may help raise systemic arterial oxygen saturation by lowering PVR and increasing PBF, with resulting increase in mixing.

4. A therapeutic balloon atrial septostomy (Rashkind procedure) may be performed to improve systemic oxygen saturation if immediate surgery is not planned. Occasionally, blade atrial septostomy may be performed for older infants and those for whom the initial balloon atrial septostomy is not successful.

5. Treatment of CHF with digitalis and diuretics may be indicated.

SURGICAL

1. As a definitive surgery, the right- and left-sided structures are switched at the atrial level (Senning operation), at the ventricular level (Rastelli operation), or at the great artery level (arterial switch operation).

a. Intraatrial repair surgeries (e.g., Senning operation) are no longer performed except in rare cases because of undesirable late complications (such as obstruction to the pulmonary or systemic venous return, TR, arrhythmias, and depressed RV function).

b. Rastelli operation, which redirects the pulmonary and systemic venous blood, is carried out at the ventricular level. It may be carried out in patients with VSD and severe PS. A valved conduit or a homograft is placed between the RV and the PA (Fig. 3-18). This procedure is less popular because of late complications and a high surgical mortality rate (10% and 29%). Two alternative procedures are now available: REV procedure and Nikaidoh procedure (see following for discussion of these procedures).

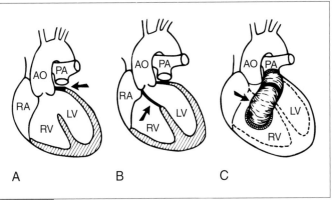

FIG. 3-18

The Rastelli operation. **A,** The PA is divided from the LV, and the cardiac end is over-sewn *(arrow)*. **B,** An intracardiac tunnel *(arrow)* is placed between the large VSD and the aorta. **C,** The RV is connected to the divided PA by an aortic homograft or a valve-bearing prosthetic conduit. AO, aorta; LV, left ventricle; PA, pulmonary artery; RA, right atrium; RV, right ventricle.

c. Arterial switch operation (ASO) is the procedure of choice (Fig. 3-19). This procedure provides anatomic correction with infrequent complications. For this procedure to be successful the LV pressure should be near systemic levels at the time of surgery, and therefore it should be performed before 3 weeks of age. Possible complications include coronary artery occlusion, supravalvular PS, supravalvular neoaortic stenosis, and AR.

d. REV procedure (réparation à l'étage ventriculaire) may be performed for patients with associated VSD and severe PS (Fig. 3-20). The procedure comprises the following: (1) infundibular resection to enlarge the VSD, (2) intraventricular baffle to direct LV output to the aorta, (3) aortic transection to perform the Lecompte maneuver (by which the right pulmonary artery [RPA] is brought anterior to the ascending aorta), and (4) direct RV-to-PA reconstruction by using an anterior patch (Fig. 3-20). Surgical mortality is 18%.

e. Nikaidoh procedure can be performed for patients with associated VSD and severe PS (Fig. 3-21). The repair consists of the following: (1) harvesting the aortic root from the RV (with attached coronary arteries in the original procedure), (2) relieving the LVOT obstruction (by dividing the outlet septum and excising the pulmonary valve), (3) reconstructing the LVOT (with posteriorly translocated aortic root and the VSD patch), and (4) reconstructing the right ventricular out-flow tract (RVOT) (with a pericardial patch or a homograft). In the modified Nikaidoh procedure, one or both coronary arteries are moved

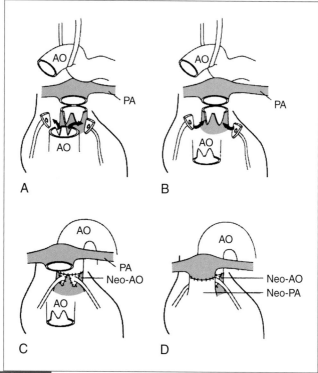

FIG. 3-19

Arterial switch operation. **A,** The aorta is transected slightly above the coronary ostia, and the main PA is transected at about the same level. The ascending aorta is lifted, and both coronary arteries are removed from the aorta with triangular buttons.
B, Triangular buttons of similar size are made at the proper position in the PA trunk.
C, The coronary arteries are transplanted to the PA. The ascending aorta is brought behind the PA and is connected to the proximal PA to form a neoaorta. **D,** The triangular defects in the proximal aorta are repaired, and the proximal aorta is connected to the PA. Note that the neopulmonary artery is in front of the neoaorta. AO, aorta; PA, pulmonary artery.

to a more favorable position as necessary (not shown) and the Lecompte maneuver is also performed (Fig. 3-21). The hospital mortality is less than 10%.

f. Damus-Kaye-Stansel operation may be performed in infants 1 to 2 years of age who have a large VSD and significant subaortic stenosis. In this procedure the subaortic stenosis is bypassed by connecting

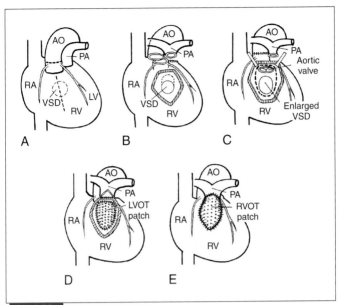

FIG. 3-20

REV procedure for patients with D-TGA + VSD + severe PS. **A,** The broken lines indicate the planned aortic and RV incision sites. The broken circle indicates a VSD. **B,** The aorta and PA have been transected and the RPA is brought anterior to the aorta (Lecompte maneuver). The proximal PA has been oversewn. The VSD is exposed through the right ventriculotomy. Dotted lines indicate the portion of the infundibular septum to be excised to enlarge the VSD. **C,** The aortic valve is well shown by retractors. The broken line indicates the planned site of a patch placement for the LV-AO connection. The transected aorta has been reconnected behind the RPA. **D,** The completed LV-to-AO tunnel is shown. The superior portion of the right ventriculotomy is sutured directly to the posterior portion of the main PA. **E,** A pericardial or synthetic patch is used to complete the RV-to-PA reconstruction. AO, aorta; LV, left ventricle; LVOT, left ventricular outflow tract; PA, pulmonary artery; RA, right atrium; RV, right ventricle; RVOT, right ventricular outflow tract; VSD, ventricular septal defect. (From Park MK: Pediatric cardiology for practitioners, ed 5, Philadelphia, 2008, Mosby.)

the proximal PA trunk to the ascending aorta. The VSD is closed, and a conduit is placed between the RV and the distal PA (Fig. 3-22). The mortality rate is considerable, ranging from 15% to 30%.

2. The indication, timing, and type of surgical treatment vary greatly from institution to institution. Figure 3-23 is a partial listing of many surgical approaches used at this time, including the timing.

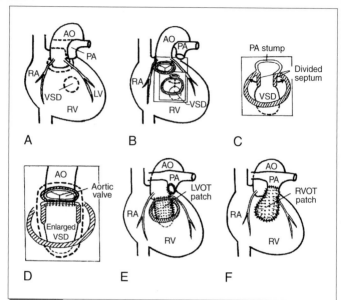

FIG. 3-21

Nikaidoh procedure (for patients with D-TGA, VSD, and severe PS). **A,** The circular broken line around the aorta is the planned incision site for aortic root mobilization. The smaller broken circle indicates a VSD. **B,** The aortic root has been mobilized by a circular incision around the aortic root, which leaves an opening in the RV free wall. The main PA is also transected. Through the opening, part of the VSD, ventricular septum, and the hypoplastic PA stump are seen. The dotted vertical line in the ventricular septum (in the smaller inset in **B**) is the planned incision through the infundibular septum. **C,** In the inset the incision in the infundibular septum has created a large opening, which includes the PA annulus and stump and the VSD. **D,** In the large inset the posterior portion of the aorta is directly sutured to the PA stump, which results in a large VSD. This completes translocation of the aorta to the original PA position. The thick, oval-shaped broken line that goes through the front of the transected aortic root is the planned site for placement of the LV outflow tract patch, which will direct the LV flow to the aorta. **E,** The completed tunnel is shown (LVOT patch, which directs the LV flow to the aorta). The distal segment of the main PA is fixed to the aorta. Some surgeons use Lecompte maneuver to bring the RPA in front of the ascending aorta (as shown here). **F,** A pericardial patch is oversewn to complete the RV-to-PA connection (RVOT patch). Abbreviations are the same as those in Figure 3-20. *(From Park MK: Pediatric cardiology for practitioners, ed 5, Philadelphia, 2008, Mosby.)*

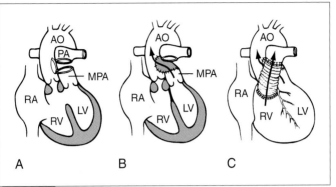

FIG. 3-22

Damus-Kaye-Stansel operation for D-TGA + VSD + subaortic stenosis. **A,** The MPA is transected near its bifurcation. An appropriately positioned and sized incision is made in the ascending aorta. **B,** The proximal MPA is anastomosed end to side to the ascending aorta, using either a Dacron tube or Gore-Tex. This channel will direct LV blood to the aorta. The aortic valve is either closed or left unclosed. **C,** Through a right ventriculotomy the VSD is closed, and a valved conduit is placed between the RV and the distal PA. This channel will carry RV blood to the PA. AO, aorta; LV, left ventricle; MPA, main pulmonary artery; PA, pulmonary artery; RA, right atrium; RV, right ventricle.

Transposition of the great arteries

- **Simple TGA** ⟶ ASO (1-3 wk)

- **TGA + other simple defects** ⟶ ASO (1-3 wk)
  (such as PDA, VSD, + Repair of other defects
  dynamic or mild PS)

- **TGA** ⟶ Shunt operation (±) ⟶ (1) VSD-AO tunnel
  + VSD (early in life) + Rastelli (>1-2 yr), or
  + severe PS (2) REV procedure (>6 mo), or
  (3) Nikaidoh operation (>1 yr)

- **TGA** ⟶ "(Initial B-T shunt [±])" ⟶ Damus-Kaye-Stansel
  + large VSD + VSD closure
  + subaortic stenosis + RV-PA connection (1-2 yr)

FIG. 3-23

Surgical approaches to TGA. ASO, arterial switch operation; BT, Blalock-Taussig; PDA, patent ductus arteriosus; PS, pulmonary stenosis; REV, réparation à l'étage ventriculaire; TGA, transposition of the great arteries; VSD, ventricular septal defect. *(From Park MK: Pediatric cardiology for practitioners, ed 5, Philadelphia, 2008, Mosby.)*

POSTSURGICAL FOLLOW-UP

1. Patients who receive an arterial switch operation need to be followed for stenosis of the anastomosis sites in the PA and AO, signs of AR, and possible coronary obstruction (such as myocardial ischemia, LV dysfunction, arrhythmias).

2. Limitation of activity may be indicated if arrhythmias or coronary insufficiency is present.

B. CONGENITALLY CORRECTED TRANSPOSITION OF THE GREAT ARTERIES (L-TGA, VENTRICULAR INVERSION)

PREVALENCE. Much less than 1% of all CHDs.

PATHOLOGY AND PATHOPHYSIOLOGY

1. Visceroatrial relationship is normal (the RA on the right of the LA). The RA empties into the anatomic LV through the mitral valve, and the LA empties into the RV through the tricuspid valve. For this to occur the LV lies to the right of the RV (i.e., ventricular inversion). The great arteries are transposed, with the aorta arising from the RV and the PA arising from the LV. The aorta lies to the left of and anterior to the PA (hence L-TGA). The final result is a functional correction in that oxygenated blood coming into the LA goes out the aorta (Fig. 3-24).

2. Theoretically, no functional abnormalities exist, but unfortunately most cases are complicated by associated defects. VSD (occurring in 80%)

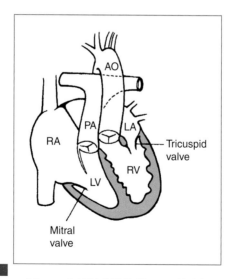

FIG. 3-24

Diagram of congenitally corrected TGA (L-TGA). AO, aorta; LA, left atrium; LV, left ventricle; PA, pulmonary artery; RA, right atrium; RV, right ventricle.

and PS (in 50%) with or without VSD are common, resulting in cyanosis. Regurgitation of the systemic AV valve (tricuspid) occurs in 30% of the patients. Varying degrees of AV block, which are sometimes progressive, and supraventricular tachycardia (SVT) are also frequent.

3. The cardiac apex is in the right chest (dextrocardia) in about 50% of patients.

CLINICAL MANIFESTATIONS

1. Patients with associated defects are symptomatic during the first few months of life with cyanosis (VSD + PS) or CHF (large VSD). Patients without associated defects are asymptomatic.

2. The S2 is single and loud. A grade 2 to 4/6 harsh holosystolic murmur along the LLSB may indicate a VSD or the systemic AV valve (tricuspid) regurgitation. A grade 2 to 3/6 systolic ejection murmur at the ULSB or URSB may indicate PS.

3. Characteristic ECG findings are the absence of Q waves in V5 and V6 and/or the presence of Q waves in V4R or V1. Varying degrees of AV block, including complete heart block, may be present. Atrial and/or ventricular hypertrophy may be present in complicated cases.

4. CXR films may show a characteristic straight left upper cardiac border (formed by the ascending aorta). Cardiomegaly and increased PVMs suggest associated VSD. Dextrocardia is frequent (50%).

5. Two-dimensional echo is diagnostic of the condition and associated defects.

6. TR develops in about 30% of patients. Progressive AV conduction disturbances, including complete heart block (up to 30%), may occur.

MANAGEMENT

MEDICAL

1. Treatment of CHF and arrhythmias is indicated, if present.

2. Antiarrhythmic agents are used to treat arrhythmias.

SURGICAL

1. Palliative procedures: PA banding for uncontrollable CHF due to a large VSD or a systemic-to-pulmonary (S-P) shunt for patients with severe PS.

2. Corrective procedures: The presence or absence of TR determines the type of corrective surgeries that can be performed, either anatomic repair or classic repair (Fig. 3-25).

a. When there is no TR, a classic repair is done that leaves the anatomic RV as the systemic ventricle.

b. When there is TR or RV dysfunction, attempts are made to make the LV as the systemic ventricle (Fig. 3-25).

c. For complex intracardiac anatomy, staged Fontan-type operation is performed.

3. Other procedures may be necessary.

a. Valve replacement for significant TR

b. Pacemaker implantation for either spontaneous or postoperative complete heart block

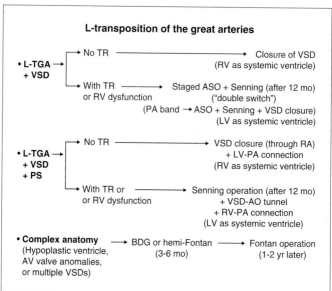

FIG. 3-25

Surgical summary of L-TGA. AO, aorta; ASO, arterial switch operation; BDG, bidirectional Glenn; LV, left ventricle; PA, pulmonary artery; RV, right ventricle; PS, pulmonary stenosis (= LV outflow tract obstruction); TGA, transposition of the great arteries; TR, tricuspid regurgitation (= left-sided AV valve regurgitation); VSD, ventricular septal defect. *(From Park MK: Pediatric cardiology for practitioners, ed 5, Philadelphia, 2008, Mosby.)*

POSTSURGICAL FOLLOW-UP
1. Follow-up every 6 to 12 months for a possible progression of AV conduction disturbances, arrhythmias, or worsening TR.
2. Routine pacemaker care if a pacemaker is implanted.
3. Varying degrees of activity restriction may be indicated depending on hemodynamic abnormalities or pacemaker status.

C. TETRALOGY OF FALLOT

PREVALENCE. 10% of all CHDs.

PATHOLOGY AND PATHOPHYSIOLOGY
1. The original description of TOF included four abnormalities: a large VSD, RVOT obstruction, RVH, and an overriding of the aorta. However, only two abnormalities are important: a VSD large enough to equalize pressures in both ventricles and an RVOT obstruction (Fig. 3-26). The

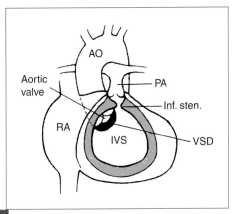

FIG. 3-26

Diagram of TOF. A large subaortic ventricular septal defect (VSD) is present through which aortic cusps are visualized. There is a pulmonary stenosis, which is either infundibular, valvular, or a combination. The right ventricular muscle is hypertrophied. An infundibular chamber and hypoplastic main pulmonary artery (PA) are evident. AO, aorta; Inf. sten., infundibular stenosis; IVS, interventricular septum; RA, right atrium. *(From Park MK: Pediatric cardiology for practitioners, ed 3, Philadelphia, 1995, Mosby.)*

RVH is secondary to the RVOT obstruction and VSD, and the overriding of the aorta varies in degree.

2. The VSD is a perimembranous defect with extension into the infundibular septum. The RVOT may be in the form of infundibular stenosis (50%), pulmonary valve stenosis (10%), or both (30%). The pulmonary annulus and the PA are usually hypoplastic. The pulmonary valve is atretic in 10% of the patients. Abnormal coronary arteries are present in about 5% of the patients, with the most common one being the anterior descending branch arising from the right coronary artery. Right aortic arch is present in 25% of the cases.

3. Because of the nonrestrictive VSD, systolic pressures in the RV and the LV are identical. Depending on the degree of the RVOT obstruction, an L-R, bidirectional, or R-L shunt is present. With a mild PS, an L-R shunt is present (acyanotic TOF). With a more severe degree of PS, a predominant R-L shunt occurs (cyanotic TOF). The heart murmur audible in cyanotic TOF originates from the RVOT obstruction, not from the VSD.

CLINICAL MANIFESTATIONS

1. Neonates with TOF with pulmonary atresia are deeply cyanotic (see the following separate heading). Most infants are symptomatic, with cyanosis, clubbing, dyspnea on exertion, squatting, or hypoxic spells. Patients with acyanotic TOF may be asymptomatic.

2. A right ventricular tap and a systolic thrill at the MLSB are usually found. An ejection click of aortic origin, a loud and single S2, and a loud (grade 3 to 5/6) systolic ejection murmur at the middle and upper left sternal border (LSB) are present (Fig. 3-27). Occasionally a continuous murmur representing PDA shunt may be audible in a deeply cyanotic neonate who has TOF with pulmonary atresia. In the acyanotic form a long systolic murmur resulting from VSD and infundibular stenosis is audible along the entire LSB, and cyanosis is absent.

3. The ECG shows RAD and RVH. BVH may be seen in the acyanotic form.

4. In cyanotic TOF, CXR films show normal heart size, decreased PVMs, and a boot-shaped heart with a concave MPA segment. Right aortic arch is present in 25% of the cases. CXRs of acyanotic TOF are indistinguishable from those of a small to moderate VSD.

5. Two-dimensional echo shows a large subaortic VSD and an overriding of the aorta. The anatomy of the RVOT, pulmonary valve, and pulmonary arteries can be imaged.

6. Children with the acyanotic form of TOF gradually change to the cyanotic form by 1 to 3 years of age. Hypoxic spells may develop in infants (see next section). Brain abscess, cerebrovascular accident, and SBE are rare complications. Polycythemia is common, but relative iron deficiency state (hypochromic) with normal hematocrit may be present. Coagulopathies are late complications of a long-standing severe cyanosis.

7. **Hypoxic spell.** Hypoxic spell (also called cyanotic spell or "tet" spell) of TOF requires timely recognition and appropriate treatment. It occurs in young infants, with peak incidence between 2 and 4 months of age. It is characterized by (1) a paroxysm of hyperpnea (rapid and deep respiration), (2) irritability and prolonged crying, (3) increasing cyanosis, and (4) decreased intensity of the heart murmur. A severe spell may lead to limpness, convulsion, cerebrovascular accident, or even death.

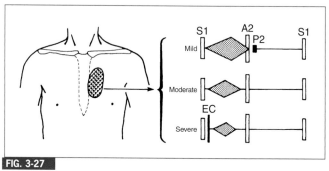

FIG. 3-27

Cardiac findings in cyanotic TOF. A long systolic ejection murmur at the MLSB and ULSB and a loud, single S2 are characteristic auscultatory findings of TOF. EC, ejection click.

a. **Pathophysiology of hypoxic spell.** In TOF the RV and LV can be viewed as a single pumping chamber because there is a large VSD equalizing pressures in both ventricles (Fig. 3-28). Lowering of the systemic vascular resistance (SVR) or increasing resistance at the RVOT will increase the R-L shunting, and this in turn stimulates the respiratory center to produce hyperpnea. Hyperpnea results in an increase in systemic venous return, which in turn increases the R-L shunt through the VSD, as there is an obstruction at the RVOT. A vicious circle becomes established (Fig. 3-29).

b. Treatment of the hypoxic spell is aimed at breaking the vicious circle. One or more of the following may be employed in decreasing order of preference.
   (1) Pick up the infant and hold in a knee-chest position.
   (2) Morphine sulfate, 0.1 to 0.2 mg/kg SC or IM, suppresses the respiratory center and abolishes hyperpnea.
   (3) Treat acidosis with sodium bicarbonate, 1 mEq/kg IV. This reduces the respiratory center–stimulating effect of acidosis.
   (4) Oxygen inhalation has only limited value because the problem is a reduced PBF, not the ability to oxygenate.

c. With these treatments the infant usually becomes less cyanotic and the heart murmur becomes louder, indicating improved PBF. If the infant is not fully responsive with the previous measures, the following may be tried.

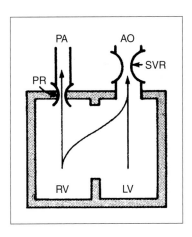

FIG. 3-28

Simplified concept of TOF that demonstrates how a change in the systemic vascular resistance (SVR) or right ventricular outflow tract obstruction (pulmonary resistance [PR]) affects the direction and magnitude of the ventricular shunt. AO, aorta; LV, left ventricle; PA, pulmonary artery; RV, right ventricle. *(From Park MK: Pediatric cardiology for practitioners, ed 5, Philadelphia, 2008, Mosby.)*

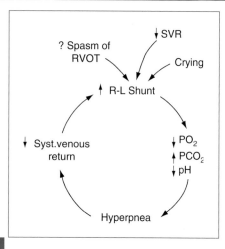

FIG. 3-29

Mechanism of hypoxic spell. R-L shunt, right-to-left shunt; RVOT, right ventricular outflow tract; SVR, systemic vascular resistance. *(From Park MK: Pediatric cardiology for practitioners, ed 5, Philadelphia, 2008, Mosby.)*

    (1) Ketamine, 1 to 3 mg/kg (average of 2 mg/kg) in a slow IV push, works well (by increasing the SVR and sedating the infant).
    (2) Propranolol, 0.01 to 0.25 mg/kg (average 0.05 mg/kg) in a slow IV push, reduces the heart rate and may reverse the spell.

MANAGEMENT
MEDICAL
1. Hypoxic spells should be recognized and treated appropriately.
2. Oral propranolol, 2 to 4 mg/kg/day, may be used to prevent hypoxic spells and delay corrective surgery. The beneficial effect of propranolol may be related to its stabilizing action on peripheral vascular reactivity (thus preventing a sudden fall of the SVR).
3. Detection and treatment of relative iron deficiency state. Anemic children are particularly prone to cerebrovascular accident.

SURGICAL
1. Palliative procedures are indicated to increase PBF in infants with severe cyanosis or uncontrollable hypoxic spells on whom the corrective surgery cannot safely be performed, and in children with hypoplastic PA on whom the corrective surgery is technically difficult. Different types of S-P shunts have been performed (Fig. 3-30).
a. The Blalock-Taussig (B-T) shunt (anastomosis between the subclavian artery and the ipsilateral PA) may be performed in older infants.

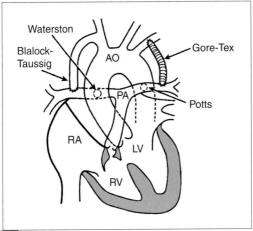

FIG. 3-30

Palliative procedures to increase pulmonary blood flow in patients with cyanosis and decreased PBF. AO, aorta; LV, left ventricle; PA, pulmonary artery; RA, right atrium; RV, right ventricle. *(From Park MK:* Pediatric cardiology for practitioners, *ed 5, Philadelphia, 2008, Mosby.)*

b. Gore-Tex interposition shunt between the subclavian artery and the ipsilateral PA (modified Blalock-Taussig [B-T] shunt) is the procedure of choice in small infants.

c. Waterston shunt (anastomosis between the ascending aorta and the right PA) is no longer performed because of many complications following the operation.

d. Potts operation (anastomosis between the descending aorta and the left PA) is no longer performed.

2. Complete repair surgery

a. Symptomatic or cyanotic infants with favorable anatomy of the RVOT and PAs may have primary repair at any time after 3 to 4 months of age. Asymptomatic and minimally cyanotic children may have repair between ages 3 and 24 months, depending on the degree of the annular and pulmonary hypoplasia. Mildly cyanotic infants who have had previous shunt surgery may have total repair at 1 to 2 years of age.

b. Total repair of the defect is carried out under cardiopulmonary bypass. The procedure includes patch closure of the VSD, widening of the RVOT by resection of the infundibular muscle tissue, and usually placement of a fabric patch to widen the RVOT (Fig. 3-31). Some centers advocate placement of a monocusp valve at the time of initial

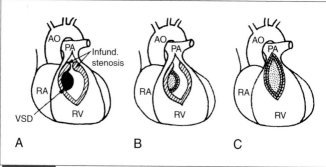

FIG. 3-31

Total correction of TOF. **A,** Anatomy of TOF showing a large ventricular septal defect (VSD) and infundibular stenosis seen through a right ventriculotomy. Note that the size of the ventriculotomy has been expanded to show the VSD. **B,** Patch closure of the VSD and resection of the infundibular stenosis. **C,** Placement of a fabric patch on the outflow tract of the right ventricle (RV). AO, aorta; PA, pulmonary artery; RA, right atrium. *(From Park MK: Pediatric cardiology for practitioners, ed 5, Philadelphia, 2008, Mosby.)*

repair, and other centers advocate pulmonary valve replacement at a later time if indicated.

c. Surgery for TOF with anomalous anterior descending coronary artery from the right coronary artery requires placement of a conduit between the RV and PA, which is usually performed after 1 year of age. A B-T shunt may be necessary to palliate the patient. Alternatively, when a small conduit is necessary between the RV and the PA, the native outflow tract should be made as large as possible through an atrial approach so that a "double outlet" (the native outlet and the conduit) results from the RV.

POSTSURGICAL FOLLOW-UP

1. Long-term follow-up every 6 to 12 months is recommended, especially for patients with residual VSD shunt, residual RVOT obstruction, residual PA stenosis, arrhythmias, or conduction disturbances.
2. Varying levels of activity limitation may be indicated.

D. TETRALOGY OF FALLOT WITH PULMONARY ATRESIA

PREVALENCE. About 10% of patients with TOF.

PATHOLOGY AND PATHOPHYSIOLOGY

1. In this extreme form of TOF the intracardiac pathology resembles that of TOF in all respects except for the presence of pulmonary atresia.
2. The PBF is more commonly through a PDA (70%) and less commonly through multiple systemic collaterals (30%), which are called multiple

aortopulmonary collateral arteries (MAPCAs). Both PDA and collateral arteries may coexist as the source of PBF. The ductus is small and long and descends vertically from the transverse arch ("vertical" ductus) and connects to the PAs, which are usually confluent. The subgroup of MAPCAs is usually associated with nonconfluent PAs, and this subgroup is designated as pulmonary atresia and ventricular septal defect.

3. The central and branch PAs are hypoplastic in most patients but more frequently in patients with MAPCAs than in those with PDA. Incomplete arborization (distribution) of one or both PAs is also more common in patients with nonconfluent PAs than those with confluent PAs.

CLINICAL MANIFESTATIONS

1. The patient is cyanotic at birth; the degree of cyanosis depends on whether the ductus is patent and how extensive the systemic collateral arteries are.
2. Usually no heart murmur is audible, but a faint, continuous murmur of PDA may be audible. The S2 is loud and single.
3. The ECG shows RAD and RVH.
4. CXR film shows normal heart size, often with a boot-shaped silhouette and a markedly decreased PVM ("black" lung field).
5. Echo studies are diagnostic of the condition, but angiocardiogram is necessary for complete delineation of the pulmonary artery anatomy and the collaterals.

MANAGEMENT
MEDICAL
1. Intravenous PGE_1 infusion is started to keep the ductus open for cardiac catheterization and in preparation for surgery (see Appendix E for the dosage).
2. Emergency cardiac catheterization is performed to delineate anatomy of the pulmonary arteries and systemic arterial collaterals.
SURGICAL
1. Primary surgical repair (closure of the VSD, conduit between the RV and the central PA) is possible only when a central PA of adequate size exists and the central PA connects without obstruction to sufficient regions of the lungs (at least equal to one whole lung). The overall hospital mortality varies between 5% and 20%.
2. Staged repair consists of the initial S-P shunts to induce the growth of the central PA before 1 or 2 years of age, followed by additional surgical procedure(s) at later times.
a. When there is a confluence of central PAs, one of the following three approaches has been used initially: (1) an S-P shunt (but this procedure often results in an iatrogenic stenosis of the PA), (2) a central end-to-side shunt (Mee procedure) for a very small confluent central PA, or (3) RVOT reconstruction with patch. The VSD may be left open, or closed with a fenestrated patch to maintain an increased PBF (Fig. 3-32, top row).

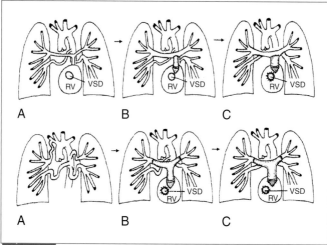

FIG. 3-32

Diagram of multiple-stage repair surgery. *Upper row*: **A,** TOF with pulmonary atresia with a hypoplastic but confluent central PA and multiple collateral arteries are shown. **B,** A small RV-to-PA connection is made with pulmonary homograft (shown in shade), with collaterals left alone. **C,** The pulmonary arteries have been grown to a larger size. Collateral arteries are now anastomosed to the originally hypoplastic PA branches. VSD may be closed at a later time, usually 1 to 3 years of age. The pulmonary homograft is usually replaced with a larger graft at this time. *Bottom row*: **A,** Pulmonary atresia and VSD with absent central pulmonary artery and MAPCAs is shown. **B,** A small pulmonary homograft (internal diameter of 6 to 8 mm, shown in shade) is used to establish RV-to-PA connection (performed at 3 to 6 months). Some collaterals are not unifocalized at this time. **C,** The homograft conduit has been replaced with a larger one. Remaining collateral arteries are anastomosed to the pulmonary homograft to complete unifocalization procedure. VSD is closed with or without fenestration, usually at 1 to 3 years of age. RV, right ventricle; VSD, ventricular septal defect. *(From Park MK: Pediatric cardiology for practitioners, ed 5, Philadelphia, 2008, Mosby.)*

b. When the central PA is nonconfluent, with multiple collaterals supplying different segments of the lungs, a surgical connection between or among the isolated regions of the lungs may be made so they might be perfused from a single source (termed *unifocalization of PBF*), with a surgical mortality rate of 5% to 15% (Fig. 3-32, bottom row). Later, a conduit between the RV and a newly created central PA can be made (Fig. 3-33).

c. Occlusion of systemic collateral arteries is done by coil embolization preoperatively or at the time of surgery.

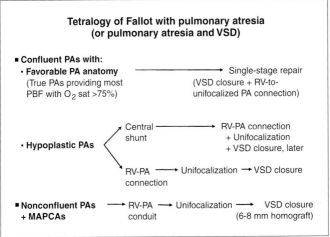

**Tetralogy of Fallot with pulmonary atresia
(or pulmonary atresia and VSD)**

■ **Confluent PAs with:**

• **Favorable PA anatomy** ————————→ Single-stage repair
(True PAs providing most   (VSD closure + RV-to-
PBF with O$_2$ sat >75%)   unifocalized PA connection)

• **Hypoplastic PAs**   ⟨   Central ————→ RV-PA connection
                            shunt   + Unifocalization
                                                     + VSD closure, later

                            RV-PA ——→ Unifocalization ——→ VSD closure
                            connection

■ **Nonconfluent PAs** ——→ RV-PA ——→ Unifocalization ——→ VSD closure
+ MAPCAs   conduit   (6-8 mm homograft)

FIG. 3-33

Surgical approaches for TOF with pulmonary atresia (or pulmonary atresia and VSD).
MAPCAs, multiple aortopulmonary collateral arteries; PA, pulmonary artery; PBF, pulmonary blood flow; RV-PA, right ventricle-to-pulmonary artery; VSD, ventricular septal
defect. (From Park MK: Pediatric cardiology for practitioners, ed 5, Philadelphia,
2008, Mosby.)

POSTSURGICAL FOLLOW-UP. Frequent follow-up is needed to assess the palliative surgery, to decide the appropriate time for further operations, and to
determine an appropriate time for conduit replacement. SBE prophylaxis is
indicated until a complete repair is accomplished. A certain level of activity
restriction is needed for most patients.

E.   TETRALOGY OF FALLOT WITH ABSENT PULMONARY VALVE

PREVALENCE. Approximately 2% to 6% of patients with TOF.

PATHOLOGY AND PATHOPHYSIOLOGY

1. The pulmonary valve leaflets are either absent or rudimentary, and the
pulmonary annulus is stenotic, usually in association with TOF. A massive
aneurysmal dilation of the PAs developing during fetal life compresses
the lower end of the developing trachea and bronchi throughout the fetal
life. Postnatally, this produces signs of airway obstruction and respiratory
difficulties. Pulmonary complications (e.g., atelectasis, pneumonia),
rather than the intracardiac defect, are the usual cause of death. In some
patients the ductus arteriosus is absent, with a more severe aneurysmal
dilation of the PAs.

2. Because the annular stenosis is only moderate, an initial bidirectional
shunt becomes predominantly an L-R shunt beyond the newborn period.

CLINICAL MANIFESTATIONS

1. Mild cyanosis may be present in the neonate, but cyanosis disappears and signs of CHF may develop when the PVR falls.

2. A to-and-fro murmur ("sawing-wood sound") at the upper and middle LSB (resulting from PS and PR) is characteristic of the condition. The S2 is loud and single, and RV hyperactivity is palpable.

3. The ECG shows RAD and RVH.

4. CXR films reveal a markedly dilated MPA and hilar PAs. The heart size is either normal or mildly enlarged, and PVMs may be slightly increased. The lung fields may show hyperinflated or atelectatic areas.

5. Echo confirms the diagnosis.

6. Most infants with severe pulmonary complications (e.g., atelectasis, pneumonia) die during infancy if treated only medically. The surgical mortality of infants with pulmonary complications is as high as 40%. Therefore, surgery should be performed in early infancy before pulmonary complications develop.

MANAGEMENT

MEDICAL. The mortality of medical management is very high. Once the pulmonary symptoms appear, neither surgical nor medical management carries good results.

SURGICAL

1. Symptomatic neonates should have corrective surgery on an urgent basis. Even asymptomatic infants should have elective primary repair surgery in early infancy. Some repairs use a homograft valve at the pulmonary valve position, and others do not.

2. Alternatively, a two-stage operation can be performed. A tight PA banding is performed to eliminate excessive pulsation of the PA, along with a B-T shunt, and a complete repair is performed later (at 2 to 4 years of age).

F. TOTAL ANOMALOUS PULMONARY VENOUS RETURN

PREVALENCE. 1% of all CHDs. There is marked male preponderance (4:1) in the infracardiac type.

PATHOLOGY AND PATHOPHYSIOLOGY

1. The PVs drain into the RA or its venous tributaries, rather than directly into the LA. The defects may be divided into the following four types (Fig. 3-34).

a. Supracardiac (50%): The common PV drains into the SVC via the left SVC (vertical vein) and the left innominate vein.

b. Cardiac (20%): The common PV drains into the coronary sinus, or the PVs enter the RA separately through four openings.

c. Infracardiac (subdiaphragmatic) (20%): The common PV drains to the portal vein, ductus venosus, hepatic vein, or IVC.

d. Mixed type (10%): A combination of different types.

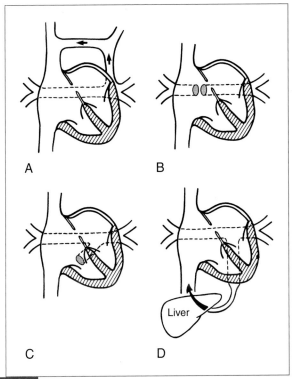

FIG. 3-34

Anatomic classification of TAPVR. **A,** Supracardiac. **B,** Cardiac, draining into the RA (only two pulmonary veins are shown). **C,** Cardiac, draining into the coronary sinus. **D,** Infracardiac.

2. An ASD is necessary for survival. The left side of the heart is relatively small. There is an obstruction of the pulmonary venous return in some cases, especially with the infracardiac type.

3. Pulmonary and systemic venous blood is completely mixed in the RA. Blood then goes to the LA through an ASD, as well as to the RV. Thus, oxygen saturations in the systemic and pulmonary circulations are the same, with resulting systemic arterial desaturation.

4. The level of systemic arterial oxygen saturation is proportional to the amount of PBF. When there is no obstruction to pulmonary venous (PV) return (as seen in most of the supracardiac and cardiac types), PV return is large and the systemic arterial blood is only minimally desaturated.

When there is obstruction to PV return (as seen in the infracardiac type), PV return is small and the patient is severely cyanotic.

CLINICAL MANIFESTATIONS *WITHOUT* PV OBSTRUCTION

1. Growth retardation, mild cyanosis, and signs of CHF (tachypnea, tachycardia, hepatomegaly) are common.
2. Hyperactive RV impulse and characteristic quadruple or quintuple rhythm are present. The S2 is widely split and fixed, and the P2 may be accentuated. A grade 2 to 3/6 systolic ejection murmur is usually present at the ULSB. A middiastolic rumble is always present at the LLSB (resulting from relative TS).
3. The ECG shows RAD, RVH (of "volume overload" type with rsR′ pattern in V1), and occasional RAH.
4. CXR films show moderate to marked cardiomegaly (involving RA and RV) with increased PVMs. A "snowman" sign is seen in older infants (rarely before 4 months of age) with the supracardiac type.
5. Two-dimensional echo may demonstrate the common PV posterior to the LA without direct communication to the LA. A markedly dilated coronary sinus protruding into the LA (seen in TAPVR to the coronary sinus) or dilated left innominate vein and SVC (seen in the supracardiac type) may be imaged. An ASD with an R-L shunt and relatively small LA and LV are imaged.
6. CHF, growth retardation, and repeated pneumonias develop by 6 months of age.

CLINICAL MANIFESTATIONS *WITH* PV OBSTRUCTION

1. Marked cyanosis and respiratory distress are present in the neonate.
2. A loud and single S2 and gallop rhythm are present. Heart murmur is usually absent. Pulmonary crackles may be audible.
3. The ECG shows RAD and RVH.
4. The heart size is usually normal on CXR films, but the lung fields reveal findings of pulmonary venous congestion or edema.
5. Two-dimensional echo shows relatively hypoplastic LA and LV. Anomalous PV return below the diaphragm can be directly imaged by 2D echo studies.
6. Patients with the infracardiac type rarely survive more than a few weeks without surgery.

MANAGEMENT OF BOTH GROUPS OF PATIENTS
MEDICAL

1. Intensive anticongestive measures with digitalis and diuretics are indicated for the nonobstructive type.
2. Oxygen and diuretics are given for pulmonary edema in infants with the obstructive type. Intubation and ventilator therapy with oxygen and positive end-expiratory pressure (PEEP) may be necessary in infants with severe pulmonary edema.
3. Balloon atrial septostomy to enlarge the interatrial communication may be beneficial at least temporarily.

SURGICAL. There is no palliative procedure. Corrective surgery is indicated for all patients with this condition. Neonates with PV obstruction are operated on soon after the diagnosis, with a surgical mortality rate of about 20%, and infants without PV obstruction are operated on by 4 to 12 months of age with a mortality rate of 5% to 10%.

1. **Supracardiac type.** A large, side-to-side anastomosis is made between the common PV and the LA. The vertical vein is ligated. The ASD is closed with a cloth patch (Fig. 3-35, *A*).

2. **TAPVR to the right atrium.** The atrial septum is excised and a patch is sewn in such a way that the pulmonary venous return is diverted to the LA (Fig. 3-35, *B*).

3. **TAPVR to the coronary sinus.** An incision is made in the anterior wall of the coronary sinus ("unroofing") to make a communication between the coronary sinus and the LA. A single patch closes the original ASD and the ostium of the coronary sinus. This results in the drainage of coronary sinus blood with low oxygen saturation into the LA (Fig. 3-35, *C*).

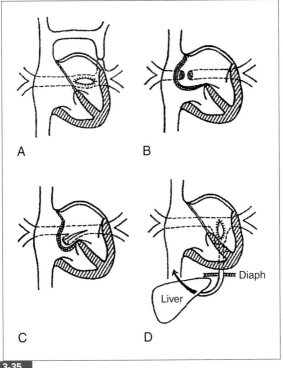

FIG. 3-35

Surgical approaches to various types of total anomalous pulmonary venous (see text).

(From Park MK: Pediatric cardiology for practitioners, ed 5, Philadelphia, 2008, Mosby.)

4. Infracardiac type. A large vertical anastomosis is made between the common PV and the LA. The common PV is ligated above the diaphragm (Fig. 3-35, *D*).

POSTSURGICAL FOLLOW-UP. Follow-up is needed for possible late development of obstruction to PV return (10%) or atrial arrhythmias, including sinus node dysfunction.

G. TRICUSPID ATRESIA

PREVALENCE. 1% to 3% of all CHDs in infancy.

PATHOLOGY AND PATHOPHYSIOLOGY

1. The tricuspid valve is absent and the RV and PA are hypoplastic, with decreased PBF. The great arteries are transposed in 30% and normally related in 70% of the cases. Associated defects such as ASD, VSD, or PDA are necessary for survival.

2. In the most common type (50%) a small VSD and PS (with hypoplasia of the PAs) are present, and the great arteries are normally related. In the second most common type the great arteries are transposed and the pulmonary valve is normal size (20%) (Fig. 3-36).

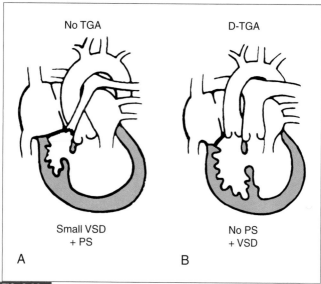

No TGA

D-TGA

Small VSD + PS

No PS + VSD

A   B

FIG. 3-36

Two most common types of tricuspid atresia. In about 50% of patients the great arteries are normally related and a small VSD and PS are present **(A).** When the great arteries are transposed (about 20% of all cases), a VSD is usually present without PS **(B).** PS, pulmonary stenosis; TGA, transposition of the great arteries; VSD, ventricular septal defect.

3. COA or interrupted aortic arch is a frequently associated anomaly, more commonly seen in cases with TGA.
4. All systemic venous return is shunted from the RA to the LA, with resulting dilation and hypertrophy of the RA. The LA and LV are large because they handle both systemic and pulmonary venous returns. The level of arterial saturation is positively related to the level of PBF.

CLINICAL MANIFESTATIONS
1. Severe cyanosis, tachypnea, and poor feeding are usual.
2. The S2 is single. A grade 2 to 3/6 systolic regurgitant murmur of VSD is usually present at the LLSB. A continuous murmur of PDA is occasionally audible. Hepatomegaly is present when there is an inadequate inter-atrial communication or CHF.
3. The ECG shows characteristic "superior" QRS axis (left anterior hemiblock), RAH or BAH, and LVH.
4. CXR film shows normal or slightly increased heart size and decreased PVMs. A boot-shaped heart with concave MPA segment may be seen. In infants with TGA, PVMs may be increased.
5. Two-dimensional echo shows atretic tricuspid valve, large LV, diminutive RV, and ASD. The presence or absence of TGA, VSD, PDA, and COA is also imaged.
6. Few infants survive beyond 6 months of life without surgical palliation. Occasionally patients with increased PBF develop pulmonary hypertension and LV failure, which preclude successful Fontan operation.

MANAGEMENT
MEDICAL
1. Intravenous PGE_1 infusion (see Appendix E for dosage) is indicated in cyanotic neonates to maintain the patency of the ductus before planned cardiac catheterization.
2. The balloon atrial septostomy (Rashkind procedure) may be performed to improve the R-L atrial shunt.
3. Rarely, patients in CHF require anticongestive measures.
4. Infants with VSD of adequate size and normal PBF need to be followed closely for decreasing oxygen saturation, which may be caused by reduction in the size of the VSD.

SURGICAL. The definitive surgery for tricuspid atresia is a Fontan-type operation. One or more palliative procedures are required to reduce the risk of the procedure. Ideal candidates for a Fontan operation have normal LV function and low PVR. Normal LV function results from prevention of excessive volume overload (by using a relatively small B-T shunt 3.5 mm for neonates) or pressure loading of the LV (by relieving LV outflow obstruction). Low PVR may result from adequate growth of PA branches (by a B-T operation), from preventing distortion of the PA (by placing a shunt into the RPA), or PA band in case of increased PBF. Because the Fontan operation is done for many other complex heart defects, a summary of the Fontan pathway is presented in Box 3-1.

BOX 3-1

FONTAN PATHWAY

Stage I. One of the following procedures is done in preparation for a future Fontan operation.

1. Blalock-Taussig shunt, when PBF is small
2. PA banding, when PBF is excessive
3. Damus-Kaye-Stansel + shunt operation (for TA + TGA + restrictive VSD)

Medical follow-up after stage I. Watch for the following:

   a. Cyanosis (O_2 saturation <75%)—cardiac catheterization or MRI to find the cause

   b. Poor weight gain (CHF from too much PBF)—tightening of PA band may be necessary

Stage II (at 3 to 6 mo)

1. BDG operation or
2. Hemi-Fontan operation

Medical follow-up after stage II. Watch for the following:

   a. A gradual decrease in O_2 saturation (<75%) may be caused by (1) opening of venous collaterals or (2) pulmonary AV fistula (due to the absence of hepatic vasoconstrictor prostaglandins reaching the pulmonary circulation).

     (1) Perform cardiac catheterization (to find and occlude venous collaterals) or

     (2) Proceed with Fontan operation.

   b. Transient hypertension 1-2 wk postoperatively—may use ACE inhibitors.

   c. Cardiac catheterization by 12 mo after stage II to assess risk factors.

   d. The following are risk factors for the Fontan operation. Presence of ≥2 risk factors is a high-risk situation.

     (1) Mean PA pressure >18 mm Hg (or PVR >2 U/m²)

     (2) LV end-diastolic pressure >12 mm Hg (or EF <60%)

     (3) AV valve regurgitation

     (4) Distorted PAs secondary to previous shunt operation

Stage III (Fontan operation)—within 1-2 yr after stage II operation

1. "Lateral tunnel" Fontan (with 4-mm fenestration); device closure of the fenestration 1-2 yr later
2. An extracardiac conduit (usually without fenestration)

BDG, bidirectional Glenn; TA, tricuspid atresia; MRI, magnetic resonance imaging.

---

1. **Stage 1.** One of the following three procedures is performed depending on the situation (Fig. 3-40).

a. A B-T shunt (3.5 mm) to the RPA, in patients with decreased PBF.

b. PA banding is rarely necessary for infants with CHF from increased PBF.

c. Damus-Kaye-Stansel and shunt operation for infants with tricuspid atresia + TGA + restrictive VSD. In this procedure the main PA is transected and the distal PA is sewn over. The proximal PA is connected end to side to the ascending aorta (see Fig. 3-22 done for patients with TGA). A B-T shunt is created to supply blood to the lungs.

2. **Stage 2.** As a stage 2 operation, either a bidirectional Glenn shunt or the hemi-Fontan operation is performed in preparation for the final Fontan operation.

a. Bidirectional Glenn operation. An end-to-side SVC-to-RPA shunt (also called bidirectional superior cavopulmonary shunt) is performed by 2.5 to 3 months of age (Fig. 3-37, *A*). Any previous B-T shunt is taken down at the time of the procedure. The azygos vein and the hemiazygos are divided. The IVC blood still bypasses the lungs. Oxygen saturation increases to about 85%. Surgical mortality rate is between 5% and 10%.

b. In the hemi-Fontan operation an anastomosis is made between the superior part of the right atrial appendage and the lower margin of the central portion of the PA. An intraatrial baffle is placed to direct SVC blood to the PAs. The B-T shunt is taken down and the native pulmonary valve is oversewn (Fig. 3-38).

3. **Stage 3.** A modified Fontan operation is the definitive procedure for patients with tricuspid atresia. In the Fontan operation the entire systemic venous return is directed to the pulmonary arteries without an intervening pumping chamber. The Fontan operation is usually completed when the child is around 2 years of age.

a. The following are risk factors for the Fontan operation: (1) a high PVR (>2 U/m^2) or high mean PA pressure (>18 mm Hg), (2) distorted or stenotic PAs secondary to previous shunt operations, (3) poor LV systolic and diastolic function (LV end-diastolic pressure >12 mm Hg or an

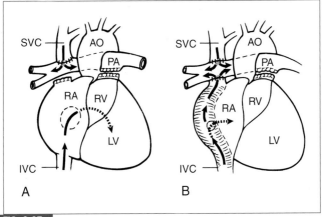

FIG. 3-37

Bidirectional Glenn operation or SVC-RPA anastomosis **(A)** and cavocaval baffle-to-PA connection with or without fenestration **(B).** AO, aorta; IVC, inferior vena cava; LV, left ventricle; PA, pulmonary artery; RA, right atrium; RV, right ventricle; SVC, superior vena cava.

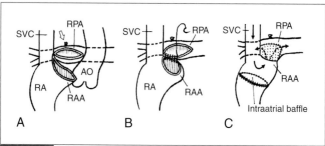

FIG. 3-38

Hemi-Fontan operation. **A,** A B-T shunt is taken down *(arrow)*. An incision is made in the superior aspect of the right atrial appendage extending it into the SVC, and a horizontal incision is made in the RPA. **B,** The lower margin of the RPA incision and the adjacent margin of the incision in the right atrial appendage (RAA) and SVC are connected. **C,** The connection is completed using pulmonary allograft. An intraatrial patch is placed to direct SVC blood to the PAs. AO, aorta; RA, right atrium; RPA, right pulmonary artery; SVC, superior vena cava. *(From Park MK:* Pediatric cardiology for practitioners, *ed 5, Philadelphia, 2008, Mosby.)*

ejection fraction <60%), and (4) AV valve regurgitation. The presence of two or more of these risk factors constitutes a high-risk situation.

b. In patients who have had a bidirectional Glenn procedure, an intraatrial tubular pathway (termed cavocaval baffle or a "lateral tunnel") is created from the orifice of the IVC to the orifice of the SVC. The cardiac end of the SVC is anastomosed to the undersurface of the RPA to complete the operation (Fig. 3-37, *B*). Some centers routinely use "fenestration" (4 to 6 mm) in the baffle, and others use it only in high-risk patients. Some centers recommend device closure of the fenestration a year or so after the Fontan procedure. However, about 20% to 40% of fenestrations will close spontaneously over the first year or two postoperatively. Alternative to the procedure just described, an extracardiac conduit may be used to complete the Fontan operation. Early survival rates have improved to more than 90%, with a 10-year survival rate of 70%.

c. In patients who had the hemi-Fontan operation, the intraatrial patch is excised and a lateral atrial tunnel is constructed, directing flow from the IVC to the previously created amalgamation of the SVC with the RPA (Fig. 3-39). Surgical approach for patients with tricuspid atresia is summarized in Figure 3-40.

4. **Complications of the Fontan-type operation.** Early complications of the Fontan operation may include the following:

a. Low cardiac output and/or heart failure.

b. Persistent pleural effusion occurring more often on the right side.

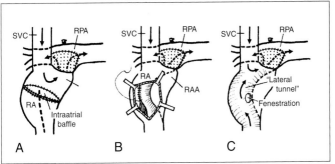

FIG. 3-39

From the hemi-Fontan to Fontan connection. **A,** A vertical incision *(heavy broken line)* is made in the anterior RA wall. **B,** The intraatrial patch is removed and a lateral tunnel is constructed to direct the IVC blood to the existing conglomerate of RA and RPA. **C,** The direction of blood flow from the SVC and IVC is shown. RA, right atrium; RAA, right atrial appendage; RPA, right pulmonary artery; SVC, superior vena cava. *(From Park MK: Pediatric cardiology for practitioners, ed 5, Philadelphia, 2008, Mosby.)*

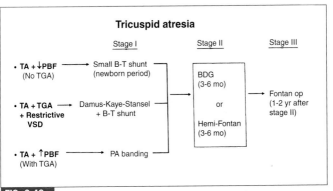

FIG. 3-40

Surgical approaches in tricuspid atresia. BDG, bidirectional Glenn; B-T, Blalock-Taussig; op, operation; PA, pulmonary artery; PBF, pulmonary blood flow; TA, tricuspid atresia; TGA, transposition of the great arteries; VSD, ventricular septal defect. *(From Park MK: Pediatric cardiology for practitioners, ed 5, Philadelphia, 2008, Mosby.)*

   c. Thrombus formation in the systemic venous pathways.
   d. Although rare, acute liver dysfunction (with ALT >1000 U/L) can occur during the first week after surgery.

POSTOPERATIVE FOLLOW-UP. Regular follow-up is necessary for general management and to detect the following late complications.

1. Patients should maintain a low-salt diet.
2. Patients should not participate in competitive, strenuous sports.
3. Antibiotic prophylaxis against SBE should be observed if a residual shunt is present.
4. Medications:
a. Some patients need continued digoxin and diuretic therapy.
b. An ACE inhibitor is generally recommended, which is an afterload reducer as well as an antithrombotic agent (by reducing synthesis of plasminogen activator inhibitor-1 [PAI-1]).
c. Aspirin (or even warfarin) is used to prevent thrombus formation in the RA.
5. Watch for late complications.
a. Prolonged hepatomegaly and ascites (which require treatment with digitalis, diuretics, and afterload-reducing agents).
b. Supraventricular arrhythmia occurs in the early postoperative period in 15% of patients. The late-onset supraventricular arrhythmia continues to increase with longer follow-up (6% at 1 year and 17% at 5 years).
c. A progressive decrease in arterial oxygen saturation (which may result from obstruction of the venous pathways, leakage in the intraatrial baffle, or development of pulmonary AV fistula).
d. Protein-losing enteropathy can result from increased systemic venous pressure that subsequently causes lymphangiectasis, occurring in 4% of survivors. The prognosis is poor (50% dying within 5 years).

H. PULMONARY ATRESIA

PREVALENCE. Less than 1% of all CHDs or 2.5% of critically ill infants with CHD.

PATHOLOGY AND PATHOPHYSIOLOGY

1. The pulmonary valve is atretic, and the interventricular septum is intact. An interatrial communication (either ASD or PFO) and PDA are necessary for survival.
2. The RV size is variable and is related to survival. In the *tripartite type,* all three (inlet, trabecular, and infundibular) portions of the RV are present and the RV is nearly normal in size (Fig. 3-41). In the *bipartite type,* the inlet and infundibular portions are present (but the trabecular portion is obliterated). In the *monopartite type,* only the inlet portion is present. In the monopartite type the RV is diminutive, and coronary sinusoids are almost always present (Fig. 3-41).
3. The high pressure in the RV is often decompressed through dilated coronary sinusoids into the left or right coronary artery. TR is commonly present. The prevalence of the sinusoids is directly related to the RV pressure and inversely related to the amount of TR. The obstruction of the proximal coronary arteries, which is often present, may cause high surgical mortality.

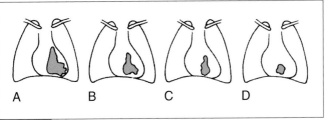

FIG. 3-41

Schematic diagram of right ventriculograms that illustrate three types of pulmonary atresia with intact ventricular septum. **A,** Normal right ventricle. **B,** Tripartite type, which shows all three portions (inlet, trabecular, and infundibular portions) of the RV. **C,** Bipartite type in which only the inlet and infundibular portions are present. **D,** Monopartite type in which only the inlet portion of the RV is present. *(From Park MK: Pediatric cardiology for practitioners, ed 5, Philadelphia, 2008, Mosby.)*

4. Pathophysiology is similar to that of tricuspid atresia. The RA hypertrophies and enlarges to shunt systemic venous return to the LA. The LA and LV handle both systemic and pulmonary venous returns and therefore they enlarge. PBF depends on the patency of PDA; closure of PDA after birth results in death.

CLINICAL MANIFESTATIONS
1. Severe and progressive cyanosis is present from birth.
2. The S2 is single. Usually no heart murmur is present. A soft, continuous murmur of PDA may be audible at the ULSB.
3. The ECG shows normal QRS axis (in contrast to the "superior" QRS axis seen in tricuspid atresia), RAH, and LVH (monopartite type) or occasional RVH (tripartite type).
4. The heart size on CXR films may be normal or large (with RA enlargement). The MPA segment is concave, with markedly decreased PVMs.
5. Two-dimensional echo usually demonstrates the atretic pulmonary valve and hypoplasia of the RV cavity and tricuspid valve. The atrial communication and PDA can be imaged and their size estimated.
6. Prognosis is exceedingly poor without neonatal PGE_1 infusion and surgery.

MANAGEMENT
MEDICAL
1. As soon as the diagnosis is suspected, intravenous PGE_1 infusion is started to maintain ductal patency (see Appendix E for the dosage).
2. Cardiac catheterization and angiocardiography are recommended for most patients to demonstrate coronary sinusoids (by RV angio) and to demonstrate possible coronary artery anomalies (by aortogram). A balloon atrial septostomy may be performed during cardiac catheterization

only when a two-ventricular repair is considered not possible (e.g., the presence of RV sinusoids or an RV cavity that is too small). The balloon atrial septostomy is not performed in patients with the tripartite type. Such patients may become candidates for RVOT patch, in which an elevated RA pressure is important to maximize RV forward output.

SURGICAL. Surgical decision for this condition depends on the RV size and the presence or absence of RV sinusoids or coronary artery anomalies. The summary of surgical approaches in pulmonary atresia with intact ventricular septum is presented in Figure 3-42.

1. Adequate RV size: In patients with tripartite or bipartite RV a connection is established between the RV and the MPA (either by transannular patch, closed transpulmonary valvotomy, or laser wire and radiofrequency-assisted valvotomy) in preparation for a possible two-ventricular repair. A B-T shunt is performed at the same time.

a. If the RV appears to have grown to an adequate size and O_2 saturation is >70% with the B-T shunt closed during cardiac catheterization, two-ventricular repair is performed.

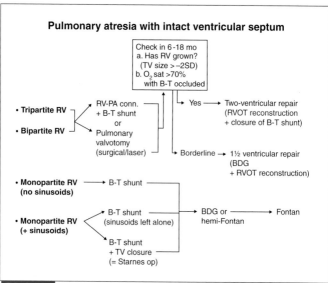

FIG. 3-42

Surgical approach to pulmonary atresia with intact ventricular septum. BDG, bidirectional Glenn; B-T, Blalock-Taussig; op, operation; RV, right ventricle; RVOT, right ventricular outflow tract; RV-PA conn., right ventricle-to-pulmonary artery connection; TV, tricuspid valve. *(From Park MK: Pediatric cardiology for practitioners, ed 5, Philadelphia, 2008, Mosby.)*

b. If the RV size is considered borderline, *one and one-half ventricular repair* may be performed. In this repair a bidirectional Glenn operation is combined with an RVOT reconstruction.

2. In patients with monopartite RV with or without coronary sinusoids, staged Fontan operation is performed (similar to that described for tricuspid atresia).

a. A B-T shunt is performed initially.

b. For patients with RV sinusoids the sinusoids may be left alone or the tricuspid valve is closed (Starnes operation).

c. A bidirectional Glenn or hemi-Fontan operation is performed at 3 to 6 months of age.

d. A Fontan-type operation is performed at 1 to 2 years of age.

POSTSURGICAL FOLLOW-UP. Most patients require close follow-up.

I.   HYPOPLASTIC LEFT HEART SYNDROME

PREVALENCE. HLHS occurs in 1% of all CHDs.

PATHOLOGY AND PATHOPHYSIOLOGY

1. Hypoplastic left heart syndrome (HLHS) includes a group of closely related anomalies characterized by hypoplasia of the LV (in association with atresia or severe stenosis of the aortic and/or mitral valves) and hypoplasia of the ascending aorta and the aortic arch. The LV is small and/or totally atretic. The atrial septum is intact with a normal patent foramen ovale. A VSD occurs in about 10% of the patients. COA frequently is an associated finding (up to 75%).

2. A high prevalence (up to 29%) of brain abnormalities has been reported, including agenesis of the corpus callosum, holoprosencephaly, microencephaly, and immature cortical mantle.

3. During fetal life the PVR is higher than the SVR, and the dominant RV maintains normal perfusion pressure in the descending aorta through the ductal R-L shunt, even in the presence of the nonfunctioning hypoplastic LV. However, difficulties arise after birth when the ductus closes and the PVR reduces. The end result is a marked decrease in systemic cardiac output and aortic pressure, resulting in circulatory shock and metabolic acidosis. An increase in PBF in the presence of the nonfunctioning LV results in an elevated LA pressure and pulmonary edema.

CLINICAL MANIFESTATIONS

1. The neonate is critically ill in the first few hours to days of life, with mild cyanosis, tachycardia, tachypnea, and pulmonary crackles.

2. Poor peripheral pulses and vasoconstricted extremities are characteristic. The S2 is loud and single. Heart murmur is usually absent. Signs of heart failure develop with hepatomegaly and gallop rhythm.

3. The ECG shows RVH. Rarely, LVH pattern is present because V5 and V6 electrodes are placed over the dilated RV.

4. CXR films show pulmonary venous congestion or pulmonary edema. The heart is only mildly enlarged.

5. Severe metabolic acidosis (caused by markedly decreased cardiac output) in the presence of slightly decreased arterial Po_2 and a normal Pco_2 is characteristic of the condition.

6. Echo findings are diagnostic and usually obviate cardiac catheterization. Severe hypoplasia of the aorta and aortic annulus and the absent or distorted mitral valve are usually imaged. The LV cavity is diminutive. The RV cavity is markedly dilated, and the tricuspid valve is large. A partially constricted PDA may be imaged.

7. Progressive hypoxemia and acidosis result in death without surgery, usually in the first month of life.

MANAGEMENT
MEDICAL

1. The patient should be intubated and ventilated appropriately with oxygen, and metabolic acidosis should be corrected.

2. An intravenous infusion of PGE_1 may produce temporary improvement by reopening the ductus arteriosus (see Appendix E for the dosage).

3. Balloon atrial septostomy may help decompress the LA and temporarily improve oxygenation.

4. A neurologic evaluation, including imaging of the head, should be obtained because of a high prevalence of neurodevelopmental abnormalities seen in this condition.

SURGICAL. Two surgical options are available in the management of these infants: the Norwood operation or cardiac transplantation. The former is more popular than the latter. The first-stage Norwood operation is performed initially and followed later by the Fontan-type operation.

1. The Norwood operation (Fig. 3-43) is performed in the neonatal period. This operation consists of (1) division of the MPA and closure of the distal stump; (2) a right-sided B-T shunt (usually a 4- to 5-mm tube) to provide PBF; (3) excision of the atrial septum (for decompression of the LA and adequate interatrial mixing); and (4) construction of a new aortic arch between the proximal MPA and the hypoplastic aortic arch, using an aortic or pulmonary artery allograft. The surgical mortality rate is as high as 25%.

2. Second-stage procedure: Either bidirectional Glenn procedure or the hemi-Fontan procedure is performed at 3 to 6 months of age (see Tricuspid Atresia for the description of these procedures). The mortality rate is less than 5%.

3. A Fontan-type operation is carried out when the patient is 12 to 18 months of age (as described under Tricuspid Atresia).

4. Cardiac transplantation is considered to be the procedure of choice in some centers. If the diameter of the ascending aorta is <2.5 mm, cardiac transplantation, rather than the Norwood operation, is believed to provide a better result. The transplantation is not a cure for the defect but creates a lifelong medical problem with the threat of infection and rejection.

POSTOPERATIVE FOLLOW-UP. Postoperative follow-up is the same as that for tricuspid atresia.

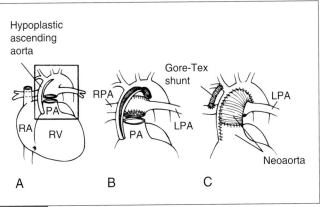

Hypoplastic
ascending
aorta

Gore-Tex
shunt

RPA

RA

RV

PA

LPA

PA

LPA

Neoaorta

A

B

C

FIG. 3-43

Schematic diagram of Norwood procedure. **A,** The heart with aortic atresia and
hypoplasia of the ascending aorta and aortic arch is shown. The MPA is transected.
B, The distal PA is closed with a patch. An incision is made in the ascending aorta
that extends around the aortic arch to the level of the ductus. The ductus is ligated.
C, A modified right Blalock-Taussig shunt is created between the right subclavian
artery and the RPA as the sole source of pulmonary blood flow. Using an aortic (or
pulmonary arterial) allograft *(shaded area)*, the PA is anastomosed to the ascending
aorta and the aortic arch to create a large arterial trunk. The procedure to widen the
atrial communication is not shown. LPA, left pulmonary artery; PA, pulmonary artery;
RA, right atrium; RPA, right pulmonary artery; RV, right ventricle.

J. EBSTEIN ANOMALY

PREVALENCE. Less than 1% of all CHDs.

PATHOLOGY AND PATHOPHYSIOLOGY

1. The septal and posterior leaflets of the tricuspid valve are displaced
into the RV cavity so that a portion of the RV is incorporated into the RA
(atrialized RV), resulting in functional hypoplasia of the RV and TR (Fig.
3-44). An interatrial communication is present, with resulting R-L atrial
shunt (and varying degree of cyanosis).
2. The RA is massively dilated and hypertrophied. The RV free wall is
often thin. Fibrosis is present in the RV and LV free walls. In addition,
Wolff-Parkinson-White (WPW) preexcitation is frequently associated with
the anomaly and predisposes to attacks of SVT.

CLINICAL MANIFESTATIONS

1. In severe cases, cyanosis and CHF develop in the first few days of life,
with some subsequent improvement. In milder cases, dyspnea, fatigue,
and cyanosis on exertion may be present in childhood.

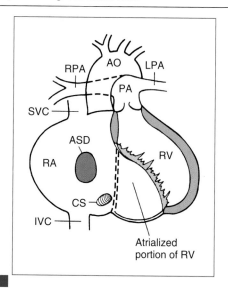

FIG. 3-44

Ebstein anomaly of the tricuspid valve. There is a downward displacement of the tricuspid valve into the RV. Part of the RV is incorporated into the RA (atrialized portion of the RV). Regurgitation of the tricuspid valve results in an enlargement of the RA. An ASD is usually present. AO, aorta; ASD, atrial septal defect; CS, coronary sinus; IVC, inferior vena cava; LPA, left pulmonary artery; PA, pulmonary artery; RA, right atrium; RPA, right pulmonary artery; RV, right ventricle; SVC, superior vena cava.

2. The S2 is widely split. Characteristic triple or quadruple rhythm, consisting of split S1, split S2, S3, and S4, is present. A soft regurgitant systolic murmur of TR is usually audible at the LLSB.
3. Characteristic ECG findings are RBBB and RAH. WPW preexcitation, SVT, and first-degree AV block are occasionally present.
4. CXR films may show extreme cardiomegaly, involving principally the RA, and decreased PVMs.
5. Two-dimensional echo shows the apical displacement of the septal leaflet of the tricuspid valve. TR, a small RV cavity, a large RA, and an ASD (with R-L shunt) are also imaged.
6. Cyanosis of neonates tends to improve as the PVR falls. Attacks of SVT are common. Other possible complications include CHF, LV dysfunction with fibrosis, and cerebrovascular accident.

MANAGEMENT
MEDICAL
1. In severely cyanotic neonates, intensive treatment with mechanical ventilation, intravenous PGE$_1$ infusion, inotropic agents, and correction of metabolic acidosis may be necessary.

2. In a less cyanotic child, anticongestive measures with digitalis and diuretics are indicated if CHF develops.

3. Acute episodes of SVT may be treated most effectively with adenosine. Beta blockers are the most appropriate agents for prevention of SVT of undetermined mechanism. For those patients with recurrent SVT due to AV reentrant mechanism, radiofrequency catheter ablation techniques may be indicated.

4. Varying degrees of activity restriction may be necessary.

SURGICAL

1. Indications. Indications for surgical intervention may include the following:

a. Critically ill neonates who show symptoms within the first week of life

b. Moderately severe or progressive cyanosis (arterial O_2 saturation of $\leq 80\%$) with polycythemia (hemoglobin level of ≥ 16 g/dL) or CHF

c. Right ventricular outflow tract obstruction by redundant tricuspid valve

d. Severe activity limitation (i.e., functional class III or IV)

e. History of paradoxic embolus

f. Repeated, life-threatening arrhythmias in patients with associated WPW syndrome

2. Procedures. Surgical approaches for this anomaly are summarized in Figure 3-45.

a. Palliative procedures are performed for critically ill neonates.

  (1) Blalock-Taussig shunt (with enlargement of ASD), especially in the presence of RVOT obstruction or stenotic or atretic tricuspid valve. A Fontan-type operation is performed later.

  (2) If the LV is "pancaked" by large RV or RA, the Starnes operation may be performed (which consists of pericardial closure of the tricuspid valve, plication of large atrialized RV, enlargement of ASD, and a Blalock-Taussig shunt using a 4-mm tube). A Fontan-type operation is performed later.

  (3) Classic Glenn anastomosis or its modification may be considered in severely cyanotic infants.

b. Two-ventricular repair (tricuspid valve repair or replacement) is indicated in children with good RV size and function.

  (1) Tricuspid valve repair surgeries (Danielson or Carpentier procedure) are preferable to valve replacement. Danielson technique plicates the atrialized portion of the RV, narrows the tricuspid orifice in a selective manner, and results in a monoleaflet tricuspid valve. ASD is closed at the time of surgery. The mortality rate of Danielson procedure is about 5%, which is lower than that for valve replacement. Carpentier technique is similar to the Danielson technique, but the valvular repair is done in a direction that is at right angles to that used by Danielson. The surgical mortality rate is 15%.

  (2) Tricuspid valve replacement (with allograft or heterograft valve) and closure of the ASD is a less desirable surgical approach but

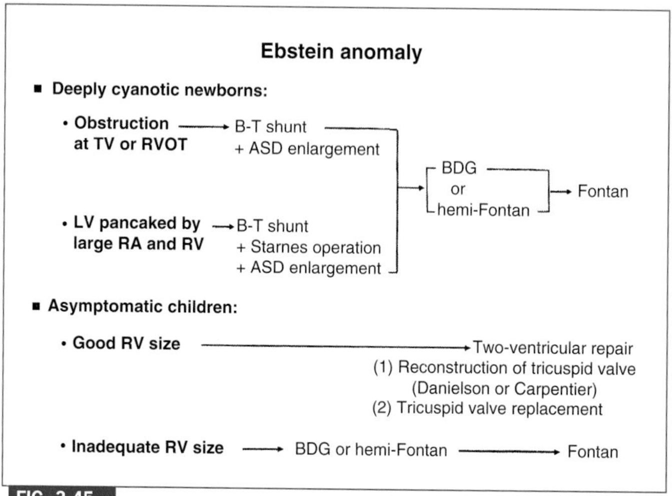

FIG. 3-45

Surgical approaches for Ebstein anomaly of the tricuspid valve. ASD, atrial septal defect; BDG, bidirectional Glenn; B-T, Blalock-Taussig; LV, left ventricle; RA, right atrium; RV, right ventricle; RVOT, right ventricular outflow tract; TV, tricuspid valve. *(From Park MK: Pediatric cardiology for practitioners, ed 5, Philadelphia, 2008, Mosby.)*

may be necessary for 20% to 30% of patients with Ebstein anomaly who are not candidates for reconstructive surgery. The surgical mortality rate ranges from 5% to 20%.
c. One-ventricular repair. For patients with inadequate size of the RV, Fontan-type operation is usually performed in stages.
d. Other procedures. For patients with WPW syndrome and recurrent SVT, surgical interruption of the accessory pathway is recommended at the time of surgery.

POSTSURGICAL FOLLOW-UP. Arrhythmias may persist even after surgery (in 10% to 20% of patients), requiring follow-up. Limitation of activities in competitive or strenuous sports may be indicated.

K. PERSISTENT TRUNCUS ARTERIOSUS

PREVALENCE. Fewer than 1% of all CHDs.
PATHOLOGY AND PATHOPHYSIOLOGY
1. Only a single arterial trunk (with a truncal valve) leaves the heart and gives rise to the pulmonary, systemic, and coronary circulations. A large VSD is always present. A right aortic arch is present in 30% of patients.
2. Collette and Edwards' classification divides this anomaly into four types (Fig. 3-46): type I (affects 60%), type II (20%), type III (10%),

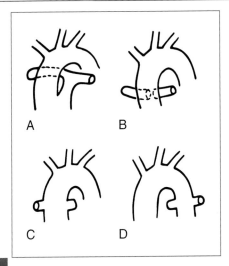

FIG. 3-46

Anatomic types of persistent truncus arteriosus. **A,** Type I. **B,** Type II. **C,** Type III.
D, Type IV, or pseudotruncus arteriosus.

and type IV (10%). Type IV is not a true persistent truncus arteriosus;
it is a severe form of TOF with pulmonary atresia with aortic collaterals
supplying the lungs.

3. Coronary artery abnormalities (stenotic coronary ostia, abnormal
branching and course) are quite common, contributing to a high surgical
mortality.

4. DiGeorge syndrome with hypocalcemia is present in about 30% of patients. Interrupted aortic arch is seen in 13% (type B interruption between the left carotid and left subclavian arteries).

5. The PBF is usually increased in type I, normal in types II and III, and
decreased in type IV. As with other cyanotic CHDs, the level of systemic
arterial oxygen saturation is directly related to the amount of PBF. Therefore, with decreased PBF, cyanosis is notable. With increased PBF, cyanosis is minimal, but CHF may develop.

CLINICAL MANIFESTATIONS

1. Cyanosis may be noted immediately after birth. Signs of CHF may develop within several weeks.

2. A grade 2 to 4/6 regurgitant systolic murmur (suggestive of VSD) is
present along the LSB. A high-pitched diastolic decrescendo murmur of
truncal valve regurgitation is occasionally present. An apical diastolic
rumble may be audible when PBF is large. Wide pulse pressure and
bounding arterial pulses may be present.

3. The ECG shows BVH (70% of patients); RVH or LVH is less common.

4. CXR films usually show cardiomegaly (biventricular and LA enlargement) and increased PVMs. A right aortic arch is seen in 30% of patients.

5. Two-dimensional echo demonstrates a large VSD directly under the truncal valve, similar to TOF. The pulmonary valve cannot be imaged (because it is absent). A large single great artery arising from the heart (truncus) and the posterior branching of the PA from the truncus may be seen.

6. Without surgery, most infants die of CHF within 6 to 12 months. Clinical improvement occurs if the infant develops PVOD. Truncal valve regurgitation, if present, worsens with time.

MANAGEMENT
MEDICAL

1. Vigorous anticongestive measures with digitalis and diuretics are required.

2. Due to the frequent association of DiGeorge syndrome, the following should be done.

a. Serum Ca and Mg levels should be obtained.

b. Only irradiated blood product should be used.

c. Because of the thymus-based immune deficiency, treatment and prophylaxis against pneumococcal and streptococcal infection are important.

d. Immunization with live vaccine should be avoided.

SURGICAL

1. PA banding may be indicated in small infants with large PBF and CHF, but the mortality is high and the result not satisfactory. Primary repair of the defect is recommended by many centers.

2. Various modifications of the Rastelli procedure are performed, ideally in the first week of life. The VSD is closed so that the LV ejects into the truncus. An aortic homograft 9 to 11 mm is placed between the RV and the PA. For types II and III a procedure to join the two PA branches is carried out before connecting the joined PAs to the distal end of the conduit. The mortality rate is as high as 30%.

3. Regurgitant truncal valve is preferably repaired rather than replaced.

POSTSURGICAL FOLLOW-UP

1. Follow-up every 4 to 12 months is required to detect late complications.

a. Progressive truncal valve insufficiency.

b. A small conduit needs to be replaced with a larger one, usually by 2 to 3 years of age.

c. Calcification of the valve in the conduit, which may occur within 1 to 5 years.

d. Ventricular arrhythmias may develop because of right ventriculotomy.

2. Restriction from competitive, strenuous sports is necessary.

L.   SINGLE VENTRICLE

PREVALENCE. Single ventricle occurs in less than 1% of all CHDs.

PATHOLOGY AND PATHOPHYSIOLOGY

1. Both AV valves empty into a common main ventricular chamber (double-inlet ventricle). A rudimentary infundibular chamber communicates with the main chamber through the bulboventricular foramen. One great artery arises from the main chamber, and the other usually arises from the rudimentary chamber. If the main chamber has anatomic characteristics of the LV (80%), it is called double-inlet LV. If the main chamber has anatomic characteristics of the RV, it is called double-inlet RV. Rarely, both atria empty via a common AV valve into the main chamber (common-inlet ventricle).

2. Either D- or L-TGA is present in 85% of patients, and pulmonary stenosis or atresia in 50% of the patients. COA and interrupted aortic arch are also common.

3. The most common form of single ventricle is double-inlet LV with L-TGA in which the aorta arises from the rudimentary chamber (Fig. 3-47).

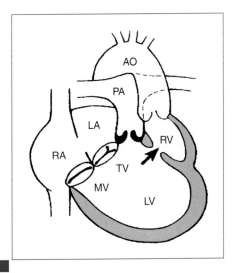

FIG. 3-47

The most common form of single ventricle. The single ventricle is anatomic LV. The great arteries have L-transposition. Stenosis of the pulmonary valve is present in about 50% of patients (shown as thick valves). The bulboventricular foramen *(thick arrow)* connects the main and the rudimentary ventricles. This type accounts for 70% to 75% of cases of single ventricle. AO, aorta; LA, left atrium; LV, left ventricle; MV, mitral valve; PA, pulmonary artery; RA, right atrium; RV, right ventricle; TV, tricuspid valve.

4. The bulboventricular foramen frequently becomes obstructive, with resulting increase in PBF and decreasing systemic flood flow. This has important hemodynamic and surgical implications (see Management).

5. A high prevalence of asplenia or polysplenia syndrome is found.

6. There is a complete mixing of systemic and pulmonary venous blood in the ventricle, and therefore the oxygen saturation in the aorta and PA is identical. The systemic oxygen saturation is proportional to the amount of PBF. With decreased PBF (seen in patients with associated PS), marked cyanosis results. In patients without PS, PBF is large and the patient is minimally cyanotic and may develop CHF.

CLINICAL MANIFESTATIONS

1. Cyanosis of a varying degree is present from birth. Symptoms and signs of CHF, failure to thrive, and bouts of pneumonia are commonly reported.

2. Physical findings depend on the magnitude of PBF. With increased PBF, physical findings resemble those of TGA with large VSD. With decreased PBF, physical findings resemble those of TOF.

3. ECG

a. An unusual ventricular hypertrophy pattern with similar QRS complexes across most or all precordial leads (RS, rS, or QR pattern) appears.

b. Abnormalities in the Q wave take one of the following forms: (1) Q waves in the right precordial leads (RPLs), (2) no Q waves in any precordial leads, or (3) Q waves in both the RPLs and left precordial leads (LPLs).

c. First- or second-degree AV block or arrhythmias may be present.

4. When PBF is increased, CXR film shows cardiomegaly and increased PVMs. When PBF is normal or decreased, the heart size is normal and the PVMs are normal or decreased.

5. Two-dimensional echo shows two distinct AV valves emptying into a single ventricular chamber. The rudimentary chamber is usually to the left of and anterior to the main chamber. The bulboventricular foramen is often obstructive (with pressure gradient >10 mm Hg).

MANAGEMENT

MEDICAL

1. Neonates with severe PS and those with COA or interrupted aortic arch require intravenous PGE_1 infusion and other supportive measures before surgery.

2. Anticongestive measures with digitalis and diuretics are indicated if CHF develops.

SURGICAL. Patients with single ventricle eventually require Fontan operation, through staged approach. Summary of surgical approach is shown in Figure 3-48.

1. Initial palliative procedures

a. A B-T shunt (for infants) or Glenn procedure (for children older than 2 years).

b. PA banding is performed in patients with uncontrollable CHF with large PBF with a high mortality (25% or higher). The banding is

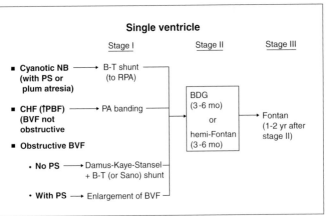

FIG. 3-48

Surgical approach for single ventricle. BDG, bidirectional Glenn; B-T, Blalock-Taussig; BVF, bulboventricular foramen; CHF, congestive heart failure; NB, newborn; PBF, pulmonary blood flow; PS, pulmonary stenosis; RPA, right pulmonary artery. *(From Park MK: Pediatric cardiology for practitioners, ed 5, Philadelphia, 2008, Mosby.)*

performed *only* when the bulboventricular foramen is *normal* or *unobstructed* because patients with obstructed bulboventricular foramen do not tolerate the banding well. These patients should be watched for the development of obstruction after the banding.

c. If the foramen is small, one of the following two alternative procedures can be performed: (1) Damus-Kaye-Stansel anastomosis (transection of the MPA and anastomosis of the proximal PA to the aorta, and a B-T shunt or a cavopulmonary shunt) or (2) enlargement of the bulbo-ventricular foramen by a transaortic approach and without cardiopulmonary bypass (surgical mortality about 15%); this procedure is performed especially when PS is present.

d. Surgery for interrupted aortic arch or COA should be performed, if present.

2. Second-stage palliative procedures. Either bidirectional Glenn operation or hemi-Fontan operation (Figs. 3-37 and 3-38) is carried out between the age of 3 months and 6 months, before proceeding with the Fontan operation.

3. The Fontan-type operation is performed at 12 to 24 months of age (see Tricuspid Atresia for more detailed discussion of the Fontan procedure).

POSTOPERATIVE FOLLOW-UP. Close follow-up is necessary for early and late complications, as discussed in Tricuspid Atresia.

M. DOUBLE-OUTLET RIGHT VENTRICLE

PREVALENCE. Less than 1% of all CHDs.

PATHOLOGY AND PATHOPHYSIOLOGY

1. The aorta and the PA arise side by side from the RV. The only outlet from the LV is a large VSD. The aortic and pulmonary valves are at the same level. Subaortic and subpulmonary conuses separate the aortic and pulmonary valves from the tricuspid and mitral valves, respectively. DORV may be subdivided according to the position of the VSD and further by the presence of PS.

a. Subaortic VSD (occurring in 50% to 70% of the patients, Fig. 3-49, *A*).

b. Subpulmonary VSD (Taussig-Bing anomaly) (Fig. 3-49, *B*).

c. PS is common (50% prevalence) in the subaortic VSD (Fig. 3-49, *C*).

d. Doubly committed VSD.

e. Remote VSD.

2. Pathophysiology of DORV is determined primarily by the position of the VSD and the presence or absence of PS.

a. With subaortic VSD (Fig. 3-49, *A*), oxygenated blood *(open arrow)* from the LV is directed to the aorta (AO), and desaturated systemic venous blood *(solid arrow)* is directed to the pulmonary artery (PA), producing mild or no cyanosis. Clinical pictures resemble those of a large VSD with pulmonary hypertension and CHF.

b. With subpulmonary VSD (Fig. 3-49, *B*), oxygenated blood from the LV is directed to the PA, and desaturated blood from the systemic vein is directed to the aorta, producing severe cyanosis. Thus, clinical pictures resemble those of TGA with CHF.

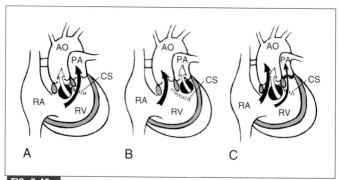

FIG. 3-49

Three representative types of DORV, viewed with the RV free wall removed. **A,** Subaortic VSD. **B,** Subpulmonary VSD (Taussig-Bing anomaly). **C,** Subaortic VSD with PS. Doubly committed and remote VSDs are not shown. AO, aorta; CS, crista supraventricularis; PA, pulmonary artery; RA, right atrium; RV, right ventricle.

c. In the presence of PS (Fallot type), clinical pictures resemble those of TOF (Fig. 3-49, C).

d. With the VSD close to both semilunar valves (doubly committed VSD) or remotely located from these valves (remote VSD), mild cyanosis is present and the PBF is increased.

CLINICAL MANIFESTATIONS

Clinical manifestations vary greatly with the location of the VSD and the presence or absence of PS.

1. Subaortic VSD without PS: Physical findings resemble those of a large VSD with pulmonary hypertension and CHF. The ECG often resembles that of ECD ("superior" QRS axis, LAH, RVH, or BVH and occasional first-degree AV block). CXR films show cardiomegaly with increased PVMs and a prominent MPA segment.

2. Subpulmonary VSD (Taussig-Bing malformation): Physical findings resemble those of TGA with severe cyanosis in newborn infants. Signs of CHF supervene later. The ECG shows RAD, RAH, and RVH. LVH may be seen during infancy. First-degree AV block is frequently present. CXR films show cardiomegaly with increased PVMs.

3. Fallot-type DORV with PS: Physical findings are similar to those seen in cyanotic TOF. The ECG shows RAD, RAH, and RVH or RBBB. CXR films show normal heart size (with upturned apex) and decreased PVMs.

4. Echo (for all types): Diagnostic 2D echo signs include (1) both great arteries arising from the RV and running a parallel course in their origin, (2) absence of the LVOT and demonstration of a VSD, and (3) the mitral-semilunar discontinuity.

MANAGEMENT

MEDICAL. Medical treatment of CHF if present.

SURGICAL

Summary of surgical approach is shown in Figure 3-50.

1. Palliative procedures

a. For infants with remote or multiple VSDs (with large PBF and CHF), a PA banding is occasionally performed. (For subaortic, subpulmonary, or doubly committed VSD, primary repair is a better choice.)

b. For infants with subpulmonary VSD, enlarging the ASD by the balloon or blade atrial septectomy is important for decompression of the LA and better mixing of pulmonary and systemic venous blood.

c. For infants with PS and decreased PBF (Fallot type), a B-T shunt may be indicated.

2. Corrective surgeries

a. Subaortic VSD and doubly committed VSD. Creation of an intraventricular tunnel between the VSD and the subaortic outflow tract in the neonatal period or at least in early infancy. The surgical mortality rate is <5%.

b. Subpulmonary VSD (Taussig-Bing malformation). There are four possible surgical approaches: (1) an intraventricular tunnel between the VSD and the PA (turning it into TGA), plus the arterial switch operation

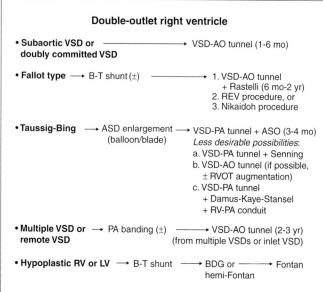

Double-outlet right ventricle

- **Subaortic VSD or** ──────────→ VSD-AO tunnel (1-6 mo)
  doubly committed VSD

- **Fallot type** ──→ B-T shunt (±) ──────→ 1. VSD-AO tunnel
  + Rastelli (6 mo-2 yr)
  2. REV procedure, or
  3. Nikaidoh procedure

- **Taussig-Bing** ──→ ASD enlargement ──→ VSD-PA tunnel + ASO (3-4 mo)
  (balloon/blade) *Less desirable possibilities:*
  a. VSD-PA tunnel + Senning
  b. VSD-AO tunnel (if possible,
  ± RVOT augmentation)
  c. VSD-PA tunnel
  + Damus-Kaye-Stansel
  + RV-PA conduit

- **Multiple VSD or** ──→ PA banding (±) ──────→ VSD-AO tunnel (2-3 yr)
  remote VSD (from multiple VSDs or inlet VSD)

- **Hypoplastic RV or LV** ──→ B-T shunt ──→ BDG or ──→ Fontan
  hemi-Fontan

FIG. 3-50

Surgical approach for DORV. AO, aorta; ASD, atrial septal defect; ASO, arterial switch operation; B-T, Blalock-Taussig; PA, pulmonary artery; REV, réparation à l'étage ventriculaire; RV, right ventricle; RVOT, right ventricular outflow tract; RV-PA, RV-to-pulmonary artery; VSD, ventricular septal defect; VSD-AO, VSD-to-aorta; VSD-PA, VSD-to-pulmonary artery. *(From Park MK: Pediatric cardiology for practitioners, ed 5, Philadelphia, 2008, Mosby.)*

during the first month of life (surgical mortality 10% to 15%); (2) as in (1) plus the Senning operation (less desirable, surgical mortality above 40%); (3) an intraventricular tunnel between the subpulmonary VSD and the aorta is desirable if technically feasible (mortality, 15%); or (4) creation of VSD-to-PA tunnel, followed by Damus-Kaye-Stansel operation and RV-to-PA conduit.

c. Fallot type. There are three surgical options: (1) an intraventricular VSD-to-aorta tunnel plus RV-to-PA homograft valved conduit at 6 months to 2 years of age, (2) REV procedure (Fig. 3-20), or (3) Nikaidoh procedure (Fig. 3-21).

d. Remote VSD. When possible, an intraventricular tunnel procedure (between inlet VSD and the aorta) is preferred (performed at age 2 to 3 years with a high mortality of 30% to 40%). PA banding is usually needed in infancy to control CHF.

POSTSURGICAL FOLLOW-UP. Long-term follow-up at 6- to 12-month intervals is necessary to detect late complications (such as the need to reoperate and ventricular arrhythmias).

N.   HETEROTAXIA (ATRIAL ISOMERISM, ASPLENIA AND POLYSPLENIA SYNDROMES)

PREVALENCE. 1% to 2% of neonates with symptomatic CHD.

PATHOLOGY AND PATHOPHYSIOLOGY

1. There is a failure of differentiation into the right- and left-sided organs in heterotaxia, with resulting congenital malformations of multiple organ systems. *Asplenia syndrome* (right atrial isomerism, Ivemark syndrome) is associated with the absence of the spleen, a left-sided organ, and a tendency to bilateral right-sidedness. In *polysplenia syndrome* (left atrial isomerism), multiple splenic tissues with a tendency for bilateral left-sidedness are present. Although the type and severity of cardiovascular malformations are somewhat different between the two syndromes, the same types of defects may be present in both conditions.
2. Noncardiac malformations may help differentiate the two syndromes.
a. In asplenia syndrome, bilateral three-lobed lungs (two right lungs) with bilateral eparterial bronchi and various gastrointestinal malformations, including a symmetrical midline liver and malrotation of the intestines, are present. The stomach may be on the right or the left.
b. In polysplenia syndrome, bilateral, bilobed lungs (two left lungs) with bilateral, hyparterial bronchi; symmetrical liver (25%); occasional absence of gallbladder; and some degree of intestinal malrotation (80%) are present.
3. Complex cardiac malformations are almost always present, especially with asplenia syndrome. Cardiovascular malformations involve all parts of the heart: systemic and pulmonary veins, the atria, the AV valves, the ventricles, and the great arteries.
a. In general, asplenia syndrome has more severe abnormalities of these structures. A normal heart or only minimal malformation of the heart is present in up to 25% of the patients with polysplenia syndrome. Bilateral SVCs are common, and anomalies of the pulmonary venous return are usually present. Single atrium, secundum ASD, and primum ASD are all common. There are either two sinus nodes (seen with asplenia) or no sinus node (seen in polysplenia). The coronary sinus is usually absent. Single AV valve is common, especially in asplenia. Either a single ventricle or VSD is usually present. TGA is usually present in asplenia syndrome (70%) and occasionally in polysplenia syndrome (15%).
b. Cardiovascular anomalies that help distinguish these two syndromes are summarized in Table 3-1. The abnormalities with asterisks are particularly helpful, but the IVC probably has the most important differential power; the IVC is almost always normal in asplenia syndrome but is interrupted (with azygous continuation) in polysplenia.
4. There is usually a complete mixing of systemic and pulmonary venous blood in the heart because of multiple cardiovascular malformations.

TABLE 3-1

CARDIOVASCULAR MALFORMATIONS IN ASPLENIA AND POLYSPLENIA
SYNDROMES

STRUCTURE	ASPLENIA SYNDROME	POLYSPLENIA SYNDROME
Systemic Veins	Normal IVC in all but may be left-sided (35%)	*Absent hepatic segment of IVC with azygos continuation, right or left (85%)
Pulmonary Veins	*TAPVR with extracardiac connection (75%), often with PV obstruction	Normal PV return (50%) Right PVs to right-sided atrium; left PVs to left-sided atrium (50%)
Atrium and Atrial Septum	Bilateral right atria (bilateral sinus node) Primum ASD (100%) + secundum ASD (66%)	Bilateral left atria (no sinus node) Single atrium, primum ASD (60%), or secundum ASD (25%)
AV Valve	*Single AV valve (90%)	Normal AV valve (50%); single AV valve (15%)
Ventricles	Single ventricle (50%); two ventricles (50%)	Two ventricles almost always present; VSD (65%); DORV (20%)
Great Arteries	*Transposition (70%) (D-TGA, L-TGA) *Stenosis (40%) or atresia (40%) of pulmonary valve	Normal great arteries (85%); transposition (15%) Normal pulmonary valve (60%); pulmonary stenosis or atresia (40%)
ECG	Normal P axis, or in the +90- to +180-degree quadrant	*Superior P axis (70%)

*Important differentiating points.

When PBF is reduced, as in asplenia, severe cyanosis results. When PBF is increased, as in polysplenia syndrome, cyanosis is not intense and CHF often develops.

CLINICAL MANIFESTATIONS
1. In asplenia syndrome, cyanosis is often severe shortly after birth. In polysplenia syndrome, signs of CHF may develop during the neonatal period. Auscultation of the heart is nonspecific, but heart murmurs of VSD and/or PS are frequently audible. A symmetrical liver (midline liver) is characteristic.
2. The ECG shows a "superior" QRS axis (due to ECD) in both conditions. An additional "superior" P axis (−30 to −90 degrees) strongly suggests polysplenia syndrome. In asplenia syndrome the P axis may be either normal or alternating between the left lower and right lower quadrants (because two sinus nodes alternate the pacemaker function). RVH,

LVH, or BVH is usually present. Complete heart block occurs in about 10% of the patients with polysplenia syndrome.

3. The heart size is normal or only slightly increased on CXR films. The PVMs are either decreased (asplenia) or increased (polysplenia). The heart is in the right or left chest or in the midline (mesocardia). A symmetrical liver (midline liver) is a striking feature of both syndromes.

4. When the systematic approach is used, 2D echo and color flow Doppler studies can detect all or most of the anomalies described under pathology.

5. There are some noncardiac clinical findings available to general physicians that may lead to the recognition of heterotaxia.

a. Symmetric "midline" liver (on palpation or x-ray films)

b. Discordant cardiac apex and stomach bubble (on chest x-ray films)

c. Biliary atresia in a neonate with congenital heart defects

d. Symmetric main-stem bronchi on chest x-rays

e. A superior P axis (or "coronary sinus rhythm") and superior QRS axis on the ECG (suggest polysplenia syndrome)

6. It is important to know which type of isomerism one has from the point of prophylaxis against bacterial infection for patients with asplenia syndrome, who have increased risk of developing sepsis.

a. Howell-Jolly and Heinz bodies seen on the peripheral smear suggest asplenia syndrome, although some normal neonates and septic infants may show these bodies.

b. A splenic scan may be useful in differentiating the two conditions in older infants but is of limited value in acutely ill neonates.

7. Without palliative surgical procedures, more than 95% of patients with asplenia syndrome die in the first year of life. Fulminating sepsis is one of the causes of death. Excessive nodal bradycardia with resulting CHF may develop in patients with polysplenia syndrome, requiring a pacemaker therapy.

MANAGEMENT
MEDICAL

1. Intravenous PGE_1 infusion (see Appendix E for dosage) to reopen the ductus is indicated for severely cyanotic newborn infants with asplenia syndrome.

2. Some patients with polysplenia syndrome may need treatment for CHF and occasionally a PA banding.

3. The risk of fulminating infection, especially by *Streptococcus pneumoniae,* is high in patients with asplenia syndrome (refer to the most recent "Red Book").

a. Oral penicillin V, 125 mg, twice a day for children <5 years, and 250 mg, twice a day for children ≥5 years, is recommended. Some experts recommend amoxicillin (20 mg/kg per day, divided into two doses). Erythromycin is an alternate choice in patients who are allergic to penicillin. Prophylactic penicillin can be discontinued at 5 years of age or continued throughout childhood and into adulthood.

b. Immunizations against *Streptococcus pneumoniae, Haemophilus influenzae* type b (Hib), and *Neisseria meningitidis* are recommended.

(1) Heptavalent pneumococcal vaccine: For children ≤5 years at diagnosis, the conjugate vaccine (PCV7) is recommended beginning at 2 months of age, times 3 every 2 months, and reimmunization at 12 to 15 months. For children >5 years, a single dose of PCV7 or 23PS is recommended.

(2) Immunization against Hib infections should be initiated at 2 months of age, as recommended for otherwise healthy children, and for previously unimmunized children with asplenia.

(3) Tetravalent meningococcal polysaccharide vaccine also should be administered to children 2 through 10 years. Meningococcal conjugate vaccine should be given to adolescents.

SURGICAL

1. For asplenia syndrome

a. A B-T shunt is usually necessary because of severe cyanosis. The surgical mortality is high, probably because of regurgitation of the common AV valve and undiagnosed obstructive TAPVR.

b. Pulmonary angiography with infusion of PGE_1 is recommended to identify patients with obstructive TAPVR.

c. Staged Fontan-type operation can be performed later as outlined under Tricuspid Atresia (but with the surgical mortality as high as 65% because of the AV valve regurgitation).

2. For polysplenia syndrome

a. Occasional PA banding is necessary for CHF.

b. In some children with polysplenia syndrome, total correction of the defect is possible. If not, a Fontan operation can be performed (with a mortality rate of about 25%).

c. Pacemaker therapy is occasionally required for excessive junctional bradycardia and CHF in children with polysplenia syndrome.

POSTSURGICAL FOLLOW-UP. As outlined under Tricuspid Atresia

O. PERSISTENT PULMONARY HYPERTENSION OF THE NEWBORN

PREVALENCE. PPHN (or persistence of the fetal circulation) occurs in approximately 1 in 1500 live births.

PATHOLOGY AND PATHOPHYSIOLOGY

1. Persistent pulmonary hypertension of the newborn (PPHN) is characterized by persistence of pulmonary hypertension, which in turn causes a varying degree of cyanosis from an R-L shunt through the PDA or PFO. No other underlying CHD is present.

2. Various causes have been identified, but they can be divided into three groups by the anatomy of the pulmonary vascular bed as shown in Box 3-2.

3. In general, pulmonary hypertension caused by the first group is relatively easy to reverse and that caused by the second group is more difficult to reverse than that caused by the first group (Box 3-2). Pulmonary hypertension caused by the third group is most difficult or impossible to reverse.

BOX 3-2

CAUSES OF PERSISTENT PULMONARY HYPERTENSION OF THE NEWBORN

Pulmonary vasoconstriction in the presence of a normally developed pulmonary vascular bed may be caused by or seen in the following:

    Alveolar hypoxia (meconium aspiration syndrome, hyaline membrane disease, hypoventilation caused by central nervous system anomalies)

    Birth asphyxia

    Left ventricular dysfunction or circulatory shock

    Infections (such as group B hemolytic streptococcal infection)

    Hyperviscosity syndrome (polycythemia)

    Hypoglycemia and hypocalcemia

Increased pulmonary vascular smooth muscle development (hypertrophy) may be caused by the following:

    Chronic intrauterine asphyxia

    Maternal use of prostaglandin synthesis inhibitors (aspirin, indomethacin) resulting in early ductal closure

Decreased cross-sectional area of pulmonary vascular bed may be seen in association with the following:

    Congenital diaphragmatic hernia

    Primary pulmonary hypoplasia

---

4. Varying degrees of myocardial dysfunction often occur in association with PPHN, manifested by a decrease in fractional shortening or TR, which are caused by myocardial ischemia and are aggravated by hypoglycemia and hypocalcemia.

CLINICAL MANIFESTATIONS

1. Full-term or postterm neonates are often affected. Symptoms begin 6 to 12 hours after birth, with cyanosis and respiratory difficulties (with retraction and grunting). History of meconium staining or birth asphyxia is often present. A history of maternal ingestion of nonsteroidal anti-inflammatory drugs (in the third trimester) may be present.

2. A prominent RV impulse and a single and loud S2 are usually found. Occasional gallop rhythm (from myocardial dysfunction) and a soft regurgitant systolic murmur of TR may be audible. Systemic hypotension may be present with severe myocardial dysfunction.

3. Arterial desaturation is found in blood samples obtained from an umbilical artery catheter. Arterial Po_2 may be lower in the umbilical artery line than in the preductal arteries (the right radial, brachial, or temporal artery) by 5 to 10 mm Hg because of an R-L ductal shunt. In severe cases, differential cyanosis may appear (with a pink upper body and a cyanotic lower body). If there is a prominent R-L intracardiac shunt (through PFO or ASD), the preductal and postductal arteries may not show a Po_2 difference.

4. The ECG usually is normal for age, but occasional RVH is present. T wave abnormalities suggestive of myocardial dysfunction may be seen.

5. CXR films reveal a varying degree of cardiomegaly with or without hyperinflation or atelectasis. The PVM may appear normal, increased, or decreased.

6. Echo and Doppler studies show no evidence of cyanotic CHD. The only structural abnormality is the presence of a large PDA with an R-L or bidirectional shunt. The atrial septum bulges toward the left due to a higher pressure in the RA, with or without an ASD or PFO. Pulmonary veins are normal (TAPVR can mimic PPHN). The LV dimension may be increased, and the fractional shortening or ejection fraction may be decreased.

MANAGEMENT

The goals of therapy are (1) to lower the PVR and PA pressure through the administration of oxygen, the induction of respiratory alkalosis, and the use of pulmonary vasodilators (such as tolazoline); (2) to correct myocardial dysfunction (by dopamine, dobutamine); and (3) to stabilize the patient and treat associated conditions (e.g., acidosis, hypocalcemia, hypoglycemia).

A high-frequency oscillatory ventilator, inhalation nitric oxide (iNO), and employment of extracorporeal membrane oxygenation (ECMO) have been shown to be effective in the management of selected patients with severe PPHN.

PROGNOSIS

1. Prognosis generally is good for neonates with mild PPHN who respond quickly to therapy. For those requiring a maximal ventilator setting for a prolonged time, the chance of survival is smaller, and many survivors develop bronchopulmonary dysplasia and other complications. Patients with developmental decreases in cross-sectional areas of the pulmonary vascular bed usually do not respond to therapy, and their prognosis is poor.

2. Neurodevelopmental abnormalities may manifest. Patients have a high incidence of hearing loss (up to 50%). An abnormal electroencephalogram (up to 80%) and cerebral infarction (45%) have been reported.

IV. MISCELLANEOUS CONGENITAL ANOMALIES

A. ANOMALOUS ORIGIN OF THE LEFT CORONARY ARTERY (BLAND-WHITE-GARLAND SYNDROME, ALCAPA SYNDROME)

The left coronary artery arises abnormally from the PA. The newborn patient is usually asymptomatic until the PA pressure falls to a critical level. Symptoms appear at 2 to 3 months of age and consist of recurring episodes of distress (anginal pain), marked cardiomegaly, and CHF. Heart murmur usually is absent. The ECG shows an anterolateral myocardial infarction pattern consisting of abnormally deep and wide Q waves; inverted T waves; and ST segment shift in leads I, aVL, and most precordial leads.

MANAGEMENT

Medical treatment alone carries a very high mortality (80% to 100%). All patients with this diagnosis need operation. The optimal operation remains controversial, but most centers prefer definitive surgery unless the patient is critically ill.

1. Palliative surgery: In critically ill infants, simple ligation of the anomalous left coronary artery close to its origin from the PA may be performed to prevent steal into the PA. This should be followed by a later elective bypass procedure.
2. Definitive surgery: One of the two-coronary system surgeries is done.
a. Intrapulmonary tunnel operation (Takeuchi repair). Initially a 5- to 6-mm aortopulmonary window is created between the ascending aorta and the MPA at the level of the takeoff of the left coronary artery. In the posterior wall of the MPA a tunnel is created that connects the opening of the aortopulmonary window and the orifice of the anomalous left coronary artery. The mortality rate is near 0% but as high as over 20% has been reported. Late complications of the procedure include supravalvular pulmonary artery stenosis (75%), baffle leak (52%) causing coronary-pulmonary artery fistula, and AR.
b. Left coronary artery implantation. In this procedure the anomalous coronary artery is excised from the PA along with a button of PA wall, and the artery is reimplanted into the anterior aspect of the ascending aorta. The early surgical mortality rate is 15% to 20%.
c. Tashiro repair. In the Tashiro procedure (1993), which was first described in adults, a narrow cuff of the MPA, including the orifice of the left coronary artery, is transected. The upper and lower edges of the cuff are closed to form a new left main coronary artery, which is anastomosed to the aorta. The divided MPA is anastomosed end to end.
d. Subclavian-to-left coronary artery anastomosis. In this technique the end of the left subclavian artery is turned down and anastomosed end to side to the anomalous left coronary artery.

B.   ARTERIOVENOUS FISTULA, CORONARY

Coronary artery fistulas occur in one of two patterns: (1) They may represent a branching tributary from a coronary artery coursing along a normal anatomic distribution (true coronary arteriovenous fistula), occurring in only 7% of patients. (2) In most patients the fistula is the result of an abnormal coronary artery system with aberrant termination (coronary artery fistula). In most cases the fistula terminates in the right side of the heart (40% in the RV, 25% in the RA, and 20% in the PA).

The patient is usually asymptomatic. A continuous murmur similar to the murmur of PDA is audible over the precordium. The ECG is usually normal, but it may show T wave inversion, RVH, or LVH if the fistula is large. CXR films usually show normal heart size. Myocardial infarction can occur.

In surgery the fistulous point is closed nearest to the entry into the cardiac chamber without compromising the coronary circulation (surgical mortality 0% to 5%). Recently, successful use of Gianturco coils or a double umbrella device has been reported in selected patients.

C. ARTERIOVENOUS FISTULA, PULMONARY

There is direct communication between the PAs and PVs, bypassing the pulmonary capillary circulation. It may take the form of either multiple tiny angiomas (telangiectasis) or a large PA-to-PV communication. About 60% of patients with pulmonary AV fistulas have Osler-Weber-Rendu syndrome. Rarely, chronic liver disease or a previous SVC-to-PA surgical connection may cause the fistula.

Cyanosis and clubbing are present, with arterial oxygen saturation ranging from 50% to 85%. A faint systolic or continuous murmur may be audible over the affected area. The peripheral pulses are not bounding. Polycythemia is usually present. CXR films show normal heart size. One or more rounded opacities of variable size may be present in the lung fields. The ECG is usually normal. Stroke, brain abscess, and rupture of the fistula with hemoptysis or hemothorax are possible complications. Following a peripheral venous injection of contrast agent, microcavitations opacify the RA and RV, then several heartbeats later, microcavitations appear in the LA and LV. The definitive diagnosis of the condition usually requires selective angiography into the affected pulmonary arteries.

Surgical resection of the lesions, with preservation of as much healthy lung tissue as possible, may be attempted in symptomatic children, but the progressive nature of the disorder calls for a conservative approach. Recently, selective embolotherapy has been proposed as an alternative to surgical resection.

D. ARTERIOVENOUS FISTULA, SYSTEMIC

There is direct communication (either a vascular channel or angiomas) between the artery and vein without the interposition of the capillary bed. The two most common sites of systemic AV fistulas are the brain and liver. In the liver, hemangioendotheliomas (densely vascular benign tumors) are more common than fistulous arteriovenous malformation. Because of decreased peripheral vascular resistance, an increase in stroke volume (with a wide pulse pressure), cardiomegaly, tachycardia, and even CHF may result.

A systolic or continuous murmur is audible over the affected organ. The peripheral pulses may be bounding. A gallop rhythm may be present with CHF. CXR films show cardiomegaly and increased PVMs. The ECG may show hypertrophy of either or both ventricles.

Most patients with large cerebral AV fistulas and CHF die as neonates, and surgical ligation of the affected artery to the brain is rarely possible without infarcting the brain. Surgical treatment of hepatic fistulas is often impossible because they are spread throughout the liver. However, hemangioendotheliomas may undergo spontaneous involution once treatment with corticosteroids, interferon, or partial embolization has begun.

E. COR TRIATRIATUM

In this rare cardiac anomaly the LA is divided into two compartments by a fibromuscular septum with a small opening, producing obstruction of pulmonary venous return. Embryologically, the upper compartment is a dilated common PV and the lower compartment is the true LA. Hemodynamic abnormalities of this condition are similar to those of MS in that both conditions produce pulmonary venous and arterial hypertension.

Important physical findings include dyspnea, basal pulmonary crackles, a loud P2, and a nonspecific systolic murmur. The ECG shows RVH and occasional RAH. CXR films show evidence of pulmonary venous congestion or pulmonary edema, prominent MPA segment, and right-sided heart enlargement. Echo demonstrates a linear structure within the LA cavity. Surgical correction is always indicated. Pulmonary hypertension regresses rapidly in survivors if the correction is made early.

F. DEXTROCARDIA AND MESOCARDIA

The terms *dextrocardia* (heart in the right side of the chest) and *mesocardia* (heart in midline of the thorax) express the position of the heart as a whole but do not specify the segmental relationship of the heart. A normally formed heart can be in the right chest because of extracardiac abnormalities. On the other hand, a heart in the right chest may be a sign of a serious cyanotic heart defect. The segmental approach is used to examine the significance of abnormal position of the heart.

1. **The segmental approach.** The heart and the great arteries can be viewed as three separate segments: the atria, the ventricles, and the great arteries. These three segments can vary from their normal positions either independently or together, resulting in many possible sets of abnormalities. Accurate mapping can be accomplished by echo and angiocardiography, but CXR and ECG are helpful also.

a. **Localization of the atria.** Chest x-ray films, the ECG, and the echo can be used to localize the atria.

   (1) CXR film
       (a) Right-sided liver shadow and left-sided stomach bubble indicate situs solitus of the atria. Left-sided liver shadow and right-sided stomach bubble indicate situs inversus of the atria.
       (b) A midline (symmetrical) liver shadow on CXR films suggests heterotaxia.
   (2) ECG: The SA node is always located in the RA. Therefore, the P axis of the ECG can be used to locate the atria. When the P axis is in the left lower quadrant (0 to +90 degrees), situs solitus of the atria is present. When the P axis is in the right lower quadrant (+90 to +180 degrees), situs inversus of the atria is present.
   (3) 2D echo: The 2D echo identifies the IVC and/or pulmonary veins. The RA is connected to the IVC, and the LA receives the pulmonary veins.

b. **Localization of the ventricles.** Ventricular localization can be accomplished noninvasively by the ECG and 2D echo.

   (1) ECG: The depolarization of the ventricular septum normally takes place from the embryonic LV to the RV, producing Q waves in the

precordial leads that lie over the anatomic LV. If Q waves are present in V5 and V6 but not in V1, D-loop of the ventricle as in normal persons is likely. If Q waves are present in V4R, V1, and V2 but not in V5 and V6, L-loop of the ventricles is likely (ventricular inversion, as seen in L-TGA).

(2) 2D echo: The tricuspid valve leaflet usually inserts on the interventricular septum more towards the apex than does the mitral septal leaflet. The ventricle that is attached to the tricuspid valve is the RV. The ventricle that has two papillary muscles is the LV.

c. **Localization of the great arteries.** Two-dimensional echo studies can locate the great arteries accurately, but the ECG is not helpful in finding them.

2. **Types of displacement.** The four most common types of dextrocardia are classic mirror-image dextrocardia, normal heart displaced to the right side of the chest, congenitally corrected TGA, and single ventricle (Fig. 3-51). Less

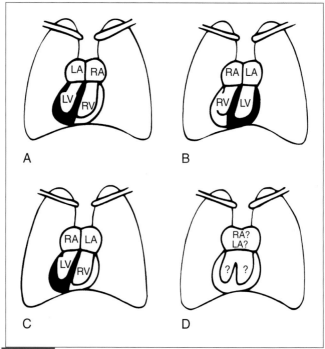

FIG. 3-51

Examples of common conditions when the apex of the heart is in the right side of the chest. LA, left atrium; LV, left ventricle; RA, right atrium; RV, right ventricle. *(From Park MK, Guntheroth WG:* How to read pediatric ECGs, *ed 4, Philadelphia, 2006, Mosby.)*

commonly, asplenia and polysplenia syndromes cause dextrocardia.
All these abnormalities may result in mesocardia. With CXR films and ECGs the segmental approach discussed earlier can be used to deduce the nature of segmental relationship in dextrocardia, as well as in mesocardia.

a. Classic mirror-image dextrocardia (Fig. 3-51, *A*) shows the liver shadow on the left on CXR films. The ECG shows the P axis between +90 and +180 degrees and Q waves in V5R and V6R.

b. Normally formed heart shifted toward the right side of the chest (dextroversion) (Fig. 3-51, *B*) shows the liver shadow on the right on CXR films, the P axis between 0 and +90 degrees, and Q waves in V5 and V6 on the ECG.

c. Congenitally corrected L-TGA with situs solitus (Fig. 3-51, *C*) shows situs solitus of abdominal viscera on CXR films. The ECG shows the P axis in the normal quadrant (0 to +90 degrees) and Q waves in V5R and V6R.

d. Undifferentiated cardiac chambers (Fig. 3-51, *D*) are often associated with complicated cardiac defects and may show midline liver on CXR films. The ECG may show shifting or superiorly oriented P axis and abnormal Q waves in the precordial leads.

G.   MITRAL STENOSIS, CONGENITAL

Isolated congenital mitral stenosis (MS) is very rare. The mitral obstruction occurs at more than one level; it may be at the valve leaflets (fusion of the leaflets), the valve ring itself (such as seen in HLHS), the papillary muscle (single papillary muscle), the chordae (thickened and fused chordae), or the supravalvar region (supravalvar mitral ring). Parachute mitral valve is a condition in which all chordae insert to a single papillary muscle, causing obstruction to the entry of blood to the LV. The mitral commissures are poorly developed. It is often part of Shone complex (which consists of LVOT obstruction, AS, aortic arch hypoplasia, and COA).

Pathophysiology is the same as in the acquired form (rheumatic MS). The patients become symptomatic during early infancy with tachypnea, feeding difficulty, and failure to thrive. They are prone to respiratory infection, such as respiratory syncytial virus infection. Echo studies are diagnostic.

Mild to moderate MS can be managed with the usual anticongestive measures. Balloon dilation of the valve may be attempted but is usually unsuccessful. For infants and children with severe MS the following may be indications for surgical intervention.

1. Symptomatic infants or children with failure to gain weight, dyspnea on exertion, pulmonary edema, or paroxysmal dyspnea may be candidates for surgery (or balloon dilation).

2. Failed balloon dilation or severe MR resulting from the balloon procedure.

3. Recurrent atrial fibrillation, thromboembolic phenomenon, and hemoptysis.

Surgically, a supravalvar ring can be removed and thickened and fused chordae can be split apart, but commissurotomy is usually not possible. Occasionally, mitral valve replacement may be necessary. A conduit from the LA to the LV is an unusual option.

H. SYSTEMIC VENOUS ANOMALIES

There are wide ranges of abnormalities of the systemic venous system, some of which have little physiologic importance. Others have surgical significance or produce cyanosis. Two well-known anomalies of systemic veins are persistent left SVC and infrahepatic interruption of the IVC with azygos continuation. Rarely, either persistent left SVC or interrupted IVC can drain into the LA, producing cyanosis.

1. Anomalies of superior vena cava

a. Persistent left SVC draining into the RA. In the most commonly encountered type, the left SVC is connected to the coronary sinus (Fig. 3-52, *A*). As a rule, persistent left SVC is part of a bilateral SVC, but rarely the right SVC is absent (Fig. 3-52, *B*). A bridging innominate vein is present in 60% of cases.

b. Isolated persistent left SVC does not produce symptoms or signs. Cardiac examination is entirely normal. CXR films may show the shadow of the left SVC along the left upper border of the mediastinum. There is a high prevalence of leftward P axis (+15 degrees or less, including "coronary sinus rhythm") on the ECG. The enlarged coronary sinus may be imaged by an echo study. Treatment for isolated persistent left SVC is not necessary.

c. Persistent left SVC draining into the LA (Fig. 3-52 *C, D*). Rarely, in the absence of the coronary sinus, persistent left SVC drains into the LA (8% of cases), resulting in systemic arterial desaturation. Associated cardiac anomalies, usually of the complex cyanotic type, are almost invariably present. Defects of the atrial septum (single atrium, secundum ASD, primum ASD) are also frequently found. Surgical correction is necessary.

2. Anomalies of the inferior vena cava

a. Interrupted IVC with azygos continuation (Fig. 3-53, *A*) has been reported in about 3% of children with CHDs. Instead of receiving the hepatic veins and entering the RA, the IVC drains via an enlarged azygos system into the right SVC and eventually to the RA. The hepatic veins connect directly to the RA. Bilateral SVC is also common. Azygos continuation of the IVC is often associated with various types of complex cyanotic heart defects. No case has been reported in association with asplenia syndrome. This defect creates difficulties in manipulating catheters during cardiac catheterization and can render surgical correction of an underlying cardiac defect more difficult. There is no need for surgical correction of this venous anomaly per se.

b. IVC connecting to the LA is an extremely rare condition in which the IVC receives the hepatic veins, curves toward the LA, and makes a

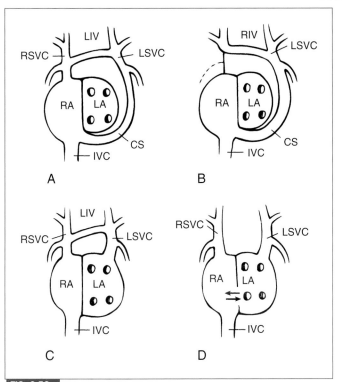

FIG. 3-52

Schematic diagram of persistent left superior vena cava (LSVC). **A,** LSVC drains via coronary sinus (CS) into the RA. The left innominate vein (LIV) and the right superior vena cava (RSVC) are adequate. **B,** Uncommonly, the RSVC may be atretic. The CS is large because it receives blood from both the right and left upper parts of the body. **C,** The coronary sinus is absent and LSVC drains directly into the LA. The atrial septum is intact. **D,** The LSVC connects to the LA, and a posterior ASD allows a predominant left-to-right atrial shunt. IVC, inferior vena cava; LA, left atrium; RA, right atrium; RIV, right innominate vein.

direct connection with the chamber (Fig. 3-53, *B*), producing cyanosis. Surgical correction is indicated.

c. There are two other extremely rare types. The lower end of the right IVC is absent and the dominant left IVC drains into the LA, producing cyanosis through (left-sided) hemiazygos system and persistent left SVC (Fig. 3-53, *C*). The lower end of the right IVC is absent, and the left IVC drains through the (right-sided) azygos system (Fig. 3-53, *D*).

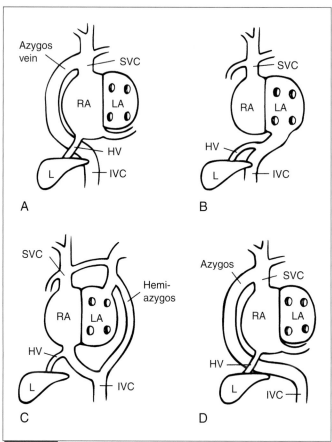

FIG. 3-53
Schematic diagram of selected abnormalities of the IVC. **A,** Interrupted IVC with azygos continuation, the most common abnormality of the IVC. The HV connects directly to the RA. **B,** Right IVC draining into the LA. **C,** Absence of the lower right IVC. The IVC drains into the left superior vena cava and LA and to the RA through the hepatic portion of the IVC. **D,** Complete absence of the right IVC, with communicating vein draining to the azygos vein. HV, hepatic veins; IVC, inferior vena cava; L, liver; LA, left atrium; RA, right atrium; SVC, superior vena cava.

I. VASCULAR RING

PREVALENCE. Vascular ring reportedly constitutes fewer than 1% of all congenital cardiovascular anomalies, but this is probably an underestimation.

PATHOLOGY AND PATHOPHYSIOLOGY

1. The vascular ring may be complete (true) or incomplete.

a. In complete vascular ring, the abnormal vascular structures form a complete circle around the trachea and esophagus. They include double aortic arch and right aortic arch with left ligamentum arteriosum.

b. Incomplete vascular ring comprises vascular anomalies that do not form a complete circle around the trachea and esophagus but do compress these structures. These include anomalous innominate artery, aberrant right subclavian artery, and anomalous left pulmonary artery (vascular sling).

2. Double aortic arch is the most common vascular ring (40%) (Fig. 3-54). The right and left aortic arches completely encircle and compress the trachea and esophagus, producing respiratory distress and feeding problems in early infancy. Both aortic arches give off two branches: the right arch giving off the right common carotid and the right subclavian and the left arch giving off the left common carotid and left subclavian arteries. The right aortic arch is usually larger than the left arch. This condition is usually an isolated anomaly but is occasionally associated with CHDs such as TGA, VSD, persistent truncus arteriosus, TOF, and COA.

3. Right aortic arch with left ligamentum arteriosum is the second most common vascular ring (30%) (Fig. 3-54). In the most common form the right aortic arch occurs with the retroesophageal left subclavian artery coursing behind the esophagus (65%) with the ligamentum arteriosum connecting the descending aorta and the left PA.

4. In anomalous innominate artery, the innominate artery takes off too far to the left from the arch or more posteriorly and compresses the trachea, producing mild respiratory symptoms (Fig. 3-54). This anomaly is commonly associated with other CHDs such as VSD.

5. In aberrant right subclavian artery, the right subclavian artery arises independently from the descending aorta and courses behind the esophagus, producing mild feeding problems (Fig. 3-54). It is the most common arch anomaly (occurring in 0.5% of the general population) without producing symptoms. It is often an isolated anomaly but may be associated with TOF with left arch, COA, or interrupted aortic arch. Its incidence is very high (38%) in Down syndrome with CHD.

6. Anomalous left PA (vascular sling) is a rare anomaly in which the left PA arises from the right PA (Fig. 3-54). To reach the left lung, the anomalous artery courses over the proximal portion of the right main-stem bronchus, behind the trachea, and in front of the esophagus to the hilum of the left lung. Therefore, both respiratory symptoms and feeding problems

	Anatomy	Ba esophagogram	Other x-ray findings	Symptoms	Treatment
Double aortic arch	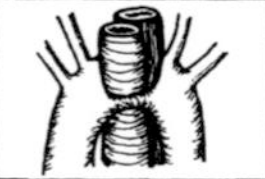	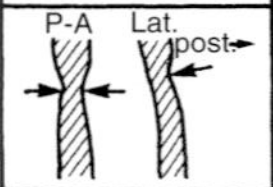	Anterior compression of trachea	Respiratory difficulty (onset <3 mo) Swallowing dysfunction	Surgical division of a smaller arch
Right aortic arch with left lig. arteriosum	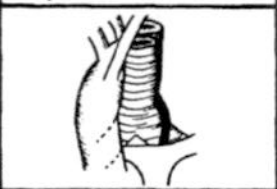	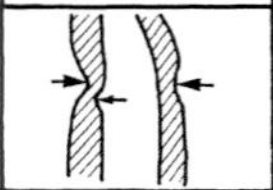		Mild respiratory difficulty (onset >1 yr) Swallowing dysfunction	Surgical division of the lig. arteriosum
Anomalous innominate artery	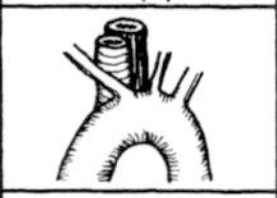	Normal	Anterior compression of trachea	Stridor and/or cough in infancy	Conservative management, or Surgical suturing of the artery to the sternum
Aberrant right subclavian artery	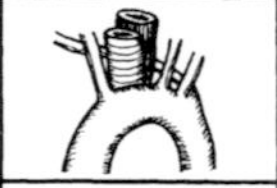	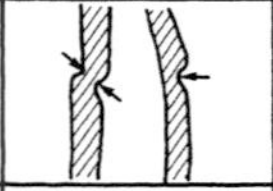		Occasional swallowing dysfunction	Usually no treatment is necessary
"Vascular sling"	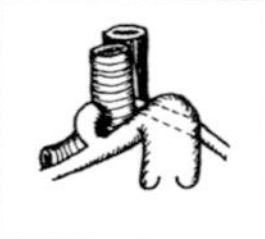	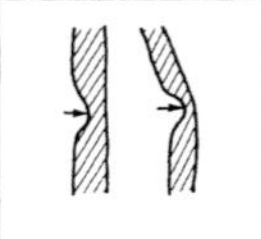	Right-sided emphysema or atelectasis Posterior compression of trachea or rt. main-stem bronchus	Wheezing and cyanotic episodes since birth	Surgical division of the anomalous LPA (from the RPA) and anastomosis to the MPA

FIG. 3-54

Summary and clinical features of vascular ring. Lat, lateral view; Lig., ligamentum; LPA, left pulmonary artery; MPA, main pulmonary artery; P-A, posteroanterior view; post, posterior; RPA, right pulmonary artery.

(such as coughing; wheezing; stridor; and episodes of choking, cyanosis, or apnea) may occur. This anomaly is often associated with other CHD, such as PDA, VSD, ASD, AV canal, and single ventricle.

CLINICAL MANIFESTATIONS

1. Respiratory distress and feeding problems of varying severity appear at varying ages. History of pneumonia is frequently elicited.
2. Physical examination is not revealing except for varying degrees of rhonchi. Cardiac examination is normal.
3. The ECGs are normal.
4. CXR films may reveal compression of the air-filled trachea, aspiration pneumonia, or atelectasis. Barium esophagogram is usually diagnostic (Fig. 3-54) except in anomalous innominate artery.
5. Echo is helpful, both for suspecting the diagnosis and excluding intra-cardiac defects and for diagnosing vascular ring.

DIAGNOSIS

1. Barium esophagogram is probably the most useful noninvasive diagnostic tool (Fig. 3-54).
   a. In double aortic arch, two large indentations are present in both sides (with the right one usually larger) in the posteroanterior (P-A) view, and a posterior indentation is seen on the lateral view.
   b. In right aortic arch with left ligamentum arteriosum a large right-sided indentation and a much smaller left-sided indentation are present. A posterior indentation, either small or large, also is present on the lateral view.
   c. Barium esophagogram is normal in anomalous left innominate artery.
   d. In aberrant right subclavian artery a small oblique indentation extends toward the right shoulder on the P-A view and a small posterior indentation on the lateral view.
   e. In vascular sling an anterior indentation of the esophagus seen in the lateral view at the level of the carina is characteristic. This is the only vascular ring that produces an anterior esophageal indentation. A right-sided indentation usually is seen on the P-A view. The right lung is either hyperlucent or atelectatic with pneumonic infiltrations.
2. Computed tomography (CT), magnetic resonance imaging (MRI), or digital subtraction angiography may provide accurate diagnosis.
3. Occasionally angiography is indicated to confirm the diagnosis.

MANAGEMENT

MEDICAL. For infants with mild symptoms, careful feeding with soft foods and aggressive treatment of pulmonary infections.

SURGICAL

1. Indications and timing. Respiratory distress and a history of recurrent pulmonary infections and apneic spells are indications for surgical intervention. Surgery may be performed during infancy.
2. Surgical procedures.

a. Double aortic arch. Division of the smaller of the two arches (usually the left) is performed through a left thoracotomy.

b. Right aortic arch and left ligamentum arteriosum. Ligation and division of the ligamentum is performed through a left thoracotomy.

c. Anomalous innominate artery. Through right anterolateral thoracotomy, the innominate artery is suspended to the posterior sternum.

d. Aberrant right subclavian artery. Surgical interruption of the artery is performed only in symptomatic patients with dysphagia.

e. Anomalous left pulmonary artery. Surgical division and reimplantation of the left PA to the main PA is performed, usually through a median sternotomy and with the use of cardiopulmonary bypass.

3. Complications. In infants who have had surgery for severe symptoms, airway obstruction may persist for weeks or months. Careful respiratory management is required in the postoperative period.

Acquired Heart Disease

In this chapter, primary myocardial disease (hypertrophic, dilated, and restrictive cardiomyopathy), cardiovascular infections (myocarditis, infective endocarditis), and acute rheumatic fever will be presented.

I. PRIMARY MYOCARDIAL DISEASE (CARDIOMYOPATHY)

Primary myocardial disease affects the heart muscle itself and is not associated with congenital, valvular, or coronary heart disease or systemic disorders. Cardiomyopathy has been classified into three types on the basis of anatomic and functional features: (1) hypertrophic, (2) dilated (or congestive), and (3) restrictive (Fig. 4-1). The three types of cardiomyopathies are functionally different from one another, and the demands of therapy are also different.

4

A. HYPERTROPHIC CARDIOMYOPATHY

In about 30% to 60% of cases, hypertrophic cardiomyopathy appears to be genetically transmitted as an autosomal dominant trait; in the remainder, it occurs sporadically. It may be seen in children with LEOPARD syndrome (see Table 1-1).

PATHOLOGY AND PATHOPHYSIOLOGY

1. A massive ventricular hypertrophy is present. Although asymmetric septal hypertrophy (ASH), formerly known as idiopathic hypertrophic subaortic stenosis (IHSS), is the most common type, a concentric hypertrophy with symmetric thickening of the left ventricle (LV) sometimes occurs. Occasionally an intracavitary obstruction may develop during systole, partly because of systolic anterior motion (SAM) of the mitral valve against the hypertrophied septum, called hypertrophic obstructive cardiomyopathy (HOCM).

2. The myocardium itself has an enhanced contractile state, but diastolic ventricular filling is impaired because of abnormal stiffness of the LV. This may lead to left atrium (LA) enlargement and pulmonary venous congestion, producing congestive symptoms (exertional dyspnea, orthopnea, paroxysmal nocturnal dyspnea).

3. A unique aspect of HOCM is the variability of the degree of obstruction from moment to moment. The obstruction to LV output worsens when LV volume is reduced (as seen with positive inotropic agents, reduced blood volume, lowering of systemic vascular resistance [SVR], and so on). The obstruction lessens when the LV systolic volume increases (negative inotropic agents, leg raising, blood transfusion, increasing SVR, and so on). About 80% of LV stroke volume occurs in the early part of systole when little or no obstruction exists, resulting in a sharp upstroke of arterial pulse.

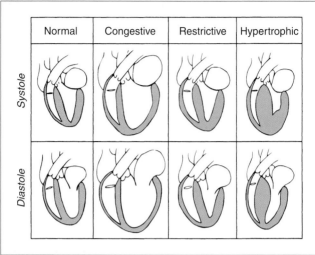

FIG. 4-1

Diagram of left anterior oblique view of heart in different types of cardiomyopathy at end-systole and end-diastole. *Congestive* corresponds to *dilated* cardiomyopathy as used in the text. *(From Goldman MR, Boucher CA: Values of radionuclide imaging techniques in assessing cardiomyopathy. Am J Cardiol 46: 1232-1236, 1980.)*

4. Anginal chest pain, syncope, and ventricular arrhythmias may lead to sudden death.
5. Infants of diabetic mothers develop hypertrophic cardiomyopathy (HCM) with or without left ventricular outflow tract (LVOT) obstruction in 10% to 20% of cases.

CLINICAL MANIFESTATIONS
1. Some 30% to 60% of cases are seen in adolescents and young adults with positive family history. Easy fatigability, dyspnea, palpitation, or anginal chest pain may be the presenting complaint.
2. A sharp upstroke of the arterial pulse is characteristic. A late systolic ejection murmur may be audible at the middle and lower left sternal border (LSB) or at the apex. A holosystolic murmur (of mitral regurgitation [MR]) is occasionally present. The intensity and even the presence of the heart murmur vary from examination to examination.
3. The ECG may show left ventricular hypertrophy (LVH), ST-T changes, abnormally deep Q waves with diminished or absent R waves in the left precordial leads (LPLs), and arrhythmias.
4. Chest x-ray (CXR) films may show mild LV enlargement with globular heart.

5. Echo demonstrates hypertrophy of the septum (ASH) and/or the LV free wall. In obstructive type, SAM of the mitral valve may be demonstrated. The Doppler examination of the mitral inflow demonstrates a decreased E velocity, an increased A velocity, and a decreased E/A ratio (Fig. 4-2).

NATURAL HISTORY

1. The obstruction may be absent, stable, or progressive (especially in genetically predisposed individuals).
2. Sudden death may occur during exercise, especially in those with episodes of ventricular tachycardia.
3. Atrial fibrillation may cause stroke.
4. Pregnancy is relatively well tolerated.

MANAGEMENT

The goal of management is to reduce LVOT obstruction (by reducing LV contractility and by increasing LV volume), increase ventricular compliance, and prevent sudden death (by preventing or treating ventricular arrhythmias).

1. General care
a. Moderate restriction of physical activity is recommended.

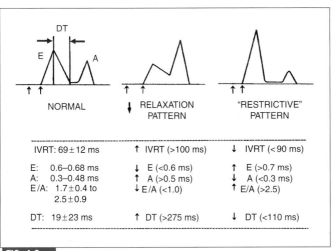

FIG. 4-2

Examples of diastolic dysfunction seen in different types of cardiomyopathy. *A*, A wave (the velocity of a second wave that coincides with atrial contraction); *DT*, deceleration time (time from the peak of the E wave to the point where the decelerating diastolic velocity reaches the baseline); *E*, E wave (the velocity of an early peak that coincides with the early ventricular filling); E/A, ratio of E wave to A wave velocity; *IVRT*, isovolumic relaxation time (measured from the cessation of ventricular outflow to the onset of the E wave, in milliseconds; between two small arrows). *(Modified from Park MK:* Pediatric cardiology for practitioners, *ed 5, Philadelphia, 2008, Mosby.)*

b. First-degree relatives and other family members should be screened.

c. Annual evaluation should be performed during adolescence with ECG and echo.

2. A β-adrenergic blocker (such as propranolol, atenolol, or metoprolol) or a calcium channel blocker (principally verapamil) is the drug of choice in the obstructive subgroup. These drugs reduce the degree of obstruction, decrease the incidence of anginal pain, and have antiarrhythmic actions. Prophylactic therapy with either β-adrenergic blockers or verapamil is controversial in patients without LVOT obstruction. In infants of diabetic mothers, β-adrenergic blockers are used when the LVOT obstruction is present. In most of these infants the hypertrophy spontaneously resolves within the first 6 to 12 months of life.

3. The following drugs are contraindicated: digitalis, other inotropic agents, and vasodilators tend to increase LVOT obstruction; diuretics may reduce LV volume and increase LVOT obstruction (but may be used in small doses to improve respiratory symptoms).

4. Morrow's myotomy-myectomy or percutaneous alcohol ablation may be considered for drug-refractory patients with LVOT obstruction.

a. Morrow's procedure. This procedure resects hypertrophied LV septum through a transaortic approach to reduce the obstruction.

b. Alcohol ablation. Absolute alcohol is injected into a target septal perforator branch of the left anterior descending coronary artery to produce a "controlled" myocardial infarction (MI).

5. Implantable cardioverter-defibrillator (ICD) has been proved to be effective in preventing sudden death. The following are risk factors for sudden death in HCM and may be indications for an ICD.

a. Prior cardiac arrest (ventricular fibrillation)

b. Spontaneous sustained ventricular tachycardia

c. Family history of premature sudden death

d. Unexplained syncope, particularly in young patients

e. LV thickness ≥30 mm

f. Nonsustained ventricular tachycardia (VT)

g. Abnormal exercise blood pressure (BP) (attenuated response or hypotension)

6. Dual-chamber pacing tends to reduce the LVOT pressure gradient.

7. Cardiac arrhythmias

a. Ventricular arrhythmias are treated with propranolol, amiodarone, and other antiarrhythmic agents.

b. Atrial fibrillation (AF) is treated with electrical cardioversion and anticoagulation with warfarin. Amiodarone is effective in preventing recurrence of AF.

B. DILATED (CONGESTIVE) CARDIOMYOPATHY

Dilated cardiomyopathy is the most common form of cardiomyopathy. The idiopathic type is most common (>60%), followed by familial cardiomyopathy, active myocarditis, and other causes. It may be the end result of myocardial damage produced by a variety of infectious, toxic, or metabolic agents or immunologic disorders. Many cases of unexplained dilated cardiomyopathy may, in fact, result from subclinical myocarditis. Other causes of dilated cardiomyopathy include hyperthyroidism and hypothyroidism, excessive catecholamines, hypocalcemia, mucopolysaccharidosis, and nutritional disorders (kwashiorkor, beriberi, carnitine deficiency). Cardiotoxic agents (doxorubicin) also can cause dilated cardiomyopathy.

PATHOLOGY AND PATHOPHYSIOLOGY

1. In dilated cardiomyopathy a weakening of systolic contraction is associated with dilation of all four cardiac chambers. Dilation of the atria is in proportion to ventricular dilation.
2. Intracavitary thrombus formation is common in the apical portion of the ventricular cavities and in atrial appendages, and it may give rise to pulmonary and systemic embolization.

CLINICAL MANIFESTATIONS

1. Fatigue, weakness, and symptoms of left heart failure (e.g., dyspnea on exertion, orthopnea) may be present.
2. On physical examination, signs of congestive heart failure (CHF) (e.g., tachycardia, pulmonary crackles, weak pulses, distended neck veins, hepatomegaly) may be present. A prominent S3 with or without gallop rhythm is present. A soft systolic murmur of MR or tricuspid regurgitation (TR) may be audible.
3. Sinus tachycardia, left ventricular hypertrophy (LVH), and ST-T changes are common ECG findings.
4. CXR films show generalized cardiomegaly, often with signs of pulmonary venous congestion.
5. Echo studies are diagnostic, and there may be unexpected findings in an asymptomatic patient. The LV and right ventricle (RV) are dilated with a reduced fractional shortening (FS) and ejection fraction (EF). Intracavitary thrombus and pericardial effusion may be present. The mitral inflow Doppler tracing demonstrates a reduced E velocity and a decreased E/A ratio (Fig. 4-2).
6. Progressive deterioration is the rule rather than the exception. About two thirds of these patients die of arrhythmias, systemic or pulmonary embolization, or CHF within 4 years of the onset of symptoms.

MANAGEMENT

1. CHF is treated with digoxin, diuretics (furosemide, spironolactone), ACE inhibitors (captopril, enalapril), bed rest, and restriction of activity. Critically ill patients may require intubation, mechanical ventilation, and administration of rapidly acting inotropic agents (dobutamine, dopamine).
2. Antiplatelet agents (aspirin) should be initiated. Anticoagulation with warfarin may be indicated. If thrombi are detected, they should be treated aggressively with heparin initially and later switched to long-term warfarin therapy.

3. Patients with arrhythmias may be treated with amiodarone or other antiarrhythmic agents. Amiodarone is effective and relatively safe in children. For symptomatic bradycardia a cardiac pacemaker may be necessary. An ICD may be considered.

4. The beneficial effects of β-adrenergic blocking agents (somewhat unorthodox, given poor contractility) have been reported in adult and pediatric patients. Carvedilol is a β-adrenergic blocker with additional vasodilating action. Recent evidence suggests that activation of the sympathetic nervous system may have deleterious cardiac effects rather than being an important compensatory mechanism as traditionally thought.

5. If carnitine deficiency is considered the cause of the cardiomyopathy, carnitine supplementation should be started.

6. A preliminary report suggests that administration of recombinant human growth hormone (0.025 to 0.04 mg/kg/day for 6 months) may improve LV ejection fraction, increase LV wall thickness, reduce the chamber size, and improve cardiac output.

7. Many of these children may become candidates for cardiac transplantation.

C. ENDOCARDIAL FIBROELASTOSIS

Endocardial fibroelastosis (EFE) is a form of dilated cardiomyopathy of unknown etiology seen in infants and children. Viral agents, especially mumps, have been implicated in the past and again recently in some cases of EFE. The condition is characterized by diffuse changes in the endocardium, with a white, opaque, glistening appearance. The left side of the heart is dilated and hypertrophied, with poor contractility. For unknown reasons the incidence of EFE has declined in the past several decades.

Symptoms and signs of CHF develop in the first 10 months of life. No heart murmur is audible in most patients, although gallop rhythm is usually present. Hepatomegaly is usually present. The ECG shows LVH with "strain." Occasionally, myocardial infarction patterns and arrhythmias are seen. CXR films show marked cardiomegaly with normal pulmonary vascular markings (PVMs) or pulmonary venous congestion patterns.

Barth syndrome consists of an infantile form of dilated cardiomyopathy (with endocardial fibroelastosis), skeletal myopathy, neutropenia (agranulocytopenia) with repeated infections, and abnormal mitochondria and has a sex-linked recessive inheritance pattern with females acting as carriers. Many patients with Barth syndrome die of cardiac failure during infancy.

Early and long-term (years) treatment with digoxin, diuretics, and afterload-reducing agents is recommended. With proper treatment about a third of the patients recover completely. Another third do not improve, and the remaining third gradually deteriorate and die.

D. DOXORUBICIN CARDIOMYOPATHY
ETIOLOGY AND PATHOLOGY

1. Doxorubicin cardiomyopathy is becoming the most common cause of chronic CHF in children. Its prevalence is nonlinearly dose related, occurring

in 2% to 5% of patients who have received a cumulative dose of 400 to 500 mg/m^2 and up to 50% of patients who have received more than 1000 mg/m^2 of doxorubicin (Adriamycin).

2. Risk factors for the cardiomyopathy include age younger than 4 years and a cumulative dose exceeding 400 to 600 mg/m^2. A dosing regimen with larger and less frequent doses has been raised as a risk factor but not proved.

3. Dilated LV, decreased contractility, and elevated LV filling pressure are present.

CLINICAL MANIFESTATIONS

1. Patients have a history of receiving doxorubicin, with the onset of symptoms 2 to 4 months, and rarely years, after completion of therapy.

2. Patients are usually asymptomatic until signs of CHF develop. Tachypnea and dyspnea made worse by exertion are the usual presenting complaints.

3. Signs of CHF may be present on physical examination.

4. CXR films show cardiomegaly with or without pulmonary congestion or pleural effusion.

5. The ECG frequently shows sinus tachycardia with occasional ST-T changes.

6. Echo studies reveal slightly increased LV size, reduced LV wall thickness, and decreased ejection fraction or fractional shortening.

7. Symptomatic patients have a high mortality rate. The 2-year survival rate is about 20%, and almost all patients die by 9 years after the onset of the illness.

MANAGEMENT

1. Attempts to reduce anthracycline cardiotoxicity have been made in three directions: (a) anthracycline dose limitation, (b) developing less cardiotoxic analogs, and (c) concurrently administering cardioprotective agents to attenuate the cardiotoxic effects of anthracycline to the heart.

a. Limiting the total cumulative dose to 400 to 500 mg/m^2 reduces the incidence of CHF to 5%, but this dose may not be effective in treating some malignancies. Continuous infusion therapy may reduce cardiac injury by avoiding peak levels, although such effects have not been observed.

b. The analog of doxorubicin, such as idarubicin and epirubicin, has not been proved to be less toxic than doxorubicin.

c. Concurrent administration of cardioprotective agents, such as dexrazoxane (an iron chelator), carvedilol (a β-receptor antagonist with antioxidant property), and coenzyme Q10, has shown some protective effects without attenuating the antimalignancy effect of the drug.

2. In symptomatic patients, the following medications are used.

a. Digoxin, diuretics, and ACE inhibitors are useful.

b. β-blockers have been shown to be beneficial in some children and adults with chemotherapy-induced cardiomyopathy. Metoprolol (starting at 0.1 mg/kg per dose twice a day and increasing to a maximum

dose of 0.9 mg/kg per day) has improved LV systolic function and alleviated symptoms.
3. Cardiac transplantation may be an option for selected patients.

E. CARNITINE DEFICIENCY

Carnitine deficiency is a rare cause of cardiomegaly in infants and small children. Carnitine deficiency leads to depressed mitochondrial oxidation of fatty acids, resulting in storage of fat in muscles and in functional abnormalities of cardiac and skeletal muscles. Carnitine is synthesized predominantly in the liver.

Primary carnitine deficiency is an uncommon inherited disorder. The condition has been classified as either systemic or myopathic. The *systemic form* of the disease may manifest with muscle weakness, cardiomyopathy (either hypertrophic or dilated), abnormal liver function, encephalopathy, and hypoglycemia during fasting in the first year of life. Low concentrations of carnitine are present in plasma, muscle, and liver. In the *myopathic form,* progressive cardiomyopathy is the most common manifestation, with or without skeletal muscle weakness that begins at 2 to 4 years of age. Biopsy reveals fatty infiltration of muscle fibers. The ECG may show bizarre T wave spiking. Those affected die suddenly, presumably from arrhythmias.

Secondary forms of carnitine deficiency have been reported in renal tubular disorders (with excessive excretion of carnitine), chronic renal failure (excessive loss of carnitine from hemodialysis), inborn errors of metabolism with increased concentrations of organic acids, and occasionally in patients who receive total parenteral nutrition. Diagnosis of the condition is established by an extremely low level of carnitine in plasma and skeletal muscle.

For both forms, oral carnitine (L-carnitine, 50 to 100 mg/kg/day, b.i.d. or t.i.d., maximum daily dose 3 g) may improve myocardial function, reduce cardiomegaly, and improve muscle weakness.

F. RESTRICTIVE CARDIOMYOPATHY
PREVALENCE, PATHOLOGY, AND PATHOPHYSIOLOGY
1. Restrictive cardiomyopathy is the least common of the three types of cardiomyopathy, occurring in 5% of cardiomyopathy cases in children.
2. The condition is characterized by an abnormal diastolic ventricular filling owing to excessively stiff ventricular walls, often caused by infiltrative disease processes (e.g., sarcoidosis, amyloidosis). The ventricles remain normal in size and maintain normal contractility, but the atria are enlarged out of proportion to the ventricles.

CLINICAL MANIFESTATIONS
1. History of exercise intolerance, weakness and dyspnea, or chest pain may be present.
2. Jugular venous distention, gallop rhythm, and a systolic murmur of MR or TR may be present.

3. CXR films show cardiomegaly, pulmonary congestion, and pleural effusion.

4. The ECG may show atrial fibrillation and paroxysms of supraventricular tachycardia (SVT).

5. Echo studies reveal characteristic biatrial enlargement, with normal cavity size of the LV and RV. LV systolic function (ejection fraction) is normal until the late stages of the disease. Atrial thrombus may be present.

MANAGEMENT

1. Diuretics are beneficial by relieving congestive symptoms. Digoxin is not indicated because systolic function is unimpaired. ACE inhibitors may reduce systemic BP without increasing cardiac output, and therefore should probably be avoided.

2. Calcium channel blockers may be used to increase diastolic compliance.

3. Anticoagulants (warfarin) and antiplatelet drugs (aspirin and dipyridamole) may help prevent thrombosis.

4. Permanent pacemaker is indicated for complete heart block.

5. Cardiac transplantation may be an option.

G.   RIGHT VENTRICULAR DYSPLASIA

RV dysplasia, or RV cardiomyopathy, is a rare abnormality of unknown etiology in which the myocardium of the RV is partially or totally replaced by fibrous or adipose tissue. The LV is usually spared. Most cases appear to be sporadic. It is prevalent in northern Italy.

The onset is in infancy, childhood, or adulthood (but usually before age 20 years), with history of palpitation, syncopal episodes, or both. Sudden death may be the first sign of the disease. Presenting manifestations may be arrhythmias (ventricular tachycardia, supraventricular arrhythmias) or signs of CHF. CXR films usually show cardiomegaly. The ECG often shows tall P waves in lead II (right atrial hypertrophy [RAH]), decreased RV potentials, T wave inversion in the right precordial leads (nonspecific), right bundle branch block (RBBB), and premature ventricular contractions (PVCs) or ventricular tachycardia of left bundle branch block (LBBB) morphology. Echo studies show selective RV enlargement with areas of akinesia or dyskinesia and extreme thinning of the RV free wall. TR and paradoxical septal motion may also be present. Cardiac magnetic resonance imaging (MRI) shows findings similar to those from echo studies. Right ventriculogram and RV biopsy may establish the diagnosis.

Various antiarrhythmic agents may be tried, but they are often unsuccessful in abolishing ventricular tachycardia. Surgical intervention (ventricular incision or complete electrical disarticulation of the RV free wall) may be tried if antiarrhythmic therapy is unsuccessful. A significant number of patients die before age 5 years of CHF and intractable ventricular tachycardia.

II. CARDIOVASCULAR INFECTIONS

A. INFECTIVE ENDOCARDITIS (SUBACUTE BACTERIAL ENDOCARDITIS)

PREVALENCE. Subacute bacterial endocarditis (SBE) affects 0.5:1000 to 1:1000 hospital patients, excluding those with postoperative endocarditis.

PATHOGENESIS AND PATHOLOGY

1. Two factors are important in the pathogenesis of infective endocarditis: (a) structural abnormalities of the heart or great arteries with a significant pressure gradient or turbulence, with resulting endothelial damage and platelet-fibrin thrombus formation and (b) bacteremia, even if transient, with adherence of the organisms and eventual invasion of the cardiac tissue.

2. Those with a prosthetic heart valve or prosthetic material in the heart are at particularly high risk for infective endocarditis. Drug addicts may develop endocarditis in the absence of known cardiac anomalies.

MICROBIOLOGY. In the past, *Streptococcus viridans,* enterococci, and *Staphylococcus aureus* were responsible for more than 90% of cases of infective endocarditis (IE). In recent years this frequency has decreased to 50% to 60%, with a concomitant increase in cases caused by fungus and HACEK organisms (*Haemophilus, Actinobacillus, Cardiobacterium, Eikenella*, and *Kingella*).

CLINICAL MANIFESTATIONS

1. Most patients are known to have an underlying heart disease. The onset is usually insidious with prolonged low-grade fever (101° F to 103° F) and various somatic complaints.

2. Heart murmur is almost always present, and splenomegaly is common (70%).

3. Skin manifestations (50%) may be present in the following forms.

a. Petechiae on the skin, mucous membranes, or conjunctivae are frequent.

b. Osler nodes (tender, pea-size red nodes at the ends of the fingers or toes) are rare in children.

c. Janeway lesions (small, painless, hemorrhagic areas on the palms or soles) are rare.

d. Splinter hemorrhages (linear hemorrhagic streaks beneath the nails) also are rare.

4. Embolic or immunologic phenomena in other organs are present in 50% of cases.

a. Pulmonary emboli or hematuria and renal failure may occur.

b. Seizures and hemiparesis occur in 20% of cases.

c. Roth spots (oval, retinal hemorrhages with pale centers located near the optic disc) occur in <5% of patients.

5. Laboratory studies

a. Positive blood cultures are obtained in more than 90% of patients in the absence of previous antimicrobial therapy.

b. Anemia and leukocytosis with a shift to the left are common. Patients with initial polycythemia may have normal hemoglobin.

c. The sedimentation rate is increased unless there is polycythemia.

d. Microscopic hematuria is found in 30% of patients.

6. Echocardiography. Although standard transthoracic echo (TTE) is sufficient in most cases, transesophageal echo (TEE) may be needed in obese
or very muscular adolescents.

a. The following echo findings are included as major criteria in the modified Duke criteria: oscillating intracardiac mass on valve or supporting
structures, in the path of regurgitation jets or on implanted material;
abscesses; new partial dehiscence of prosthetic valve; and new valvular regurgitation.

b. The absence of vegetations on echo does not in itself rule out IE. False-
negative diagnosis is possible if vegetations are small or have already
embolized. A false-positive diagnosis is possible. An echogenic mass may
represent a sterile thrombus, sterile prosthetic material, normal anatomic
variation, an abnormal uninfected valve (previous scarring, severe myxomatous changes), or improper gain of the echo machine. Echo evidence
of vegetation may persist for months or years after bacteriologic cure.

c. Certain echo features suggest a high-risk case or a need for surgery:
(1) large vegetations (greatest risk when the vegetation is >10 mm),
(2) severe valvular regurgitation, (3) abscess cavities, (4) pseudoaneu-
rysm, or (5) valvular perforation or dehiscence.

DIAGNOSIS. The diagnosis of infective endocarditis is challenging. The
modified Duke criteria are used in the diagnosis. There are three categories
of diagnostic possibilities using the modified Duke criteria: definite, possible, and rejected. A diagnosis of "definite" IE is made either by pathologic
evidence or fulfillment of certain clinical criteria (Box 4-1). Box 4-2 shows
definitions of major and minor clinical criteria.

MANAGEMENT

1. Blood cultures are indicated for all patients with fever of unexplained
origin and a pathologic heart murmur, a history of heart disease, or previous endocarditis.

a. Usually three blood cultures are drawn by separate venipunctures over
24 hours, unless the patient is very ill. In 90% of cases the causative
agent is recovered from the first two cultures.

b. If there is no growth by the second day of incubation, two more cultures
may be obtained. There is no value in obtaining more than five blood
cultures over 2 days unless the patient received prior antibiotic therapy.

c. Aerobic incubation alone suffices because it is rare for IE to be caused
by anaerobic bacteria.

2. Consultation from a local infectious disease specialist is highly
recommended.

3. Initial empirical therapy is started with the following antibiotics while
awaiting the results of blood cultures.

a. The usual initial regimen is an antistaphylococcal semisynthetic
penicillin (nafcillin, oxacillin, or methicillin) and an aminoglycoside

---

BOX 4-1

DEFINITION OF INFECTIVE ENDOCARDITIS ACCORDING TO THE MODIFIED DUKE CRITERIA

DEFINITE INFECTIVE ENDOCARDITIS

A. PATHOLOGIC CRITERIA

1. Microorganisms demonstrated by culture or histological examination of a vegetation, a vegetation that has embolized, or an intracardiac abscess specimen; or
2. Pathological lesions; vegetation or intracardiac abscess confirmed by histological examination showing active endocarditis

B. CLINICAL CRITERIA

1. Two major criteria; or
2. One major criterion and three minor criteria; or
3. Five minor criteria

POSSIBLE IE

1. One major criterion and one minor criterion; or
2. Three minor criteria

REJECTED

1. Firm alternative diagnosis explaining evidence of IE; or
2. Resolution of IE syndrome with antibiotic therapy for <4 days; or
3. No pathologic evidence of IE at surgery or autopsy, with antibiotic therapy for <4 days; or
4. Does not meet criteria for possible IE as shown previously

From Baddour LM, Wilson WR, Bayer AS et al: Infective endocarditis: diagnosis, antimicrobial therapy, and management of complications: a statement for healthcare professionals from the Committee on Rheumatic Fever, Endocarditis, and Kawasaki Disease, Council on Cardiovascular Disease in the Young, and the Councils on Clinical Cardiology, Stroke, and Cardiovascular Surgery and Anesthesia, American Heart Association, *Circulation* 111(23):e394-e433, 2005.

(gentamicin). This combination covers against *S. viridans, S. aureus,* and gram-negative organisms.

b. If a methicillin-resistant *S. aureus* is suspected, vancomycin should be substituted for the semisynthetic penicillin.

c. Vancomycin can be used in place of penicillin or a semisynthetic penicillin in penicillin-allergic patients.

4. The final selection of antibiotics for native valve IE depends on the organism isolated and the results of an antibiotic sensitivity test.

a. Streptococcal infective endocarditis

   (1) For highly sensitive *S. viridans,* IV penicillin (or ceftriaxone given once daily) for 4 weeks is sufficient. Alternatively, penicillin, ampicillin, or ceftriaxone combined with gentamicin for 2 weeks may be used.

   (2) For penicillin-resistant streptococci, 4 weeks of penicillin, ampicillin, or ceftriaxone combined with gentamicin for the first 2 weeks are recommended.

b. Staphylococcal endocarditis

BOX 4-2

DEFINITION OF MAJOR AND MINOR CLINICAL CRITERIA FOR THE DIAGNOSIS OF INFECTIVE ENDOCARDITIS

MAJOR CRITERIA

A. BLOOD CULTURE POSITIVE FOR IE

1. Typical microorganisms consistent with IE from two separate blood cultures: *Streptococcus viridans, Streptococcus bovis,* HACEK group, *Staphylococcus aureus,* or community-acquired enterococci in the absence of a primary focus

2. Microorganisms consistent with IE from persistently positive blood cultures defined as follows: at least two positive cultures of blood samples drawn >12 hr apart, or all of three or a majority of at least four separate cultures of blood (with first and last sample drawn at least 1 hr apart)

3. Single positive blood culture for *Coxiella burnetii* or antiphase-1 IgG antibody titer >1:800

B. EVIDENCE OF ENDOCARDIAL INVOLVEMENT

Echocardiogram positive for IE (transesophageal echo [TEE] recommended for patients with prosthetic valves, rated at least "possible IE" by clinical criteria, or complicated IE [paravalvular abscess]; transthoracic echo [TTE] as first test in other patients) defined as follows:

1. Oscillating intracardiac mass on valve or supporting structures, in the path of regurgitant jets, or on implanted material in the absence of an alternative anatomic explanation; or

2. Abscess; or

3. New partial dehiscence of prosthetic valve; or

4. New valvular regurgitation (worsening or changing or preexisting murmur not sufficient)

MINOR CRITERIA

1. Predisposition, predisposing heart condition, or injection drug users

2. Fever, temperature >38° C

3. Vascular phenomena: major arterial emboli, septic pulmonary infarcts, mycotic aneurysm, intracranial hemorrhage, conjuctival hemorrhages, and Janeway lesions

4. Immunologic phenomena: glomerulonephritis, Osler nodes, Roth spots, and rheumatoid factor

5. Microbiologic evidence: positive blood culture but does not meet a major criterion as noted previously* or serologic evidence or active infection with organisms consistent with IE

From Baddour LM, Wilson WR, Bayer AS et al: Infective endocarditis: diagnosis, antimicrobial therapy, and management of complications: a statement for healthcare professionals from the Committee on Rheumatic Fever, Endocarditis, and Kawasaki Disease, Council on Cardiovascular Disease in the Young, and the Councils on Clinical Cardiology, Stroke, and Cardiovascular Surgery and Anesthesia, American Heart Association, *Circulation* 111(23):e394-e433, 2005.
*Excludes single positive cultures for coagulase-negative staphylococci and organisms that do not cause endocarditis.

(1) For methicillin-susceptible staphylococci IE, one of the semisynthetic β-lactamase-resistant penicillins (nafcillin, oxacillin, and methicillin) for a minimum of 6 weeks (with or without gentamicin for the first 3 to 5 days) is used.

(2) For patients with methicillin-resistant IE, vancomycin for 6 weeks (with or without gentamicin for the first 3 to 5 days) is used.

c. Enterococcus-caused endocarditis usually requires a combination of IV penicillin or ampicillin together with gentamicin for 4 to 6 weeks. If patients are allergic to penicillin, vancomycin combined with gentamicin for 6 weeks is required.

d. For HACEK organisms, ceftriaxone or another third-generation cephalosporin alone or ampicillin plus gentamicin for 4 weeks is recommended. IE caused by other gram-negative bacteria (such as *E. coli, Pseudomonas aeruginosa,* or *Serratia marcescens*) is treated with piperacillin or ceftazidime together with gentamicin for a minimum of 6 weeks.

e. For fungal IE, amphotericin B is the most effective agent.

f. In culture-negative endocarditis, treatment is directed against staphylococci, streptococci, and the HACEK organisms using ceftriaxone and gentamicin. When staphylococcal IE is suspected, nafcillin should be added to the above therapy.

5. Patients with prosthetic valve endocarditis should be treated for 6 weeks on the basis of the organism isolated and the results of the sensitivity test. Operative intervention may be necessary before the antibiotic therapy is completed if the clinical situation warrants (such as progressive CHF, significant malfunction of prosthetic valves, persistently positive blood cultures after 2 weeks' therapy). Bacteriologic relapse after an appropriate course of therapy also calls for operative intervention.

PROGNOSIS. The overall recovery rate is 80% to 85%; it is 90% or better for *S. viridans* and enterococci and about 50% for *Staphylococcus* organisms. Fungal endocarditis is associated with a very poor outcome.

PREVENTION

Recently the American Heart Association (AHA) made a major change in the antibiotic prophylaxis against IE (Wilson W et al. Circulation. 2007 Oct 9;116(15):1736-54). The following are the main reasons for the change.

1. An exceedingly small number of IE cases could be caused by bacteremia-producing dental procedures. Estimated frequency of bacteremia during routine daily activities (such as chewing, toothbrushing, flossing, use of toothpicks, use of water irrigation devices, and other activities) far exceeds that occurring during dental procedures. For example, toothbrushing and flossing results in bacteremia 20% to 40% of the time and chewing food, 7% to 51% of the time. Cumulative risk over time of bacteremia from routine daily activities is estimated to be greater than 100,000 times compared with that resulting from dental procedures.

2. Besides, the ability of antibiotic therapy to prevent or reduce bacteremia is controversial, and nonfatal adverse reactions (such as rash, diarrhea, and gastrointestinal upset) occur frequently.

3. Therefore, emphasis should be placed on maintaining good oral hygiene and eradicating dental disease to decrease the frequency of bacteremia from routine daily activities. Antibiotic prophylaxis is recommended only for cardiac conditions listed in Box 4-3. Procedures for which antibiotic prophylaxis is recommended and those for which it is not recommended are listed in Box 4-4. Regimens for dental procedures are given in Table 4-1.

SPECIAL SITUATIONS

1. Patients already receiving antibiotics
a. Rheumatic fever prophylaxis: Rather than using a higher dose of the same antibiotic, use other antibiotics, such as clindamycin, azithromycin, or clarithromycin.
b. If possible, delay a dental procedure until at least 10 days after completion of the antibiotic therapy.
2. Patients who undergo cardiac surgery. A careful preoperative dental evaluation is recommended so that required dental treatment may be completed whenever possible before cardiac valve surgery or replacement or repair of congenital heart disease (CHD). Prophylaxis at the time of surgery should be directed primarily against staphylococci and should be of short duration. Prophylaxis should be initiated immediately before the operative procedure, repeated during prolonged procedures to maintain serum concentrations intraoperatively, and continued for no more than 48 hours postoperatively.

B. MYOCARDITIS

PREVALENCE. Myocarditis severe enough to be recognized clinically is rare, but the prevalence of mild and subclinical cases is probably much higher.

BOX 4-3

CARDIAC CONDITIONS FOR WHICH PROPHYLAXIS WITH DENTAL PROCEDURES IS RECOMMENDED

1. Prosthetic cardiac valve
2. Previous infective endocarditis
3. Congenital heart disease (CHD)*
   a. Unrepaired cyanotic CHD, including palliative shunts and conduits
   b. Completely repaired CHD with prosthetic material or device, whether placed by surgery or by catheter intervention, during the first 6 months after the procedure[†]
   c. Repaired CHD with residual defects at the site or adjacent to the site of a prosthetic patch or prosthetic device (which inhibits endothelialization)
4. Cardiac transplantation recipients who develop cardiac valvulopathy

---

*Except for conditions listed above, antibiotic prophylaxis is no longer recommended for any other form of CHD.

[†]Prophylaxis is recommended because endothelialization of prosthetic material occurs within 6 months after the procedure.

BOX 4-4

PROCEDURES FOR WHICH ENDOCARDITIS PROPHYLAXIS IS RECOMMENDED

1. Dental procedures. *All dental procedures* that involve manipulation of gingival tissue of the periapical region of teeth or perforation of the oral mucosa. Antibiotic choices and dosages for dental procedures are shown in Table 4-1.
2. Respiratory tract procedures
   a. Recommended for procedures that involve incision or biopsy of the respiratory mucosa, such as tonsillectomy and adenoidectomy
   b. Not recommended for bronchoscopy (unless it involves incision of the mucosa, such as for abscess or empyema)
3. Gastrointestinal (GI) and genitourinary (GU) procedures
   a. No prophylaxis for diagnostic esophagogastroduodenoscopy or colonoscopy.
   b. Prophylaxis is reasonable in patients with infected GI or GU tract (with amoxicillin or ampicillin to cover against enterococci).
4. Skin, skin structure, or musculoskeletal tissue
   a. Recommended for surgical procedures that involve infected skin, skin structure, or musculoskeletal tissue (with antibiotics against *Staphylococcus* and β-hemolytic *Streptococcus,* such as antistaphylococcal penicillin or a cephalosporin).
   b. Vancomycin or clindamycin is administered if unable to tolerate β-lactam or if infection is caused by methicillin-resistant *Staphylococcus*.

TABLE 4-1

REGIMENS FOR DENTAL PROCEDURES

SITUATION	AGENT	SINGLE DOSE 30-60 MIN BEFORE PROCEDURE	
		CHILDREN	**ADULTS**
Oral	Amoxicillin	50 mg/kg	2 g
Unable to take oral medications	Ampicillin, or	50 mg/kg (IM, IV)	2 g (IM, IV)
	Cefazolin or ceftriaxone	50 mg/kg (IM, IV)	1 g (IM, IV)
Allergic to penicillin or ampicillin—oral	Cephalexin*†, or	50 mg/kg	2 g
	Clindamycin, or	20 mg/kg	600 mg
	Azithromycin or clarithromycin	15 mg/kg	500 mg
Allergic to penicillin or ampicillin and unable to take oral medication	Cefazolin, or ceftriaxone, or	50 mg/kg (IM, IV)	1 g (IM, IV)
	Clindamycin	20 mg/kg	600 mg

*Or other first- or second-generation oral cephalosporin in equivalent adult or pediatric dosage.
†Cephalosporins should not be used in an individual with a history of anaphylaxis, angioedema, or urticaria with penicillin or ampicillin.

ETIOLOGY

1. Infections: Viruses (such as adenovirus, coxsackieviruses, echoviruses, and many other viruses) are the most common cause of myocarditis in North America. A cell-mediated immunologic reaction, not merely myocardial damage from viral replication, appears important in viral myocarditis. In South America, Chagas disease (caused by *Trypanosoma cruzi,* a protozoan) is far more common. Rarely, bacteria, rickettsia, fungi, protozoa, and parasites are the causative agents.
2. Immune-mediated diseases: acute rheumatic fever, Kawasaki disease.
3. Collagen vascular diseases.
4. Toxic myocarditis (drug ingestion, diphtheria exotoxin, and anoxic agents).

CLINICAL MANIFESTATIONS

1. History of an upper respiratory infection may be present in older children. The onset of illness may be sudden in neonates and small infants, causing anorexia, vomiting, lethargy, and occasionally circulatory shock. In older children a gradual onset of CHF and arrhythmia is commonly seen.
2. A soft, systolic ejection murmur and irregular rhythm caused by supraventricular or ventricular ectopic beats may be audible. Hepatomegaly (evidence of viral hepatitis) may be present.
3. The ECG may show any one or combination of the following: low QRS voltages; ST-T changes; prolongation of the QT interval; and arrhythmias, especially premature contractions.
4. Cardiomegaly on CXR films is the most important clinical sign of myocarditis.
5. Echo studies reveal cardiac chamber enlargement and impaired LV function. Occasionally, LV thrombi are found.
6. Cardiac troponin levels (I and T) and myocardial enzymes (creatine kinase [CK], MB isoenzyme of CK [CK-MB]) may be elevated. Troponin levels may be more sensitive than the cardiac enzymes. The normal value of cardiac troponin I in children is 2.0 ng/mL or less. Radionuclide scanning (after administration of gallium-67 or technetium-99m pyrophosphate) may identify inflammatory and necrotic changes characteristic of myocarditis. Myocarditis can be confirmed by an endomyocardial biopsy.
7. The mortality rate is as high as 75% in symptomatic neonates with acute viral myocarditis. Most infected children, especially those with mild inflammation, recover completely. Some patients develop subacute or chronic myocarditis with persistent cardiomegaly with or without signs of CHF and ECG evidence of LVH or biventricular hypertrophy (BVH). Clinically, these patients are indistinguishable from those with dilated cardiomyopathy. Myocarditis may be a precursor to idiopathic dilated cardiomyopathy.

MANAGEMENT

1. Virus identification by viral cultures from the blood, stool, or throat washing should be attempted, and comparison of acute and convalescent sera may be made for serologic titer rise.

2. Bed rest and limitation of activities are recommended during the acute phase.

3. Beneficial effects of high-dose γ-globulin (2 g/kg over 24 hours) have been reported (with better survival and better LV function by echo), as in Kawasaki disease.

4. Anticongestive measures include rapid-acting diuretics (e.g., furosemide or ethacrynic acid), rapid-acting inotropic agents (e.g., isoproterenol, dobutamine, or dopamine), administration of oxygen, and bed rest. An ACE inhibitor (e.g., captopril) may be beneficial in the acute phase. Later, digoxin may be given cautiously, using half of the usual digitalizing dose, as some patients with myocarditis are exquisitely sensitive to digoxin.

5. Arrhythmias should be treated aggressively and may require the use of IV amiodarone.

6. The role of corticosteroids is unclear except in the treatment of severe rheumatic carditis.

7. Specific therapies include the use of antitoxin in diphtheric myocarditis.

C. PERICARDITIS
ETIOLOGY

1. Viral infection is probably the most common cause, particularly in infancy.

2. Acute rheumatic fever is a common cause of pericarditis in older children in certain parts of the world.

3. Bacterial infection (purulent pericarditis). Commonly encountered are *S. aureus, Streptococcus pneumoniae, Haemophilus influenzae, Neisseria meningitidis,* and streptococci.

4. Tuberculosis (an occasional cause of constrictive pericarditis with insidious onset).

5. Heart surgery (postpericardiotomy syndrome; see Chapter 7).

6. Collagen disease such as rheumatoid arthritis.

7. A complication of oncologic disease or its therapy, including radiation.

8. Uremia (uremic pericarditis).

PATHOLOGY AND PATHOPHYSIOLOGY

1. Pericardial effusion may be serofibrinous, hemorrhagic, or purulent. Effusion may be completely reabsorbed or may result in pericardial thickening or chronic constriction (constrictive pericarditis).

2. Symptoms and signs of pericardial effusion are determined by two factors: speed of fluid accumulation and competence of the myocardium. A slow accumulation of a large amount of fluid may be well tolerated by stretching of the pericardium, if the myocardium is intact. A rapid accumulation of even a small amount of fluid in the presence of myocarditis can produce circulatory embarrassment.

3. With the development of pericardial tamponade, several compensatory mechanisms are called on: systemic and pulmonary venous constriction (to improve diastolic filling), an increase in the SVR (to raise falling blood pressure), and tachycardia (to improve cardiac output).

CLINICAL MANIFESTATIONS

1. Precordial pain (dull, aching, or stabbing) with occasional radiation to the shoulder and neck may be a presenting complaint. The pain may be relieved by leaning forward and made worse by supine position or deep inspiration.
2. Pericardial friction rub is the cardinal physical sign. The heart is hypodynamic, and heart murmur is usually absent. In children with purulent pericarditis, septic fever (101° F to 105° F, or 38° C to 41° C), tachycardia, chest pain, and dyspnea are almost always present. Signs of cardiac tamponade may be present (distant heart sounds, tachycardia, pulsus paradoxus, hepatomegaly, neck vein distention, and occasional hypotension with peripheral vasoconstriction).
3. The ECG may show a low-voltage QRS complex, ST segment shift, and T wave inversion.
4. CXR films may show a varying degree of cardiomegaly. Water bottle–shaped heart and increased pulmonary venous markings are seen with large effusion.
5. Echo is the most useful tool in establishing the diagnosis of pericardial effusion. It appears as an echo-free space between the epicardium (visceral pericardium) and the parietal pericardium.
   a. Small pericardial effusion first appears posteriorly in the dependent portion of the pericardial sac. A small amount of fluid, which appears only in systole, is normal. With larger effusion, the fluid also appears anteriorly. With very large effusions, the swinging motion of the heart may be imaged.
   b. The following are helpful 2D echo findings of cardiac tamponade.
      (1) Collapse of the right atrium (RA) in late diastole (Fig. 4-3) (because the pressure in the pericardial sac exceeds the pressure within the right atrium at end-diastole when the atrium has emptied)

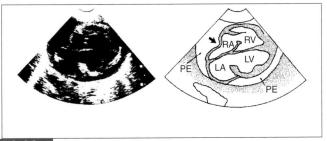

FIG. 4-3

Subcostal four-chamber view demonstrating pericardial effusion (PE) and collapse of the right atrial wall *(arrow)*, a sign of cardiac tamponade. *LA,* left atrium; *LV,* left ventricle; *RA,* right atrium; *RV,* right ventricle.

(2) Collapse or indentation of the RV free wall, especially the outflow tract

MANAGEMENT

1. Pericardiocentesis or surgical drainage to identify the cause of the pericarditis is mandatory, especially when purulent or tuberculous pericarditis is suspected. A drainage catheter may be left in place with intermittent low-pressure drainage.

2. Pericardial fluid studies include cell counts and differential, glucose, and protein concentrations; histologic examination of cells; Gram and acid-fast stains; and viral, bacterial, and fungal cultures.

3. For cardiac tamponade, urgent decompression by surgical drainage or pericardiocentesis is indicated. In preparation for the procedure, fluid push with Plasmanate should be given to increase central venous pressure and thereby improve cardiac filling, which can provide temporary emergency stabilization.

4. Urgent surgical drainage of the pericardium is indicated when purulent pericarditis is suspected. This must be followed by IV antibiotic therapy for 4 to 6 weeks.

5. There is no specific treatment for viral pericarditis.

6. Salicylates are given for precordial pain in patients with nonbacterial or rheumatic pericarditis.

7. Corticosteroid therapy may be indicated in children with severe rheumatic carditis or postpericardiotomy syndrome.

8. Digitalis is contraindicated in cardiac tamponade because it blocks tachycardia, a compensatory response to impaired venous return.

D. CONSTRICTIVE PERICARDITIS

Although rare in children, constrictive pericarditis may be associated with an earlier viral pericarditis, tuberculosis, incomplete drainage of purulent pericarditis, hemopericardium, mediastinal irradiation, neoplastic infiltration, or connective tissue disorders. In this condition a fibrotic, thickened, and adherent pericardium restricts diastolic filling of the heart.

Clinical findings that suggest the diagnosis are as follows:

1. Signs of elevated jugular venous pressure occur. Hepatomegaly with ascites and systemic edema may be present. Diastolic pericardial knock, which resembles the opening snap, is often heard along the left sternal border in the absence of heart murmur.

2. CXR films may show calcification of the pericardium, enlargement of the superior vena cava (SVC) and LA, and pleural effusion.

3. The ECG may show low QRS voltages, T wave inversion or flattening, and left atrial hypertrophy (LAH). Atrial fibrillation occasionally is seen.

4. M-mode echo may reveal two parallel lines representing the thickened visceral and parietal pericardia or multiple dense echoes. Two-dimensional echo shows (a) a thickened pericardium, (b) dilated inferior vena cava (IVC) and hepatic vein, and (c) paradoxical septal motion and abrupt displacement of the interventricular septum during early diastolic filling

("septal bounce") (not specific for this condition). Doppler examination of the mitral inflow reveals findings of diastolic dysfunction (Fig. 4-2) and a marked respiratory variation in diastolic inflow tracings.

5. Cardiac catheterization may document the presence of constrictive physiology.

a. The RA and LA pressures, ventricular end-diastolic pressures, and pulmonary artery (PA) wedge pressure are all elevated and usually equalized.

b. Ventricular pressure waveforms demonstrate the characteristic "square root sign" (in which there is an early rapid fall in diastolic pressure followed by a rapid rise to an elevated diastolic plateau).

6. The treatment for constrictive pericarditis is complete resection of the pericardium; symptomatic improvement occurs in 75% of patients.

III. KAWASAKI DISEASE

ETIOLOGY AND EPIDEMIOLOGY

1. The cause of Kawasaki disease is not known. It may be related to abnormalities of the immune system initiated by the infectious insult.

2. It peaks in winter and spring in the United States. It occurs primarily in young children; 80% of the patients are younger than age 4 years, 50% are younger than age 2 years, and cases in children older than 8 years and younger than 3 months are rarely reported.

PATHOLOGY

1. During the first 10 days after the onset of fever, a multisystem vasculitis develops that has the greatest predilection for the coronary arteries. Other arteries, such as iliac, femoral, axillary, and renal, are less frequently involved.

2. Coronary artery aneurysm may develop in 15% to 20% of patients during the period of 1 to 3 weeks of illness.

3. There is also pancarditis, involving the atrioventricular (AV) conduction system (which can produce AV block), myocardium (myocardial dysfunction, CHF), pericardium (pericardial effusion), and endocardium (with AV valve involvement).

4. Late changes (after 40 days) consist of healing and fibrosis in the coronary arteries, with thrombus formation and stenosis in the postaneurysmal segment and myocardial fibrosis from old myocardial infarction.

5. The elevated platelet count seen in this condition contributes to coronary thrombosis.

CLINICAL MANIFESTATIONS

The clinical course of the disease may be divided into three phases: acute, subacute, and convalescent.

1. Acute phase (first 10 days)

a. Six signs that comprise the principal clinical features of Kawasaki disease are present during the acute phase (Box 4-5).

   (1) Abrupt onset, with fever usually >39° C (102° F) and often >40° C (104° F); fever persists for a mean of 11 days without treatment

   (2) Bilateral conjunctivitis without exudate, which resolves rapidly

(3) Changes in the lips and oral cavity: erythema, dryness, fissuring, and bleeding of the lips; "strawberry tongue"; and diffuse erythema of the oropharynx

(4) Changes in extremities: erythema of the palms and soles, firm edema, and sometimes painful induration (desquamation of hands and feet occurs within 2 to 3 weeks)

(5) Diffuse maculopapular eruption involving the trunk, extremities, and perineal region; desquamation usually occurs by days 5 to 7

(6) Unilateral cervical lymphadenopathy, usually >1.5 cm, in approximately 50% of patients

b. Cardiovascular abnormalities include some or all of the following: tachycardia, gallop rhythm, and/or other signs of heart failure, MR murmur, and cardiomegaly on CXR films. The ECG may show arrhythmias, prolonged PR interval (occurring in up to 60% of patients), nonspecific ST-T change, or abnormal Q waves (wide and deep) suggestive of myocardial infarction.

c. Echocardiography

(1) Coronary artery aneurysm rarely occurs before day 10 of illness. Echo studies may show coronary artery abnormalities at the end of the first week through the second week of illness. According to the new guidelines, aneurysms are classified as *saccular* (nearly equal axial and lateral diameters), *fusiform* (symmetric dilation with gradual proximal and distal tapering), and *ectatic* (dilated without segmental aneurysm). "Giant" aneurysm is present when the diameter of the aneurysm is ≥8 mm.

(2) Normal data on the size of the proximal coronary arteries are shown in Appendix D (Table D-8). A coronary dimension that is greater than +3SD in one of the three segments (left main coronary artery [LMCA], left anterior descending [LAD], and right coronary artery [RCA]) or one that is greater than +2.5SD in two proximal segments is considered abnormal.

(3) During the first 10 days of illness before coronary aneurysm appears, other echo findings suggestive of cardiac involvement may appear: LV enlargement with decreased LV systolic function, mild MR, and pericardial effusion.

d. Involvement of other organ systems is also frequent during the acute phase.

(1) Arthritis or arthralgia of multiple joints (30%)

(2) Sterile pyuria (60%)

(3) Abdominal pain with diarrhea (20%), liver dysfunction (40%), hydrops of the gallbladder (10%, demonstrable by abdominal ultrasound) with jaundice

(4) Irritability, lethargy or semicoma, and aseptic meningitis (25%)

e. Laboratory studies. Even though laboratory results are nonspecific, they provide diagnostic support of the disease during the acute phase. For example, Kawasaki disease is unlikely if acute phase reactants and platelet counts are normal after 7 days of the illness.

(1) Marked leukocytosis with a shift to the left and anemia are common.

(2) Acute phase reactant levels (C-reactive protein [CRP] levels, erythrocyte sedimentation rate [ESR]) are always elevated, which is uncommon with viral illnesses. An elevated sedimentation rate (but not CRP) can be caused by intravenous immune globulin (IVIG) infusion per se.

(3) Thrombocytosis (usually >450,000/mm^3) occurs after day 7 of the illness, sometimes reaching 600,000 to >1 million/mm^3 during the subacute phase. Low platelet count suggests viral illnesses.

(4) Elevated liver enzymes (>2 times the upper limit of normal) in 40% of patients. Hypoalbuminemia and mild hyperbilirubinemia may be present in 10%.

2. Subacute phase (11 to 25 days after onset). The following clinical findings are seen during the subacute phase.

a. Desquamation of the tips of the fingers and toes is characteristic.

b. Rash, fever, and lymphadenopathy disappear.

c. Significant cardiovascular changes, including coronary aneurysm (seen in approximately 20%), pericardial effusion, CHF, and myocardial infarction, can occur in this phase.

d. Thrombocytosis also occurs during this period (peaking at 2 weeks or more after the onset of the illness).

3. Convalescent phase. This phase lasts until the elevated erythrocyte sedimentation rate and platelet count return to normal. Deep transverse grooves (Beau lines) may appear across the fingernails and toenails.

NATURAL HISTORY. It is a self-limited disease for most patients. However, coronary aneurysm occurs in 15% to 25% of patients and is responsible for myocardial infarction (fewer than 5%) and mortality (1% to 5%). If the coronary artery remains normal throughout the first month after onset, subsequent development of a coronary lesion is extremely unusual. Coronary aneurysm has a tendency to regress within a year in about 50% of patients, but these arteries do not dilate in response to exercise or coronary vasodilators. In some patients, stenosis, tortuosity, and thrombosis of the coronary arteries result.

DIAGNOSIS

The diagnosis of Kawasaki disease is based on clinical findings. Box 4-5 lists the principal clinical features that establish the diagnosis. Fever of ≥5 days and at least four of the five diagnostic criteria establish the diagnosis.

It is necessary to rule out diseases with similar manifestations through appropriate cultures and laboratory tests. Measles and group A β-hemolytic streptococcal infection most closely mimic Kawasaki disease. Other differential diagnoses of Kawasaki disease include the following: viral infections (e.g., measles, adenovirus, enterovirus, Epstein-Barr virus), scarlet fever, staphylococcal calded skin syndrome, toxic shock syndrome, bacterial cervical lymphadenopathy, drug hypersensitivity reaction, Stevens-Johnson syndrome, juvenile rheumatoid arthritis, and Rocky Mountain spotted fever.

BOX 4-5

PRINCIPAL CLINICAL FEATURES FOR DIAGNOSTIC CRITERIA OF KAWASAKI DISEASE

PRINCIPAL CLINICAL FEATURES

1. Fever persisting at least 5 days
2. Presence of at least four of the following principal features
    a. Changes in extremities
        (1) Acute: erythema of palms and soles; edema of hands and feet
        (2) Subacute: periungual peeling of fingers and toes in weeks 2 and 3
    b. Polymorphous exanthema
    c. Bilateral bulbar conjunctival injection without exudate
    d. Changes in the lips and oral cavity: erythema, lips cracking, strawberry tongue, diffuse injection of oral and pharyngeal mucosa
    e. Cervical lymphadenopathy (>1.5 cm in diameter), usually unilateral
3. Exclusion of other diseases with similar findings (see text)

DIAGNOSIS OF KAWASAKI DISEASE

1. Diagnosis of Kawasaki disease is made in the presence of ≥5 days of fever and at least four of the five principal clinical features listed under No. 2 above.
2. Patients with fever ≥5 days and fewer than four principal criteria can be diagnosed with Kawasaki disease when coronary artery abnormalities are detected by 2D echo or angiography.
3. In the presence of at least four principal criteria plus fever, Kawasaki disease diagnosis can be made on day 4 of illness.

Modified from Newburger JW, Takahashi M, Gerber MA et al: Diagnosis, treatment, and long-term management of Kawasaki disease: a statement for health professionals from the Committee on Rheumatic Fever, Endocarditis, and Kawasaki Disease, Council on Cardiovascular Disease in the Young, American Heart Association, *Pediatrics* 114:1708-1733, 2004.

MANAGEMENT

Two goals of therapy are reduction of inflammation within the coronary artery and prevention of thrombosis by inhibition of platelet aggregation.

1. A high-dose (2 g/kg), single infusion of IVIG with aspirin (80 to 100 mg/kg per day), given within 10 days (preferably within 7 days) of illness, is considered the treatment of choice. Following IVIG infusion, two thirds of patients become afebrile by 24 hours after completion of infusion; 90% are afebrile by 48 hours.

2. A repeat dose (2 g/kg) of IVIG is indicated in children with a persistent fever. IVIG given before 5 days of illness appears no more likely to prevent coronary aneurysm but is associated with increased need for retreatment with gamma globulin for persistent or recrudescent fever. Gamma globulin should be given even after day 10 of illness if the patient has persistent fever, aneurysms, or ongoing systemic inflammation (by ESR or CRP).

3. Aspirin is reduced to 3 to 5 mg/kg/day in a single dose after the child has been afebrile for 48 to 72 hours. Some physicians continue the high-dose aspirin until day 14 of illness. Aspirin is continued until the patient shows no evidence of coronary changes by 6 to 8 weeks after the onset of illness. For children who develop coronary abnormalities, aspirin may be continued indefinitely.

4. The usefulness of steroids in the initial treatment of Kawasaki disease is not well established at this time. However, steroids may be used along with IVIG for patients who continue to be febrile despite two or more courses of IVIG.

5. In patients with coronary artery aneurysm, antiplatelet agents with or without an anticoagulant are indicated, depending on the severity of the involvement.

a. For mild and stable disease, low-dose aspirin may be appropriate.

b. For more severe coronary involvement, aspirin combined with other antiplatelet agents (e.g., dipyridamole [Persantine], clopidogrea [Plavix]) may be used.

c. For giant aneurysm or the combination of stenosis and aneurysm, low-dose aspirin together with warfarin (with INR maintained at 2.0 to 2.5) should be used.

6. Serial follow-up is important for evaluation of the cardiac status. The recommendations of the AHA are shown in Table 4-2.

IV. ACUTE RHEUMATIC FEVER

ETIOLOGY. Acute rheumatic fever is a delayed sequela of group A hemolytic streptococcal infection of the pharynx (but not of the skin). The peak incidence is at 8 years (range 6 to 15 years).

CLINICAL MANIFESTATIONS

1. The patient may have had streptococcal pharyngitis 1 to 5 weeks (average 3 weeks) before the onset of symptoms. The latent period may be as long as 2 to 6 months (average 4 months) in cases of isolated chorea.

2. Clinical manifestations of acute rheumatic fever may be grouped into five major criteria, four minor criteria, and supporting evidence of preceding streptococcal infection (Box 4-6).

3. Major manifestations

a. Arthritis involving large joints (knees, ankles, elbows, wrists) is the most common manifestation (60% to 85%). Often more than one joint, either simultaneously or in succession, is involved, with the characteristic migratory nature of the arthritis. Swelling, heat, redness, severe pain, tenderness, and limitation of motion are common. The arthritis responds dramatically to antiinflammatory salicylate therapy; if patients treated with salicylates do not improve within 48 hours, the diagnosis of acute rheumatic fever probably is incorrect. Arthritis subsides in a few days to weeks even without treatment and does not cause permanent damage.

TABLE 4-2

FOLLOW-UP RECOMMENDATIONS ACCORDING TO THE DEGREE OF CORONARY ARTERY INVOLVEMENT

RISK LEVEL	PHARMACOLOGIC THERAPY	PHYSICAL ACTIVITY	FOLLOW-UP AND DIAGNOSTIC TESTING	INVASIVE TESTING
I. No coronary artery changes at any stage of illness	None beyond first 6-8 wk (aspirin for first 6-8 wk only)	No restrictions beyond first 6-8 wk	Cardiovascular risk assessment, counseling at 5-yr intervals	None recommended
II. Transient coronary artery ectasia disappears within first 6-8 wk	None beyond first 6-8 wk (aspirin for first 6-8 wk only)	No restrictions beyond first 6-8 wk	Cardiovascular risk assessment and counseling at 3- to 5-yr intervals	None recommended
III. One small to medium coronary artery aneurysm/major coronary artery	Low-dose aspirin (3-5 mg/kg/day), at least until aneurysm regression documented	For patients <11 yr, no restrictions beyond first 6-8 wk Patients 11-20 yr old, physical activity guided by stress test or myocardial perfusion scan every 2 yr Contact or high-impact sports discouraged for patients taking antiplatelet agents	Annual cardiology follow-up with echocardiogram + ECG Cardiovascular risk assessment and counseling Stress test with myocardial perfusion scan every 2 yr in patients >10 yr	Angiography, if noninvasive test suggests ischemia

Risk level	Pharmacologic therapy	Physical activity	Follow-up	Invasive testing
IV. One or more large or giant coronary artery aneurysm, or multiple or complex aneurysms in same coronary artery without obstruction	Long-term aspirin (3-5 mg/kg/day) and warfarin (target: INR 2.0-2.5) or low-molecular heparin (target: antifactor Xa level 0.5-1.0 U/mL) should be combined in giant aneurysm	Contact or high-impact sports should be avoided because of risk of bleeding. Other physical activity recommendations guided by annual stress test or myocardial perfusion evaluation	Cardiology follow-up with echocardiogram + ECG every 6 mo. Annual stress test with myocardial perfusion evaluation. For females of childbearing age, reproductive counseling recommended	First angiography at 6-12 mo or sooner if clinically indicated. Repeat angiography if noninvasive test, clinical, or laboratory findings suggest ischemia. Elective repeat angiography under some circumstances (atypical anginal pain, inability to do stress testing, etc.)
V. Coronary artery obstruction	Long-term low-dose aspirin (3-5 mg/kg/day). Warfarin or low-molecular-weight heparin if giant aneurysm persists. Consider use of β-blocker to reduce myocardial oxygen consumption	Contact or high-impact sports should be avoided because of risk of bleeding. Other physical activity recommendations guided by stress test or myocardial perfusion scan	Cardiology follow-up with echocardiogram with ECG every 6 mo. Annual stress test or myocardial perfusion scan. For females of childbearing age, reproductive counseling is recommended	Angiography recommended to address therapeutic options of bypass grafting or catheter intervention

Modified from Newburger JW, Takahashi M, Gerber MA et al: Diagnosis, treatment, and long-term management of Kawasaki disease: a statement for health professionals from the Committee on Rheumatic Fever, Endocarditis, and Kawasaki Disease, Council on Cardiovascular Disease in the Young, American Heart Association, *Pediatrics* 114:1708-1733, 2004.

BOX 4-6

GUIDELINES FOR THE DIAGNOSIS OF INITIAL ATTACK OF RHEUMATIC FEVER (JONES CRITERIA, 1992)

MAJOR MANIFESTATIONS	MINOR MANIFESTATIONS
Carditis	**CLINICAL FINDINGS**
Polyarthritis	Arthralgia
Chorea	Fever
Erythema marginatum	**LABORATORY FINDINGS**
Subcutaneous nodule	Elevated acute-phase reactants (ESR, C-reactive protein)
	Prolonged PR interval

PLUS

SUPPORTING EVIDENCE OF ANTECEDENT GROUP A STREPTOCOCCAL INFECTION

Positive throat culture or rapid streptococcal antigen test

Elevated or rising streptococcal antibody titer

If supported by evidence of preceding group A streptococcal infection, the presence of two major manifestations or one major and two minor manifestations indicates a high probability of acute rheumatic fever.

From Special Writing Group of the Committee on Rheumatic Fever, Endocarditis, and Kawasaki Disease of the Council on Cardiovascular Disease in the Young, American Heart Association: Guidelines for the diagnosis of rheumatic fever: Jones criteria, updated 1992, *Circulation* 87:302-307, 1993.
ESR, erythrocyte sedimentation rate.

---

b. Carditis affects 40% to 50% of patients. Mild carditis disappears rapidly in weeks, but severe carditis may last for months. Only carditis can cause permanent cardiac damage. Signs of carditis include some or all of the following:

(1) Tachycardia (out of proportion for the degree of fever).

(2) A heart murmur of MR and/or aortic regurgitation (AR) is frequently present. Although the Jones criteria require the presence of audible MR and/or AR murmur to make the diagnosis of acute rheumatic carditis, hemodynamically significant echo abnormalities (such as gross prolapse of the mitral valve or posterolateral MR jet) may be present in the absence of audible heart murmur.

(3) Pericarditis (friction rub, pericardial effusion, chest pain, and ECG changes).

(4) Cardiomegaly on CXR film (caused by pericarditis, pancarditis, or CHF).

(5) Signs of CHF (gallop rhythm, distant heart sounds, and cardiomegaly).

c. Erythema marginatum (10%), with the characteristic nonpruritic serpiginous or annular erythematous rashes, is most prominent on the trunk and the inner proximal portions of the extremities. The rashes are evanescent, disappearing with exposure to cold and reappearing after a hot shower or when the patient is covered with a warm blanket.

d. Subcutaneous nodules (2% to 10%) are hard, painless, nonpruritic, freely movable swellings, 0.2 to 2 cm in diameter. They are usually found symmetrically, singly or in clusters, on the extensor surfaces of both large and small joints, over the scalp, or along the spine. They are not transient, lasting for weeks, and have a significant association with carditis. They are also found in conditions other than rheumatic fever (such as rheumatoid arthritis and systemic lupus erythematosus).

e. Sydenham chorea, or St. Vitus dance (15%), is found more often in prepubertal (8 to 12 years) girls than in boys. It is a neuropsychiatric disorder consisting of both neurologic disorders (choreic movement and hypotonia) and psychiatric components (such as emotional lability, hyperactivity, separation anxiety, obsessions, and compulsions). It begins initially with emotional lability and personality changes, soon (in 1 to 4 weeks) replaced by the characteristic spontaneous, purposeless movement of chorea, which is followed by motor weakness. The choreic movements last for an average of 7 months (and up to 17 months) before slowly waning in severity. It is often an isolated manifestation; the patient may have no fever, and ESR and antistreptolysin O (ASO) titers may be normal. Recently, elevated titers of "antineuronal antibodies" recognizing basal ganglion tissues have been found in over 90% of patients, suggesting that chorea may be related to dysfunction of basal ganglia and cortical neuronal components.

4. Minor manifestations include fever, arthralgia, elevated acute-phase reactants (elevated ESR and CRP), and prolonged PR interval (Box 4-6).

5. Evidence of antecedent group A streptococcal infection

a. History of sore throat or scarlet fever, positive throat culture, or rapid streptococcal antigen tests (Streptozyme test) for group A streptococci are less reliable than the antibody test.

b. Specific antibody tests are the most reliable laboratory evidence of antecedent streptococcal infection capable of producing acute rheumatic fever. An ASO titer above 333 Todd units in children or above 250 Todd units in adults is considered significant. Antideoxyribonuclease B titer of 240 Todd units or more in children or 120 Todd units or more in adults is considered elevated.

DIAGNOSIS

Diagnosis of acute rheumatic fever is highly probable in the presence of either two major manifestations or one major plus two minor manifestations plus evidence of antecedent streptococcal infection. The absence of supporting evidence of a preceding group A streptococcal infection makes the diagnosis doubtful. Arthralgia or a prolonged PR interval cannot be used as a minor manifestation in the presence of arthritis and carditis, respectively.

The following are exceptions to the Jones criteria: (1) Chorea may occur as the only manifestation of rheumatic fever, (2) indolent carditis may be the only manifestation in a patient who seeks medical attention months after the onset of rheumatic fever, and (3) occasionally, patients with rheumatic fever recurrences may not fulfill the Jones criteria.

MANAGEMENT

1. When acute rheumatic fever is suspected, the following laboratory studies are obtained: complete blood count, acute phase reactants (ESR, CRP), throat culture, ASO titer, CXR film, and ECG. Cardiology consultation is recommended early to clarify any cardiac involvement; 2D echo and Doppler studies are usually performed at that time.

2. Benzathine penicillin G, 0.6 million to 1.2 million units, is administered IM to eradicate *Streptococcus* (and also every 28 days for prevention of recurrence). In patients allergic to penicillin, erythromycin, 40 mg/kg/day in two to four doses for 10 days, may be substituted for penicillin.

3. It is important to impress on the patient and parents the necessity of preventing subsequent streptococcal infection through continuous antibiotic prophylaxis.

4. Bed rest of different levels is recommended (Table 4-3), followed by a period of indoor ambulation, before the child is allowed to go back to school. Full activity is allowed later, when the ESR returns to normal, except for children with significant cardiac involvement.

5. Therapy with antiinflammatory agents should be started as soon as the diagnosis of acute rheumatic fever has been established.

a. For arthritis, aspirin therapy is continued for 2 weeks and gradually withdrawn over the following 2 to 3 weeks. Rapid resolution of joint symptoms with aspirin within 24 to 36 hours is supportive evidence of acute rheumatic fever.

b. For mild to moderate carditis, aspirin alone is recommended in a dose of 90 to 100 mg/kg/day in four to six divided doses (target blood level of salicylate 20 to 25 mg/100 mL).

c. For severe carditis, prednisone, 2 mg/kg/day in four divided doses, may be added to aspirin therapy for 2 to 6 weeks.

6. Management of Sydenham chorea

a. Reduce physical and emotional stress and use protective measures as indicated.

b. Give benzathine penicillin G, 1.2 million units, initially for eradication of *Streptococcus* and also every 28 days for prevention of recurrence, just as in patients with other rheumatic manifestations.

TABLE 4-3
GENERAL GUIDE FOR BED REST AND AMBULATION

	ARTHRITIS ALONE	MILD CARDITIS	MODERATE CARDITIS	SEVERE CARDITIS
Bed Rest	1-2 wk	2-4 wk	4-6 wk	As long as CHF is present
Ambulation	1-2 wk	3-4 wk	4-6 wk	2-3 mo

Mild carditis, questionable cardiomegaly; *moderate carditis,* definite but mild cardiomegaly; *severe carditis,* marked cardiomegaly or heart failure.

c. Antiinflammatory agents are not needed in patients with isolated chorea.

d. For severe cases, any of the following drugs may be used: phenobarbital, haloperidol, valproic acid, chlorpromazine (Thorazine), diazepam (Valium), or steroids.

e. Results of plasma exchange (to remove antineuronal antibodies) and IVIG therapy (to inactivate the effects of the antineuronal antibodies) are promising in decreasing the severity of chorea.

PREVENTION

1. Any patient with a documented history of rheumatic fever, including those with isolated chorea and those without evidence of rheumatic heart disease, must receive prophylaxis.

2. Benzathine penicillin G, 600,000 units for patients under 60 lb (27 kg) and 1.2 million units for patients over 60 lb, given IM every 28 days (not once a month), is the method of choice. Although less effective, the following alternative drugs may be used.

a. Oral penicillin V, 250 mg twice daily.

b. Oral sulfadiazine, 1 g or sulfisoxazole 0.5 g once daily.

c. If the patient is allergic to penicillin, erythromycin, 250 mg twice daily, may be used.

3. Recommended duration of prophylaxis for rheumatic fever is summarized in Table 4-4.

V. VALVULAR HEART DISEASE

Most acquired valvular heart diseases are of rheumatic etiology. They are, however, rare in industrialized countries, although they still occur frequently in less developed countries. Among rheumatic heart disease, mitral valve involvement occurs in about three fourths and aortic valve involvement in about one fourth of the cases. Stenosis and regurgitation of the same valve usually occur together. Isolated aortic stenosis (AS) of rheumatic origin without mitral valve involvement is extremely rare. Rheumatic involvement of the tricuspid and pulmonary valves almost never occurs.

TABLE 4-4	
RECOMMENDED DURATION OF PROPHYLAXIS FOR RHEUMATIC FEVER	
CATEGORY	**DURATION**
Rheumatic fever without carditis	At least for 5 years or until 21 years of age, whichever is longer
Rheumatic fever with carditis but without residual heart disease (no valvular disease)	At least 10 years or well into adulthood, whichever is longer
Rheumatic fever with carditis and residual heart disease (persistent valvular disease)	At least 10 years since last episode and at least until age 40 years; sometimes lifelong prophylaxis

From Dajani A, Taubert K, Ferrieri P et al: Treatment of acute streptococcal pharyngitis and prevention of rheumatic fever: a statement for health professionals, *Pediatrics* 96:758-764, 1995.

A. MITRAL STENOSIS

PREVALENCE. Mitral stenosis (MS) of rheumatic origin is rare in children (because it requires 5 to 10 years from the initial attack to develop the condition), but it is the most common valvular involvement in adult rheumatic patients in areas where rheumatic fever is still prevalent.

PATHOLOGY AND PATHOPHYSIOLOGY

1. In rheumatic MS, thickening of the leaflets and fusion of the commissures dominate the pathologic findings. Calcification with immobility of the valve results over time.

2. A significant MS results in the enlargement of the LA, pulmonary venous hypertension, and pulmonary artery hypertension with resulting enlargement and hypertrophy of the right side of the heart.

3. In patients with severe MS, pulmonary congestion and edema, fibrosis of the alveolar walls, hypertrophy of the pulmonary arterioles, and loss of lung compliance result.

CLINICAL MANIFESTATIONS

1. Children with mild MS are asymptomatic. With significant MS, dyspnea with or without exertion is the most common symptom in older children. Orthopnea, nocturnal dyspnea, or palpitation is present in more severe cases.

2. Neck veins are distended if right-sided heart failure supervenes. A loud S1 at the apex and a narrowly split S2 with accentuated P2 are audible if pulmonary hypertension is present (Fig. 4-4). An opening snap (a short snapping sound accompanying the opening of the mitral valve) and a low-frequency mitral diastolic rumble may be present at the apex. A crescendo presystolic murmur may be audible at the apex. Occasionally, a high-frequency diastolic murmur of PR (Graham Steell murmur) is present at the upper left sternal border (ULSB) in patients with pulmonary hypertension.

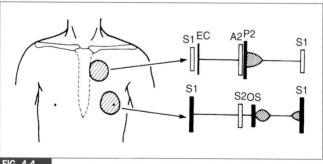

FIG. 4-4

Cardiac findings of MS. Abnormal sounds are shown in black and include a loud S1, an ejection click (EC), a loud S2, and an opening snap (OS). Also note the middiastolic rumble and presystolic murmur. The murmur of pulmonary insufficiency indicates long-standing pulmonary hypertension.

3. The ECG may show right axis deviation (RAD), LAH, and right ventricular hypertrophy (RVH) (caused by pulmonary hypertension). Atrial fibrillation is rare in children.

4. CXR films show enlargement of the LA and RV. The main PA segment is usually prominent. Lung fields show pulmonary venous congestion, interstitial edema shown as Kerley B lines (dense, short, horizontal lines most commonly seen in the costophrenic angles), and redistribution of pulmonary blood flow with increased pulmonary vascularity to the upper lobes.

5. Echo studies provide accurate diagnosis of MS.

a. Echo studies show dilated LA, RV, and RA and prominent main PA.

b. A mean Doppler gradient of <4 to 5 mm Hg results from mild stenosis, 6 to 12 mm Hg from moderate stenosis, and >13 mm Hg from severe stenosis.

c. RV systolic pressure can be estimated from the TR jet velocity.

NATURAL HISTORY

1. Most children with mild MS are asymptomatic but become symptomatic with exertion.

2. Atrial flutter or fibrillation and thromboembolism (related to the chronic atrial arrhythmias) are rare in children.

3. Hemoptysis can develop from the rupture of small vessels in the bronchi as a result of long-standing pulmonary venous hypertension.

MANAGEMENT

MEDICAL

1. Mild to moderate MS is managed with digoxin and diuretics.

2. Balloon dilation is an effective and safe option for children with rheumatic mitral stenosis.

3. If atrial fibrillation develops, digoxin is the initial treatment to slow the AV conduction. Intravenous procainamide may be used for conversion to sinus rhythm in hemodynamically stable patients. For patients with chronic atrial fibrillation, anticoagulation with warfarin should be started 3 weeks before cardioversion to prevent systemic embolization of atrial thrombus. Anticoagulation is continued for 4 weeks after restoration of sinus rhythm. Quinidine may prevent recurrence.

4. Varying degrees of restriction of activity may be indicated.

5. Recurrence of rheumatic fever should be prevented with penicillin or sulfonamide (see Acute Rheumatic Fever).

SURGICAL

1. Indications. The American College of Cardiology (ACC)/American Heart Association (AHA) 2006 guidelines for surgical indications are as follows:

a. Surgery is indicated in symptomatic patients (NYHA functional class III or IV) and mean Doppler MV gradient >10 mm Hg. (Symptoms may include angina, syncope, or dyspnea on exertion.)

b. Surgery is reasonable in mildly symptomatic patients (NYHA functional class II) and mean Doppler MV gradient >10 mm Hg.

c. Surgery is reasonable in asymptomatic patients with pulmonary artery pressure ≥50 mm Hg and mean MV gradient ≥10 mm Hg.

2. Procedures and mortality
a. For rheumatic MS, if balloon dilation is unsuccessful, closed or open mitral commissurotomy remains the procedure of choice for those with pliable mitral valves without calcification or MR. The operative mortality rate is <1%.
b. Mitral valve replacement. A prosthetic valve (Starr-Edwards, Bjork-Shiley, St. Jude) is inserted either in the annulus or in a supraannular position. The surgical mortality is 0% to 19%. All mechanical valves require anticoagulation with warfarin. Bioprostheses (porcine valve, heterograft valve) do not require anticoagulation therapy but require low-dose aspirin. Bioprostheses tend to deteriorate more rapidly due to calcific degeneration in children.
3. Postoperative follow-up
a. Regular checkups every 6 to 12 months with echo and Doppler studies should be done for possible dysfunction of the repaired or replaced valve.
b. When there are no risk factors after replacement with a mechanical valve, warfarin is indicated to achieve an INR of 2.5 to 3.5. Low-dose aspirin is also indicated. When there are risk factors after replacement with a bioprosthesis, warfarin is also indicated. When there are no risk factors after bioprosthesis placement, antiplatelet dose of aspirin alone is indicated. Risk factors include atrial fibrillation, previous thromboembolism, LV dysfunction, and hypercoagulable state.

B. MITRAL REGURGITATION

PREVALENCE. MR of rheumatic origin is rare, but it is the most common valvular involvement in children with rheumatic heart disease.

PATHOLOGY
1. In rheumatic heart disease, mitral valve leaflets are shortened because of fibrosis, resulting in MR.
2. With increasing severity of MR, dilation of the LA and LV results, and the mitral valve ring may become dilated. Pulmonary hypertension may eventually develop but is less common than with MS.

CLINICAL MANIFESTATIONS
1. Patients are usually asymptomatic with mild MR. A history of fatigue and palpitation may be present.
2. The S2 may split widely as a result of shortening of the LV ejection and early closure of the aortic valve. A loud S3 is common. The hallmark of MR is a grade 2 to 4/6 regurgitant systolic murmur at the apex, with good transmission to the left axilla (best demonstrated in the left decubitus position). A short, low-frequency diastolic rumble may be present at the apex (Fig. 4-5).
3. The ECG is normal in mild cases. With moderate to severe MR, LVH (or LV dominance) with or without LAH may be present. Atrial fibrillation is rare in children but frequent in adults.
4. CXR films may show LA and LV enlargement. Pulmonary venous congestion may develop if CHF supervenes.

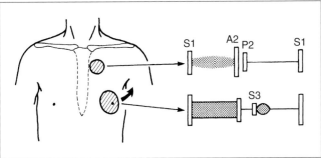

FIG. 4-5

Cardiac findings of MR. Arrow near the apex indicates the direction of radiation of the murmur toward the axilla.

5. Two-dimensional echo shows dilated LA and LV; the degree of the dilation is related to the severity of MR. Color flow mapping of the regurgitant jet into the LA and Doppler studies can assess the severity of the regurgitation. The MR is central with rheumatic MR (and eccentric with congenital cleft mitral valve).

6. Patients are relatively stable for a long time with MR. LV failure and consequent pulmonary hypertension may develop in adult life.

MANAGEMENT

MEDICAL

1. Prophylaxis against recurrence of rheumatic fever is important.

2. Activity need not be restricted in mild cases.

3. Afterload-reducing agents (such as ACE inhibitors) are particularly beneficial.

4. Anticongestive therapy (with diuretics and digoxin) is provided if CHF develops.

5. If atrial fibrillation develops (rare in children), digoxin is indicated to slow the ventricular response.

SURGICAL

1. Indications. Indications for valve surgery in adolescents and young adults with severe MR are as follows, according to the ACC/AHA 2006 guidelines.

a. Symptomatic patients with severe MR with NYHA functional class III or IV.

b. Asymptomatic patients with severe MR and LV systolic dysfunction (EF ≤0.6).

c. Surgery may be considered in patients with preserved LV function if the likelihood of successful repair without residual MR is great.

d. Some centers consider an LV diastolic dimension of 60 mm in adults an indication for mitral valve replacement. For children, intractable CHF, progressive cardiomegaly with symptoms, and pulmonary hypertension may be indications.

2. Procedures and mortality

a. Valve repair surgery is preferred over valve replacement in pediatric patients. For central regurgitation with dilated annulus, annuloplasty is performed by commissuroplasty. Valve repair has a lower mortality rate (<1%), and anticoagulation is not necessary.

b. Valve replacement is rarely necessary for unrepairable regurgitation. Frequently used low-profile prostheses are the Bjork-Shiley tilting disk and the St. Jude pyrolytic carbon valve. The surgical mortality rate is 2% to 7% for valve replacement. If a prosthetic valve is used, anticoagulation therapy must be continued.

3. Postoperative follow-up

a. Valve function (of either the repaired natural valve or the replacement valve) should be checked by echo and Doppler studies every 6 to 12 months.

b. When there are no risk factors after replacement with a mechanical valve, warfarin is indicated to achieve an INR of 2.5 to 3.5, along with a low-dose aspirin. When there are no risk factors after replacement with a bioprosthesis, aspirin alone is indicated. If there are risk factors (which include atrial fibrillation, previous thromboembolism, LV dysfunction, and hypercoagulable state), warfarin is also indicated.

C. AORTIC REGURGITATION

PREVALENCE AND PATHOLOGY. Sclerosis of the aortic valve results in distortion and retraction of the cusps with regurgitation of the valve. AR of rheumatic origin is almost always associated with mitral valve involvement.

CLINICAL MANIFESTATIONS

1. Patients with mild regurgitation are asymptomatic. Exercise tolerance is reduced with more severe AR.

2. With moderate or severe AR, hyperdynamic precordium is present. A wide pulse pressure and a bounding water-hammer pulse may be present with severe AR. The S2 may be normal or single. A high-pitched diastolic decrescendo murmur, best audible at the third or fourth left intercostal space, is the auscultatory hallmark (Fig. 4-6). This murmur is more easily audible with the patient sitting and leaning forward. The longer the murmur, the more severe the regurgitation. A middiastolic mitral rumble (Austin Flint murmur) may be present at the apex when the AR is severe.

3. The ECG is normal in mild cases. In severe cases, LVH usually is present with or without LAH.

4. CXR films show cardiomegaly of varying degrees involving the LV.

5. Echo studies demonstrate an increased LV dimension. The LV diastolic dimension is proportional to the severity of AR. Color flow and Doppler examination can estimate the severity of AR. LV systolic dysfunction develops at a later stage in severe AR.

6. Patients with mild to moderate AR remain asymptomatic for a long time, but once symptoms begin to develop, many patients deteriorate

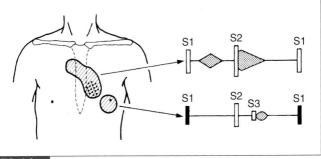

FIG. 4-6

Cardiac findings of AR. The S1 is abnormally soft *(black bar)*. The predominant murmur is a high-pitched, diastolic decrescendo murmur at the third left intercostal space.

rapidly. Anginal pain, CHF, and multiple PVCs are unfavorable signs occurring with severe AR.

MANAGEMENT

MEDICAL

1. Antibiotic prophylaxis (with penicillin or sulfonamide) to prevent the recurrence of rheumatic fever is indicated.
2. Varying degrees of activity restriction may be indicated. Aerobic exercise is a better form of exercise (weight-lifting exercise is discouraged).
3. ACE inhibitors have been shown to reduce the dilation and hypertrophy of the LV in children with AR.
4. If CHF develops, digoxin, diuretics, and ACE inhibitors may be temporarily beneficial.

SURGICAL

1. Indications. According to ACC/AHA 2006 guidelines, the following are surgical indications in adolescent and adult patients with chronic severe AR.
a. Symptomatic patients (with angina, syncope, or dyspnea on exertion)
b. Asymptomatic patients with LV systolic dysfunction (EF <0.5) on serial studies 1 to 3 months apart
c. Asymptomatic patients with progressive LV enlargement (end-diastolic dimension > mean + 4SD)
2. Procedure and mortality. Aortic valve repair is favored over valve replacement whenever possible. The mortality rate for valve repair is near zero and that for valve replacement is about 2% to 5%.
a. Valve repair may include repair of simple tears or valvuloplasty for prolapsed cusps.
b. Valve replacement surgery: The antibiotic-sterilized aortic homograft appears to be the device of choice. The porcine heterograft has the risk of accelerated degeneration. The Bjork-Shiley and St. Jude prostheses require anticoagulation therapy and are less suitable for young patients.

c. A pulmonary root autograft (Ross procedure) may be an attractive alternative to the conventional valve replacement surgery (see Fig. 3-14). The surgical mortality rate is near zero. This procedure does not require anticoagulant therapy, the autograft may last longer than a porcine bioprosthesis, and there is a growth potential for the autograft pulmonary valve.

3. Postoperative follow-up

a. Perform regular follow-up every 6 to 12 months with echo and Doppler studies.

b. Anticoagulation is needed after a prosthetic mechanical valve replacement. INR should be maintained between 2.5 and 3.5 for the first 3 months and 2.0 to 3.0 beyond that time. Low-dose aspirin (81 mg per day for adolescents) is also indicated in addition to warfarin.

c. After aortic valve replacement with bioprosthesis, low-dose aspirin (81 mg) is indicated if there are no risk factors, but warfarin is not indicated. When there are risk factors (which include atrial fibrillation, previous thromboembolism, LV dysfunction, and hypercoagulable state), warfarin is indicated to achieve an INR of 2.0 to 3.0.

d. Following Ross procedure, anticoagulation is not indicated.

D. MITRAL VALVE PROLAPSE

PREVALENCE. The reported incidence of mitral valve prolapse (MVP) of 2% to 5% in the pediatric population probably is an overestimate. The prevalence of MVP increases with age. This condition is more common in adults than in children and in females than in males.

PATHOLOGY

1. MVP is primary in most cases and is due to an inherited (autosomal dominant) abnormality of the mitral valve leaflets and their supporting chordae tendineae.

2. Thick and redundant mitral valve leaflets bulge into the mitral annulus (caused by myxomatous degeneration of the valve leaflets and/or the chordae). The posterior leaflet is more commonly and more severely affected than the anterior leaflet.

3. MVP is often associated with heritable disorders of connective tissue disease, such as Marfan syndrome, Ehlers-Danlos syndrome, and Stickler syndrome. Nearly all patients with Marfan syndrome have MVP, progressive with advancing age.

4. MVP is sometimes seen in patients with secundum atrial septal defect (ASD).

CLINICAL MANIFESTATIONS

1. MVP usually is asymptomatic, but a history of nonexertional chest pain, palpitation, and, rarely, syncope may be elicited. There may be a family history of MVP.

2. An asthenic build with a high incidence of thoracic skeletal anomalies (80%), including pectus excavatum (50%), straight back (20%), and scoliosis (10%), is common.

3. The midsystolic click with or without a late systolic murmur audible at the apex is the hallmark of the condition (Fig. 4-7). The presence or absence of the click and murmur, as well as their timing, varies from one examination to the next.

a. The click and murmur may be brought out by held expiration, left decubitus position, sitting, standing, or leaning forward.

b. Various maneuvers can alter the timing of the click and the murmur.

   (1) The click moves toward the S1 and the murmur lengthens with maneuvers that decrease the LV volume, such as standing, sitting, Valsalva's strain phase, tachycardia, and the administration of amyl nitrite.

   (2) The click moves toward the S2 and the murmur shortens with maneuvers that increase the LV volume, such as squatting, hand grip exercise, Valsalva's release phase, bradycardia, and the administration of pressor agents or propranolol.

4. The ECG is usually normal but may show flat or inverted T waves in II, III, and aVF (in 20% to 60%) and, rarely, SVT, premature atrial contractions (PACs), PVCs, first-degree AV block, or RBBB.

5. CXR films are unremarkable except for LA enlargement seen in patients with severe MR. Thoracoskeletal abnormalities (e.g., straight back, pectus excavatum, and scoliosis) may be present.

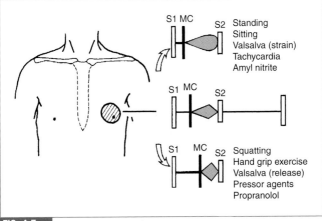

FIG. 4-7

Diagram of auscultatory findings in MVP and the effect of various maneuvers on the timing of the midsystolic click (MC) and the murmur. The maneuvers that reduce ventricular volume enhance leaflet redundancy and move the click and murmur earlier in systole. An increase in LV dimension has the opposite effect.

6. Two-dimensional echo shows the following:

a. In adult patients, prolapse of the mitral valve leaflet(s) superior to the plane of the mitral valve seen in the parasternal long-axis view is diagnostic. The superior displacement seen only on the apical four-chamber view is not diagnostic because it occurs in more than 30% of normal individuals due to the "saddle-shaped" mitral valve ring.

b. Some pediatric patients with characteristic body build and auscultatory findings of the condition do not show the adult echo criterion of MVP because MVP is a progressive disease with the full manifestations occurring in the adult life.

NATURAL HISTORY

1. The majority of patients are asymptomatic, particularly during childhood.

2. Rare complications reported in adult patients, although rare in childhood, include infective endocarditis, spontaneous rupture of chordae tendineae, progressive MR, CHF, arrhythmias, conduction disturbances, and sudden death (probably from ventricular arrhythmias).

MANAGEMENT

1. Asymptomatic patients require no treatment or restriction of activity.

2. β-Adrenergic blockers (propranolol or atenolol) are often used in the following situations.

a. Patients who are symptomatic (with palpitation, light-headedness, dizziness, or syncope) secondary to ventricular arrhythmias; symptomatic patients suspected to have arrhythmias should undergo ambulatory ECG monitoring and/or treadmill exercise testing

b. Patients with self-terminating episodes of SVT

c. Patients with chest discomfort

3. Reconstructive surgery or mitral valve replacement rarely may be indicated in patients with severe MR.

VI. CARDIAC TUMORS

PREVALENCE. Cardiac tumors are extremely rare among children.

PATHOLOGY

The most common cardiac tumor among children is rhabdomyoma. In infants younger than 1 year old, more than 75% of tumors are rhabdomyomas and teratomas, and in children ages 1 to 15 years, 80% of cardiac tumors are rhabdomyomas, fibromas, and myxomas. More than 90% of primary tumors are benign. Myxomas are extremely rare in children, although the LA myxoma is the most common type of cardiac tumor in adults. Myxomas can produce hemodynamic disturbances by interfering with mitral valve function or cause thromboembolic phenomena in the systemic circulation.

CLINICAL MANIFESTATIONS

1. Clinical manifestations of cardiac tumors are nonspecific, and they vary primarily with the location of the tumor. Tumors near cardiac valves may produce heart murmurs of stenosis or regurgitation of the valves. Tumors involving the conduction tissue may manifest with arrhythmias or conduction disturbances. Intracavitary tumors may produce inflow or outflow obstruction or thromboembolic phenomena. Invasion of the myocardium by the tumor (mural tumors) may result in heart failure or cardiac arrhythmias. Pericardial tumors, which may signal malignancy, may produce pericardial effusion and cardiac tamponade or features simulating infective pericarditis. Occasionally, for unknown reasons, fever and general malaise may manifest, especially with myxomas.
2. The ECG may show nonspecific ST-T changes, an infarctlike pattern, low-voltage QRS complexes, Wolff-Parkinson-White (WPW) preexcitation, arrhythmias, or conduction disturbances.
3. CXR film may occasionally reveal altered contour of the heart with or without changes in pulmonary vascular markings.
4. Echo and Doppler studies are diagnostic and can determine the hemodynamic significance of the tumor. Cardiac tumors are often found on a routine echo study without suspicion of the diagnosis, especially in neonates and small infants.
   a. Multiple intraventricular tumors are most likely rhabdomyomas in infants and children.
   b. A solitary tumor of varying size arising from the ventricular septum or the ventricular wall is likely to be fibroma.
   c. Left atrial tumors, especially when pedunculated, are usually myxomas.
   d. An intrapericardial tumor arising near the great arteries is most likely a teratoma.
   e. Pericardial effusion suggests a possibility of a secondary malignant tumor.

TREATMENT

Surgery is indicated for inlet or outlet obstruction and for symptoms of cardiac failure or ventricular arrhythmias refractory to medical treatment.
1. A successful complete resection of a fibroma is possible.
2. In asymptomatic patients with multiple rhabdomyomas, surgery should be delayed because of the possibility of spontaneous regression of the tumor.
3. Surgical removal of myxomas has a favorable outcome.
4. If there is an extensive myocardial involvement, surgical treatment is not possible. Cardiac transplantation may be an option in such cases.

Arrhythmias and Atrioventricular Conduction Disturbances

5

Normal heart rate varies with age: the younger the child, the faster the heart rate. Therefore, the definitions used for adults of bradycardia (fewer than 60 beats/min) and tachycardia (more than 100 beats/min) have little significance for children. A child has tachycardia when the heart rate is beyond the upper limit of normal for age, and bradycardia when the heart rate is slower than the lower limit of normal (see Table 1-9).

I. BASIC ARRHYTHMIAS

A. RHYTHMS ORIGINATING IN THE SINUS NODE

All rhythms that originate in the sinoatrial (SA) node (sinus rhythm) have two important characteristics (Fig. 5-1).

1. A P wave is present in front of each QRS complex with a regular PR interval. (The PR interval may be prolonged, as in first-degree atrioventricular [AV] block.)

2. The P axis is between 0 and +90 degrees, often a neglected criterion. This produces upright P waves in lead II and inverted P waves in aVR (see Figs. 1-14 and 1-15).

REGULAR SINUS RHYTHM

1. **Description:** The rhythm is regular and the rate is normal for age. Two characteristics of sinus rhythm described previously are present (Fig. 5-1).

2. **Significance:** This rhythm is normal at any age.

3. **Treatment:** No treatment is required.

SINUS TACHYCARDIA

1. **Description:** The characteristics of sinus rhythm are present. A rate above 140 beats/min in children and above 170 beats/min in infants may be significant. In sinus tachycardia the heart rate is usually lower than 200 beats/min (Fig. 5-1).

2. **Causes:** Anxiety, fever, hypovolemia, circulatory shock, anemia, congestive heart failure (CHF), catecholamines, thyrotoxicosis, and myocardial disease are possible causes.

3. **Significance:** Increased cardiac work is well tolerated by the healthy myocardium.

4. **Treatment:** The underlying cause is treated.

227

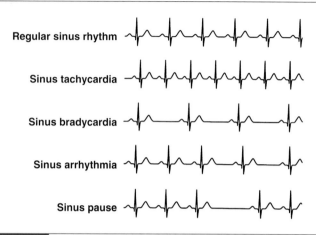

FIG. 5-1

Normal and abnormal rhythms originating in the sinoatrial node. *(From Park MK, Guntheroth WG:* How to read pediatric ECGs, *ed 4, Philadelphia, 2006, Mosby.)*

SINUS BRADYCARDIA

1. **Description:** The characteristics of sinus rhythm are present. A rate below 80 beats/min in newborn infants and below 60 beats/min in older children may be significant (Fig. 5-1).
2. **Causes:** Sinus bradycardia may occur in trained athletes. Vagal stimulation, increased intracranial pressure, hypothyroidism, hypothermia, hypoxia, and drugs such as digitalis and β-adrenergic blockers are possible causes.
3. **Significance:** Some patients with marked bradycardia do not maintain normal cardiac output.
4. **Treatment:** The underlying cause is treated.

SINUS ARRHYTHMIA

1. **Description:** There is a phasic variation in the heart rate, increasing during inspiration and decreasing during expiration, and the two characteristics of sinus rhythm are maintained (Fig. 5-1).
2. **Causes:** This normal phenomenon is due to a phasic variation in the firing rate of cardiac autonomic nerves with the phase of respiration.
3. **Significance:** There is no hemodynamic significance.
4. **Treatment:** No treatment is indicated.

SINUS PAUSE

1. **Description:** In *sinus pause,* there is a momentary cessation of sinus node pacemaker activity, resulting in the absence of P wave and QRS complex for a relatively short duration. *Sinus arrest* lasts longer and usually results in an escape beat (such as nodal escape).

2. **Causes:** Increased vagal tone, hypoxia, digitalis toxicity, and sick sinus syndrome (see next section).

3. **Significance:** No hemodynamic significance is present.

4. **Treatment:** Treatment is rarely indicated except in sick sinus syndrome and digitalis toxicity.

SINOATRIAL EXIT BLOCK

1. **Description:** A P wave is absent from the normally expected P wave, resulting in a long RR interval. The duration of the pause is a multiple of the basic PP interval. An impulse formed within the sinus node fails to depolarize the atria.

2. **Causes:** Excessive vagal stimulation; myocarditis or fibrosis involving the atrium; and drugs such as quinidine, procainamide, or digitalis.

3. **Significance:** It is usually transient and has no hemodynamic significance.

4. **Treatment:** The underlying cause is treated.

SINUS NODE DYSFUNCTION (SICK SINUS SYNDROME)

1. **Description:** The sinus node fails to function as the dominant pacemaker of the heart or performs abnormally slowly, producing a variety of arrhythmias. The arrhythmias may include profound sinus bradycardia, sinus arrest with junctional escape, and ectopic atrial or nodal rhythm. When these arrhythmias are accompanied by symptoms such as dizziness or syncope, sinus node dysfunction is referred to as sick sinus syndrome.

2. **Causes:** Extensive cardiac surgery involving the atria (e.g., the Fontan operation); arteritis; myocarditis; antiarrhythmic drugs; hypothyroidism; congenital heart disease (CHD), such as sinus venosus atrial septal defect (ASD) or Ebstein anomaly; and occasionally idiopathic occurring in an otherwise normal heart.

3. **Significance:** Bradytachyarrhythmia is the most worrisome rhythm. Profound bradycardia following a period of tachycardia (overdrive suppression) can cause syncope and even death.

4. **Treatment:** Severe bradycardia is treated with atropine (0.02 to 0.04 mg/kg, IV, every 2 to 4 hours) or isoproterenol (0.05 to 0.5 mcg/kg, IV) or both. Chronic medical treatment with various drugs has not been successful uniformly. Permanent pacemaker implantation is the treatment of choice in symptomatic patients. Either atrial demand, dual-chambered demand or triggered, or ventricular demand pacemakers may be used.

B.   RHYTHMS ORIGINATING IN THE ATRIUM

Atrial arrhythmias (Fig. 5-2) are characterized by the following:

1. P waves of unusual contour (abnormal P axis) and/or an abnormal number of P waves per QRS complex

2. QRS complexes of normal duration (but with occasional wide QRS duration caused by aberrancy)

PREMATURE ATRIAL CONTRACTION

1. **Description:** In premature atrial contraction (PAC) the QRS complex occurs prematurely with abnormal P wave morphology. There is an incomplete

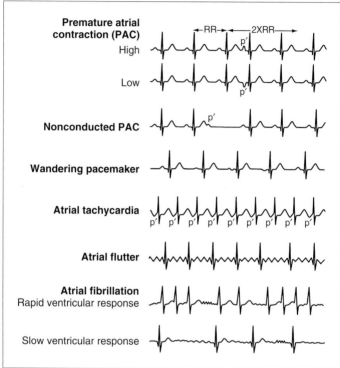

FIG. 5-2

Arrhythmias originating in the atrium. *(From Park MK, Guntheroth WG: How to read pediatric ECGs, ed 4, Philadelphia, 2006, Mosby.)*

compensatory pause; that is, the length of two cycles including one premature beat is less than the length of two normal cycles. An occasional PAC is not followed by a QRS complex (i.e., a nonconducted PAC) (Fig. 5-2). A nonconducted PAC is differentiated from a second-degree AV block by the prematurity of the nonconducted P wave (p´ in Fig. 5-2). The P´ wave occurs earlier than the anticipated normal P rate, and the resulting PP´ interval is shorter than the normal PP interval for that individual. In second-degree AV block the P wave that is not followed by the QRS complex occurs at the anticipated time, maintaining a regular PP interval.

2. **Causes:** Follows cardiac surgery and digitalis toxicity; also appears in healthy children, including newborn infants.

3. **Significance:** There is no hemodynamic significance.

4. **Treatment:** Usually no treatment is indicated except in cases of digitalis toxicity.

WANDERING ATRIAL PACEMAKER

1. **Description:** Gradual changes in the shape of P waves and PR intervals occur. The QRS complex is normal.
2. **Causes:** This is seen in otherwise healthy children. It is the result of a gradual shift of impulse formation in the atria through several cardiac cycles.
3. **Significance:** There is no clinical significance.
4. **Treatment:** No treatment is indicated.

ECTOPIC ATRIAL TACHYCARDIA

1. **Description:** There is a narrow QRS complex tachycardia (in the absence of aberrancy or preexisting bundle branch block) with visible P waves at an inappropriately rapid rate. The P axis is different from that of sinus rhythm. When the ectopic focus is near the sinus node, the P axis may be the same as in sinus rhythm. The usual heart rate in older children is between 110 and 160 beats/min, but the tachycardia rate varies substantially during the course of a day, reaching 300 beats/min with sympathetic stimuli. It represents about 20% of supraventricular tachycardia (SVT). This arrhythmia is sometimes difficult to distinguish from the reentrant AV tachycardia and thus it is included under "supraventricular tachycardia."
2. **Causes:** This arrhythmia is believed to be secondary to increased automaticity of nonsinus atrial focus or foci. Myocarditis, cardiomyopathies, atrial dilation, atrial tumors, and previous cardiac surgery involving atria (such as Fontan procedure) may be the cause. Most patients have a structurally normal heart (idiopathic).
3. **Significance:** CHF is common in chronic cases. There is a high association with tachycardia-induced cardiomyopathy.
4. **Treatment:** It is refractory to medical therapy and cardioversion. Drugs that are effective in reentrant atrial tachycardia (such as adenosine) do not terminate the tachycardia. Cardioversion is ineffective because the ectopic rhythm resumes immediately. The goal may be to slow the ventricular rate (using digoxin or β-blockers) rather than to try to convert the arrhythmia to sinus rhythm. Intravenous amiodarone may achieve rate control relatively quickly. Long-term oral antiarrhythmic drugs (such as flecainide or amiodarone) are the mainstay of therapy in patients not undergoing radiofrequency ablation. Radiofrequency ablation may prove to be effective in nearly 90% of cases.

MULTIFOCAL (OR CHAOTIC) ATRIAL TACHYCARDIA

1. **Description:** There are three or more distinct P wave morphologies. The PP and RR intervals are irregular with variable PR intervals. The arrhythmia resembles atrial fibrillation. Mechanism of this arrhythmia has been poorly defined. The onset of the arrhythmia may coincide with respiratory illness.

2. **Causes:** Young infants with (30% to 50%) or without various CHDs.

3. **Significance:** CHF may develop. Sudden death has been reported in up to 17% while on therapy. Long duration of the arrhythmia may cause left ventricle (LV) systolic dysfunction. Spontaneous resolution frequently occurs.

4. **Management:** Ineffectiveness of adenosine is a useful diagnostic sign of the condition. Drugs that slow AV conduction (propranolol or digoxin) and those that decrease automaticity (such as class IA or IC or class III) may be useful. Amiodarone (IV followed by PO) may be effective. This arrhythmia is refractory to cardiac pacing, cardioversion, and adenosine.

ATRIAL FLUTTER

1. **Description:** Atrial flutter is characterized by a fast atrial rate (F waves with saw-tooth configuration) of about 300 beats/min, the ventricle responding with varying degrees of block (e.g., 2:1, 3:1, 4:1), and normal QRS complexes (Fig. 5-2).

2. **Causes:** Structural heart disease with dilated atria, myocarditis, thyrotoxicosis, previous surgery involving atria, and digitalis toxicity are possible causes. However, most fetuses and neonates with atrial flutter have a normal heart.

3. **Significance:** The ventricular rate determines the eventual cardiac output; a too-rapid ventricular rate may decrease the cardiac output.

4. **Treatment:** In acute situations, synchronized cardioversion is the treatment of choice. Adenosine is not effective. It is important to rule out intracardiac thrombus by echo (preferably transesophageal echo) before cardioversion because it may lead to cerebral embolization. If a thrombus is found or suspected, anticoagulation with warfarin (with INR 2 to 3) is started and cardioversion delayed for 2 to 3 weeks. Warfarin is continued for an additional 3 to 4 weeks after conversion to sinus rhythm. To control the ventricular rate, calcium channel blockers, propranolol, or digoxin may be used. Amiodarone may be more effective than digoxin in treating atrial flutter. Quinidine may prevent the recurrences. For refractory cases, antitachycardia pacing or radiofrequency ablation may be indicated.

ATRIAL FIBRILLATION

1. **Description:** Atrial fibrillation is characterized by an extremely fast atrial rate (f wave at 350 to 600 beats/min) and an irregular ventricular response with normal QRS complexes (Fig. 5-2).

2. **Causes:** Same as those for atrial flutter.

3. **Significance:** Atrial fibrillation usually suggests a significant pathology. Rapid ventricular rate and the loss of coordinated contraction of the atria and ventricles decrease cardiac output. Atrial thrombus formation is quite common.

4. **Treatment:** Treatment of atrial fibrillation is similar to that described under atrial flutter. If atrial fibrillation has been present more than 48 hours, the patient should receive anticoagulation with warfarin for 3 to 4 weeks to prevent systemic embolization of atrial thrombus, if the conversion can be delayed. Anticoagulation is continued for 4 weeks after restoration of sinus

rhythm. If cardioversion cannot be delayed, heparin should be started with subsequent oral anticoagulation. Digoxin is given to slow the ventricular rate. Propranolol (1.0 to 4.0 mg/kg/day, orally in three or four doses) may be added. Class I antiarrhythmic agents (e.g., quinidine, procainamide, flecainide) and the class III agent amiodarone may be used. In patients with chronic atrial fibrillation, anticoagulation with warfarin should be considered to reduce the incidence of thromboembolism. Quinidine may prevent recurrence.

SUPRAVENTRICULAR TACHYCARDIA

1. **Description:** Three groups of tachycardia are included in SVT: atrial, nodal, and AV reentrant tachycardias. The great majority of SVTs are due to reentry AV tachycardia rather than to rapid firing of a single focus in the atria (atrial tachycardia) or in the AV node (nodal tachycardia). The heart rate is extremely rapid and regular (usually 240 ± 40 beats/min) (Fig. 5-3). The P wave is usually invisible, but when it is visible, it has an abnormal P axis and either precedes or follows the QRS complex. The QRS duration is usually normal, but occasionally aberrancy will prolong the QRS, making differentiation of this arrhythmia from ventricular tachycardia difficult.

a. *AV reentrant tachycardia* is the most common tachyarrhythmia seen among children. It used to be called paroxysmal atrial tachycardia because its onset and termination were characteristically abrupt. In SVT, due to reentry, two pathways are involved, at least one of which is the AV node and the other is an accessory pathway. The accessory pathway may be an anatomically separate bypass tract such as the bundle of Kent (which produces *accessory reciprocating AV tachycardia*) or only functionally separate, as in a dual AV node pathway (which produces *nodal reciprocating AV tachycardia*). Patients with the bundle of Kent frequently have Wolff-Parkinson-White (WPW) preexcitation.

b. *Ectopic*, or *nonreciprocating, atrial tachycardia* is a rare mechanism of SVT in which rapid firing of a single focus in the atrium is responsible for the tachycardia (see a previous section). In contrast to reciprocating atrial tachycardia, in ectopic atrial tachycardia the heart rate

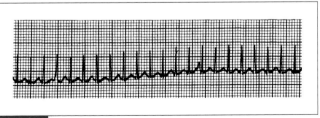

FIG. 5-3

Rhythm strip of SVT. The heart rate is 300 beats/min. *(From Park MK, Guntheroth WG: How to read pediatric ECGs, ed 4, Philadelphia, 2006, Mosby.)*

varies substantially during the course of a day, and second-degree AV block may develop. (The latter will terminate reentrant tachycardia.)

c. *Nodal tachycardia* may superficially resemble atrial tachycardia because the P wave is buried in the T waves of the preceding beat and becomes invisible in the latter, but the rate of nodal tachycardia is relatively slower (120 to 200 beats/min) than the rate of atrial or reentry tachycardia.

2. **Causes**

a. No heart disease is found in about half of patients. This idiopathic type of SVT occurs more commonly in young infants than in older children.

b. WPW preexcitation is present in 10% to 20% of cases and is evident only after conversion to sinus rhythm.

c. Some congenital heart defects (e.g., Ebstein anomaly, single ventricle, L-TGA) are more prone to this arrhythmia.

d. SVT may occur following cardiac surgeries.

3. **Significance:** It may decrease cardiac output and result in CHF in infants (with irritability, tachypnea, poor feeding, and pallor). When CHF develops, the infant's condition can deteriorate rapidly. Older children and adults may express a fairly unique complaint of "pounding sensation" in the neck, probably caused by cannon waves when the atrium contracts against a simultaneously contracting ventricle.

4. **Treatment**

a. Vagal stimulatory maneuvers (e.g., carotid sinus massage, gagging, and pressure on an eyeball) may be effective in older children, but they are rarely effective in infants. Placing an ice bag on the face (up to 10 seconds) is often successful in infants (by diving reflex). In children a headstand often successfully interrupts the SVT.

b. Adenosine is considered the drug of choice. It has negative chronotropic, dromotropic, and inotropic actions with a very short duration of action (half-life < 10 seconds) and minimal hemodynamic consequences. Adenosine is given by rapid intravenous bolus followed by a saline flush, starting at 50 mcg/kg, increasing in increments of 50 mcg/kg, every 1 to 2 minutes. The usual effective dose is 100 to 150 mcg/kg with maximum dose of 250 mcg/kg. Adenosine is effective for almost all reciprocating SVT (in which the AV node forms part of the reentry circuit) and for both narrow- and wide-complex *regular* tachycardia. It is not effective for irregular tachycardia. It is not effective for nonreciprocating atrial tachycardia, atrial flutter/fibrillation, and ventricular tachycardia.

c. If the infant is in severe CHF, an immediate cardioversion may be carried out. The initial dose of 0.5 joule/kg is increased in steps up to 2 joule/kg. Alternatively, in infants in CHF, one may start with digoxin (to treat CHF), but if WPW preexcitation is found, digoxin should be switched to propranolol when the infant's heart failure improves. Verapamil can also be used, but it should be used with caution in patients with poor LV function and in young infants.

d. Intravenous administration of propranolol is usually successful in treating SVT in the presence of WPW syndrome. Intravenous verapamil should be avoided in infants younger than 12 months of age because it may produce extreme bradycardia and hypotension.

e. For postoperative atrial tachycardia (which requires rapid conversion), intravenous amiodarone may provide excellent results.

f. Overdrive suppression (by transesophageal pacing or by atrial pacing) may be effective in children who have been digitalized.

5. Preventing recurrence of SVT

a. In infants without WPW preexcitation, oral propranolol for 12 months is effective. In children beyond infancy, verapamil can also be used. Digoxin, although still commonly used, is less effective.

b. In infants or children with WPW preexcitation on the ECG, propranolol or atenolol is used in long-term management. In the presence of WPW preexcitation, digoxin or verapamil may increase the rate of antegrade conduction of the impulse through the accessory pathway, and therefore should be avoided.

c. In adolescent patients, catheter ablation may be an effective alternative to long-term drug therapy.

C. RHYTHMS ORIGINATING IN THE AV NODE

Rhythms originating in the AV node (Fig. 5-4) are characterized by the following:

1. The P wave may be absent, or inverted P waves may follow the QRS complex.

2. The QRS complex is usually normal in duration and configuration.

NODAL PREMATURE BEATS

1. **Description:** A normal QRS complex occurs prematurely. P waves are usually absent, but inverted P waves may follow QRS complexes. The compensatory pause may be complete or incomplete (Fig. 5-4).

2. **Causes:** Usually idiopathic in an otherwise normal heart but may result from cardiac surgery or digitalis toxicity.

3. **Significance:** Usually no hemodynamic significance.

4. **Treatment:** Treatment is not indicated unless the cause is digitalis toxicity.

NODAL ESCAPE BEAT

1. **Description:** When the sinus node impulse fails to reach the AV node, the node-His (NH) region of the AV node will initiate an impulse (nodal or junctional escape beat). The QRS complex occurs later than the anticipated normal beat. The P wave may be absent, or an inverted P wave may follow the QRS complex (Fig. 5-4).

2. **Causes:** It may follow cardiac surgery involving the atria (e.g., Fontan operation) or may be seen in otherwise healthy children.

3. **Significance:** Little hemodynamic significance.

4. **Treatment:** Generally no specific treatment is required.

NODAL OR JUNCTIONAL RHYTHM

1. **Description:** If there is a persistent failure of the sinus node, the AV node may function as the main pacemaker of the heart with a relatively

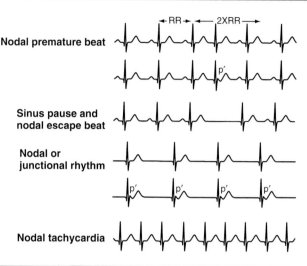

FIG. 5-4

Arrhythmias originating in the atrioventricular node. *(From Park MK:* Pediatric cardiology for practitioners, *ed 5, Philadelphia, 2008, Mosby.)*

slow rate (40 to 60 beats/min). Either P waves are absent or inverted P waves follow QRS complexes (Fig. 5-4).

2. **Causes:** It may be seen in an otherwise normal heart, after cardiac surgery, in conditions of an increased vagal tone (e.g., increased intracranial pressure, pharyngeal stimulation), and with digitalis toxicity. Rarely, it may be seen in children with polysplenia syndrome.

3. **Significance:** The slow heart rate may significantly decrease the cardiac output and produce symptoms.

4. **Treatment:** No treatment is indicated if the patient is asymptomatic. Atropine or electric pacing is indicated for symptoms. Treatment is directed to digitalis toxicity if caused by digitalis.

ACCELERATED NODAL RHYTHM

1. **Description:** In the presence of normal sinus rate and AV conduction, if the AV node (NH region) with enhanced automaticity captures the pacemaker function (60 to 120 beats/min), the rhythm is called accelerated nodal (or AV junctional) rhythm. Either P waves are absent or inverted P waves follow QRS complexes.

2. **Causes:** Idiopathic, digitalis toxicity, myocarditis, or previous cardiac surgery.

3. **Significance:** Little hemodynamic significance.

4. **Treatment:** No treatment is necessary unless the cause is digitalis toxicity.

NODAL TACHYCARDIA

1. **Description:** The ventricular rate varies from 120 to 200 beats/min. Either P waves are absent or inverted P waves follow QRS complexes. The QRS complex is usually normal, but aberration may occur. Nodal tachycardia is difficult to separate from atrial tachycardia. Therefore, both arrhythmias are grouped under SVT (Fig. 5-4).
2. **Causes:** Similar to those of atrial tachycardia.
3. **Significance:** Too fast a rate may decrease cardiac output.
4. **Treatment:** Treatment is not indicated if the rate is slower than 130 beats/min. Digoxin, β-blockers, and calcium channel blockers are generally ineffective. Amiodarone has been the most successful drug, especially in postoperative patients. Cooling (to 31° C to 34° C) has been shown to be effective in postoperative patients.

D. RHYTHMS ORIGINATING IN THE VENTRICLE

Ventricular arrhythmias (Fig. 5-5) are characterized by the following:
1. Bizarre and wide QRS complexes with T waves pointing in opposite directions
2. QRS complexes randomly related to P waves, if visible

PREMATURE VENTRICULAR CONTRACTION

1. **Description**
   a. A bizarre, wide QRS complex appears earlier than anticipated, and the T wave points in the opposite direction. A full compensatory pause usually appears; that is, the length of two cycles, including the premature beat, is the same as that of two normal cycles (Fig. 5-5).
   b. Premature ventricular contractions (PVCs) may be classified into several types, depending on their interrelationship, similarities, timing, and coupling intervals.

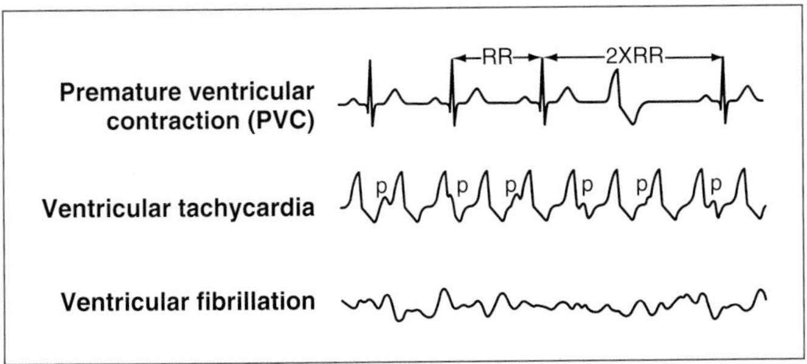

FIG. 5-5

Ventricular arrhythmias. *(From Park MK, Guntheroth WG:* How to read pediatric ECGs, *ed 4, Philadelphia, 2006, Mosby.)*

   (1) By interrelationship of PVCs

      (a) Ventricular *bigeminy* or *coupling*: Each abnormal QRS complex alternates with normal QRS complex regularly.

      (b) Ventricular *trigeminy:* Each abnormal QRS complex follows two normal QRS complexes regularly.

      (c) *Couplets:* Two abnormal QRS complexes come in sequence.

      (d) *Triplets:* Three abnormal QRS complexes come in sequence. Three or more successive PVCs arbitrarily are termed ventricular tachycardia.

   (2) By similarity among abnormal QRS complexes

      (a) Uniform (monomorphic or unifocal) PVCs: Abnormal QRS complexes have the same configuration in a single lead. It is assumed that they originate from a single focus.

      (b) Multiform (polymorphic or multifocal) PVCs: Abnormal QRS complexes have different configurations in a single lead. It is assumed that they originate from different foci.

   (3) Coupling interval

      (a) Fixed coupling. PVCs appear at a constant interval after the QRS complex of the previous cardiac cycle. This suggests ventricular reentry within the Purkinje system as the underlying mechanism. Most PVCs in children have a fixed coupling interval and a uniform left bundle branch block (LBBB) morphology.

      (b) Varying coupling. When coupling intervals vary by more than 80 ms, the PVCs may result from parasystole. If the intervals between ectopic beats can be factored so that each interval is a multiple of a single basic interval (within 0.08 seconds), ventricular parasystole is diagnosed. (Ventricular parasystole consists of an impulse-forming focus in the ventricle that is independent of the sinus node–generated impulse and is protected from depolarization [entrance block] by sinus impulses.)

2. **Causes:** PVCs may be seen in otherwise healthy children. Left ventricular false tendon, myocarditis, myocardial injury or infarction, cardiomyopathy (dilated or hypertrophic), cardiac tumors, right ventricular dysplasia (right ventricle [RV] cardiomyopathy), long QT syndrome, preoperative or postoperative congenital or acquired heart disease, digitalis toxicity, certain drugs (such as catecholamines, theophylline, caffeine, amphetamines, and some anesthetic agents), and mitral valve prolapse (MVP) are also possible causes.

3. **Significance**

a. Occasional PVCs are benign in children, particularly if they are uniform and disappear or decrease in frequency with exercise.

b. PVCs are more likely to be significant if (1) they are associated with underlying heart disease (e.g., preoperative or postoperative status, MVP, cardiomyopathy), (2) there is a history of syncope or a family history of sudden death, (3) they are precipitated by or increase in frequency with activity, (4) they are multiform, particularly couplets,

(5) there are runs of PVC with symptoms, or (6) there are incessant or frequent episodes of paroxysmal ventricular tachycardia.

4. **Management**
a. Some or all of the following tools are used in the investigation of PVCs and other ventricular arrhythmias.
   (1) ECGs are used to detect QTc prolongation or ST-T changes.
   (2) Echo studies detect structural heart disease or functional abnormalities.
   (3) Twenty-four-hour Holter monitoring or event recorder detects the frequency and severity of the arrhythmia.
   (4) Exercise stress testing: Arrhythmias that are potentially related to exercise are significant and require documentation of the relationship. The induction or exacerbation of arrhythmia with exercise may be an indication of underlying heart disease. In children, PVCs characteristically are reduced or eliminated by exercise.
   (5) Cardiac catheterization if arrhythmogenic RV dysplasia is suspected.
   (6) Electrophysiologic studies and endomyocardial biopsy.
b. In children with otherwise normal hearts, occasional isolated uniform PVCs that are suppressed by exercise do not require extensive investigation or treatment. ECG, echo studies, and 24-hour Holter monitoring suffice.
c. Children with uniform PVCs, including ventricular bigeminy and trigeminy, do not need to be treated if the echo and exercise stress tests are normal.
d. Asymptomatic children with multiform PVCs and ventricular couplets should have 24-hour Holter monitoring, even if they have structurally normal hearts, to detect the severity and extent of ventricular arrhythmias.
e. All children with symptomatic ventricular arrhythmias and those with complex PVCs (multiform PVCs, ventricular couplets, unsustained ventricular tachycardia) should be treated.
   (1) β-blockers (such as atenolol, 1 to 2 mg/kg orally in a single daily dose) are effective for cardiomyopathy and occasionally for RV dysplasia.
   (2) Other antiarrhythmic drugs, such as phenytoin sodium (Dilantin) and mexiletine, may be effective. Antiarrhythmic agents that prolong the QT interval, such as those of class IA (quinidine, procainamide), class IC (encainide, flecainide), and class III (amiodarone, bretylium), should be avoided.
f. For patients with symptomatic ventricular arrhythmias or sustained ventricular tachycardia and seemingly normal hearts, cardiac catheterization may be indicated to investigate for RV dysplasia. Occasionally, invasive electrophysiologic studies and RV endomyocardial biopsy may be indicated.
g. Children with multiform PVCs and runs of PVCs (ventricular tachycardia) with or without symptoms need to be evaluated by an electrophysiologist.

ACCELERATED VENTRICULAR RHYTHM

1. **Description:** There is a wide QRS complex rhythm of short duration (usually several beats but can be longer than 100 beats). The QRS morphology is LBBB pattern in the great majority. The ventricular rate approximates the patient's sinus rate, within ±10% to 15% of the sinus rate *(isochronicity)*. The isochronicity with sinus rhythm is more important than the rate per minute. The ventricular rate is usually ≤120 beats/min in children and 140 to 180 beats/min in newborns.

2. **Causes:** Accelerated ventricular rhythm (AVR) is usually an isolated finding. Rarely, it may be associated with underlying heart disease, such as CHD, myocarditis, digitalis toxicity, hypertension, cardiomyopathy, metabolic abnormalities, postoperative state, or myocardial infarction (MI) (in adults). The mechanism of AVR is unknown: ectopic ventricular focus may accelerate its rate enough to overcome sinus rate.

3. **Significance:** Usually asymptomatic and hemodynamically insignificant. Exertional sinus tachycardia usually converts it to sinus rhythm. Rarely seen in patients with syncope, presyncope, or palpitation or found in routine ECG or Holter monitoring.

4. **Treatment:** In children, AVR is generally considered benign. AVR is notably resistant to antiarrhythmic agents (no treatment is required).

VENTRICULAR TACHYCARDIA

1. **Description:** Ventricular tachycardia (VT) is a series of three or more PVCs with a heart rate of 120 to 200 beats/min. QRS complexes are wide and bizarre, with T waves pointing in opposite directions. QRS contours during the VT may be unchanging (uniform, monomorphic) or may vary randomly (multiform, polymorphous, or pleomorphic). Torsades de pointes (meaning "twisting of the points") is a distinct form of polymorphic VT characterized by a paroxysm of VT during which there are progressive changes in the amplitude and polarity of QRS complexes separated by a narrow transition QRS complex. Torsades de pointes occurs in patients with marked QT prolongation. VT is sometimes difficult to differentiate from SVT with aberrant conduction. However, wide QRS tachycardia in an infant or child must be considered VT until proved otherwise.

2. **Causes**

a. Structural heart diseases (such as tetralogy of Fallot [TOF], aortic stenosis [AS], cardiomyopathies, or MVP).

b. Postoperative CHDs (such as TOF, D-TGA, or double-outlet right ventricle [DORV]).

c. Myocarditis, pulmonary hypertension, arrhythmogenic RV dysplasia, Brugada syndrome (young men from Southeast Asia), Chagas disease (trypanosomiasis, in South America), myocardial tumors, myocardial ischemia, and MI.

d. Metabolic causes (hypoxia, acidosis, hyperkalemia, hypokalemia, and hypomagnesemia).

e. Mechanical irritation—intraventricular catheter

f. Pharmacologic or chemical causes (catecholamine infusion, digitalis toxicity, cocaine, and organophosphate insecticides). Most antiarrhythmic drugs (especially classes IA, IC, and III) are also proarrhythmic.

g. Torsades de pointes may be seen in patients with long QT syndrome. A partial list of drugs that may prolong the QT interval is shown in Box 5-1. Classes IA, IC, and III antiarrhythmic drugs prolong the QTc interval, but classes II and IV agents do not.

h. Benign VT may occur in healthy children who have a structurally and functionally normal heart. This group is discussed under a separate heading (see following).

3. **Significance**

a. VT usually signifies a serious myocardial pathology or dysfunction and can cause sudden death. Cardiac output may decrease notably and may deteriorate to ventricular fibrillation.

b. Patients may present with dizziness, syncope, palpitation, or chest pain.

c. Most patients with arrhythmogenic RV dysplasia present with LBBB QRS pattern (because the tachycardia arises in the RV). Patients with Brugada syndrome present with right bundle branch block (RBBB) and striking ST segment elevation in V1 and V2.

4. **Treatment**

a. Prompt synchronized cardioversion (0.5 to 1.0 joules/kg) if the patient is unconscious or if there is evidence of low cardiac output.

b. If the patient is conscious, an IV bolus of lidocaine, 1 mg/kg over 1 to 2 minutes, followed by an IV drip of lidocaine, 20 to 50 μg/kg/min, may be effective.

c. One should search for and correct reversible conditions (such as hypokalemia and hypoxemia) that could contribute to the initiation and maintenance of VT.

d. An IV bolus injection of magnesium sulfate, 2 g, has recently been reported to be very effective and safe for torsades de pointes in adult patients.

e. Intravenous amiodarone is used in patients with drug-refractory ventricular tachycardia, particularly that seen in postoperative patients.

f. Patients with long QT syndrome are treated with β-blockers, which alleviate symptoms in 75% to 80%. Implantable cardioverter-defibrillator (ICD) is sometimes recommended as initial therapy.

g. Some incessant ventricular tachycardias are amenable to surgical or radiofrequency ablation.

h. ICD has become the established standard for treating many, if not most, forms of ventricular tachycardia, which are potentially lethal.

i. Recurrence may be prevented with administration of propranolol, atenolol, diphenylhydantoin, or quinidine. A combination of 24-hour Holter monitoring and treadmill exercise testing is the best noninvasive means of evaluating drug effectiveness.

BOX 5-1

ACQUIRED CAUSES OF QT PROLONGATION

DRUGS

Antibiotics: erythromycin, clarithromycin, telithromycin, azithromycin, trimethoprim-sulfamethoxazole

Antifungal agents: fluconazole, itraconazole, ketoconazole

Antiprotozoal agents: pentamidine isethionate

Antihistamines: astemizole, terfenadine (Seldane) (Seldane has been removed from the market for this reason)

Antidepressants: tricyclics such as imipramine (Tofranil), amitriptyline (Elavil), desipramine (Norpamin), and doxepin (Sinequan)

Antipsychotics: haloperidol, risperidone, phenothiazines such as thioridazine (Mellaril) and chlorpromazine (Thorazine)

Antiarrhythmic agents

    Class 1A (sodium channel blockers): quinidine, procainamide, disopyramide

    Class III (prolong depolarization): amiodarone (rare), bretylium, dofetilide, N-acetyl-procainamide, sotalol

Lipid-lowering agents: probucol

Antianginals: befpridil

Diuretics (through K loss): furosemide (Lasix), ethacrynic acid (Edecrine)

Oral hypoglycemic agents: glibenclamide, glyburide

Organophosphate insecticides

Promotility agents: cisapride

Vasodilators: prenylamine

ELECTROLYTE DISTURBANCES

Hypokalemia: diuretics, hyperventilation

Hypocalcemia

Hypomagnesemia

UNDERLYING MEDICAL CONDITIONS

Bradycardia: complete atrioventricular block, severe bradycardia, sick sinus syndrome

Myocardial dysfunction: anthracycline cardiotoxicity, congestive heart failure, myocarditis, cardiac tumors

Endocrinopathy: hyperparathyroidism, hypothyroidism, pheochromocytoma

Neurologic: encephalitis, head trauma, stroke, subarachnoid hemorrhage

Nutritional: alcoholism, anorexia nervosa, starvation

A more exhaustive updated list of medications that can prolong QTc interval is available at the University of Arizona Center for Education and Research on Therapeutics website (www.torsades.org or www.qtdrugs.org).

VENTRICULAR ARRHYTHMIAS IN CHILDREN WITH NORMAL HEARTS

Although recurrent sustained VT usually signals an organic cause of the arrhythmia, some VTs are seen in healthy adolescents and young adults with structurally and functionally normal hearts. The prognosis is good.

1. **Right ventricular outflow tract (RVOT) ventricular tachycardia.** This special form of VT originates from the RV conal septum and thus has inferior QRS axis and LBBB morphology (Fig. 5-6). This is usually benign tachycardia. It may manifest as frequent PVCs or short runs or salvos of VT, but many children are asymptomatic or minimally symptomatic. Exercise stress may not completely abolish the tachycardia. β-blockers are sufficient for treatment. Verapamil and other agents may also prove to be effective. Radiofrequency ablation can be curative.

2. **RBBB ventricular tachycardia (Belhassen's tachycardia).** It appears to arise from the septal surface of the LV and is less common than RVOT VT. It is characterized by RBBB morphology and superior QRS axis. It is sensitive to verapamil or adenosine. When refractory to medical therapy, radiofrequency ablation or surgery is effective. The long-term outcome is excellent.

Aberration. When a supraventricular impulse prematurely reaches the AV node or bundle of His, it may find one bundle branch excitable and the other still refractory. Therefore, the resulting QRS complex resembles a bundle branch block pattern. The right bundle branch usually has a longer refractory period than the left, producing QRS complexes similar to those

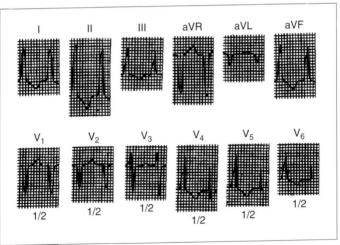

FIG. 5-6

Tracing from a 4-year-old girl who is asymptomatic even while having the ventricular tachycardia. The child was on atenolol. In this child the ventricular tachycardia rate was 160 beats/min. The QRS complexes have LBBB morphology indicating the RV as the ectopic focus and the axis of VT is directed inferiorly. Spontaneous temporary interruption of VT occurred while recording V4, V5, and V6 leads. (*From Park MK: Pediatric cardiology for practitioners, ed 5, Philadelphia, 2008, Mosby.*)

of RBBB. The following features are helpful in differentiating aberrant ventricular conduction from ectopic ventricular impulses.

a. An rsR′ pattern in V1, resembling QRS complexes of RBBB, suggests aberration. In a ventricular ectopic beat, the QRS morphology is bizarre and does not resemble the classic form of RBBB or LBBB.

b. Occasional wide QRS complexes following P waves with regular PR intervals suggest an aberration.

c. The presence of a ventricular fusion complex is a reliable sign of ventricular ectopic rhythm.

VENTRICULAR FIBRILLATION

1. **Description:** Ventricular fibrillation is characterized by bizarre QRS complexes of varying sizes and configurations. The rate is rapid and irregular (Fig. 5-5).

2. **Causes:** Postoperative state, severe hypoxia, hyperkalemia, digitalis or quinidine toxicity, myocarditis, myocardial infarction, and drugs (catecholamines, anesthetics, etc.) are possible causes.

3. **Significance:** It is usually fatal because it results in ineffective circulation.

4. **Treatment:** Immediate cardiopulmonary resuscitation, including electric defibrillation at 2 joules/kg, is required. ICDs are often indicated in patients who survived ventricular fibrillation.

E. LONG QT SYNDROME

Long QT syndrome (LQTS) is a disorder of ventricular repolarization characterized by a prolonged QT interval on the ECG and ventricular arrhythmias, usually torsades de pointes, that may result in sudden death.

The QT prolongation may be congenital or acquired.

1. Congenital long QT syndrome is caused by mutations of cardiac ion channel genes. The following subgroups are known.

a. Jervell and Lange-Nielsen syndrome (autosomal recessive mode) consists of a prolonged QTc interval, congenital deafness, syncopal spells, and a family history of sudden death.

b. Romano-Ward syndrome (autosomal dominant mode) has all the features of Jervell and Lange-Nielsen syndrome but without deafness.

c. Sporadic form of Romano-Ward syndrome (with normal hearing) with a negative family history of the syndrome.

d. In Anderson-Tawil syndrome, the QU interval (rather than QT interval) is prolonged; also characteristic of this syndrome are muscle weakness (periodic paralysis), ventricular arrhythmias, and developmental abnormalities.

e. Timothy syndrome is associated with webbed fingers and toes and a prolonged QTc interval.

2. Acquired prolongation of the QT interval can be caused by a number of drugs, electrolyte disturbances, and other underlying medical conditions (Box 5-1). In the acquired type of long QT syndrome, a similar ionic mechanism may be involved as is observed in congenital LQTS. This discussion will focus on congenital LQTS.

CLINICAL MANIFESTATIONS

1. Positive family history is present in about 60% and deafness in 5% of patients.
2. Presenting symptoms may be syncope (26%), seizure (10%), cardiac arrest (9%), presyncope, or palpitation (6%). The majority of these symptoms occur during exercise or with emotion.
3. Syncope occurs in the setting of intense adrenergic arousal, intense emotion, and during or following rigorous exercise. Swimming appears to be a particular trigger. A loud doorbell, alarm clock, telephone, or security alarm can trigger symptoms.
4. The ECG shows the following:
a. A prolonged QTc interval usually >0.46 seconds. The upper limit of normal QTc is 0.44 seconds.
b. Abnormal T wave morphology (bifid, diphasic, or notched) is frequent.
c. Bradycardia (20%), second-degree AV block, multiform PVCs, and monomorphic or polymorphic VT may be present.
5. Echo studies usually show a structurally and functionally normal heart.
6. A treadmill exercise test results in a highly significant prolongation of the QTc interval, with the maximal prolongation present after 1 to 2 minutes of recovery. Ventricular arrhythmias may develop during the test in up to 30% of patients.
7. Holter monitoring reveals prolongation of the QTc interval, major changes in the T wave configuration (T wave alternation), and ventricular arrhythmias. The QTc interval on Holter monitor may be longer than that recorded on a standard ECG (see a later section).

DIAGNOSIS

A correct diagnosis and proper treatment can save lives, but the diagnosis of this disease should not be made lightly because it implies a high-risk disease with a lifelong commitment to treatment.

1. Accurate measurement of the QTc interval is essential in the diagnosis of long QT syndrome.
a. Lead II (with q waves) and precordial leads (V1, V3, or V5, with well-defined T waves) are good leads in measuring the QT interval.
b. In patients with sinus arrhythmia the QT interval immediately following the shortest RR interval has been recommended for use in calculating the QTc interval. However, the QTc measurement during sinus arrhythmia may not be reliable because Bazett's formula is reliable only for the steady state but sinus arrhythmia is not a steady state.
c. The QTc interval is longer during sleep; therefore, Holter monitoring may show the QTc interval to be 0.05 seconds longer than the interval on a standard ECG.
d. In patients with wide QRS complexes (such as BBB) the JTc interval may be a more sensitive predictor of repolarization abnormalities than the QTc. Rate correction is accomplished by the use of Bazett's formula. Normal JTc interval (mean ± SD) is 0.32 ± 0.02 seconds (with the upper limit of normal 0.34 seconds).

2. Schwartz diagnostic criteria. The diagnosis of long QT syndrome is clear-cut when there is a marked prolongation of the QTc interval with positive family history of the syndrome. However, many cases are borderline, making it difficult to make or reject the diagnosis. Schwartz et al. refined diagnostic criteria using a point system (Table 5-1) as follows:

a. ≤1 point ≡ low probability of LQTS

b. 2 to 3 points ≡ intermediate probability of LQTS

c. ≥4 points ≡ high probability of LQTS

3. Initially, five steps are considered in making the diagnosis of LQTS.

a. History of presyncope, syncope, seizure, or palpitation and family history are carefully examined.

b. Causes of acquired LQTS are excluded.

c. The ECG is examined for the QTc interval and morphology of the T waves. ECGs are also obtained from immediate family members.

d. The LQTS score is calculated (Table 5-1) and the diagnostic possibility is graded as described previously.

e. Patients with an LQTS score ≥4 or an abnormal exercise test are considered to have LQTS, while an LQTS score ≤1 is excluded from the diagnosis. Those patients with an LQTS score of 2 or 3 are followed up for possible LQTS.

4. For borderline cases, additional testing, such as Holter monitoring, exercise testing, pharmacologic test, or electrophysiology study, may be performed. However, their diagnostic utility remains unclear.

TABLE 5-1

SCHWARTZ DIAGNOSTIC CRITERIA FOR LONG QT SYNDROME

ECG Findings	
(in the absence of medications or disorders known to prolong the QTc interval)	
QTc	
>480 ms	3
460-470 ms	2
450 (male) ms	1
Torsades de pointes	2
T wave alterans	1
Notched T waves in three leads	1
Low heart rate for age (<2nd percentile)	0.5
Clinical History	
Syncope with stress	2
Syncope without stress	1
Congenital deafness	0.5
Family History	
Family member with definite LQTS	1
Unexplained sudden cardiac death <30 yr among immediate family members	0.5

Adapted from Schwartz PJ, Moss AJ, Vincent GM et al: Diagnostic criteria for the long QT syndrome: an update, *Circulation* 88:782-784, 1993.

MANAGEMENT

1. The following are known risk factors for sudden death, and they should be considered when making a treatment plan.
   a. Bradycardia for age (sinus bradycardia, junctional escape rhythm, or second-degree AV block)
   b. An extremely long QTc interval (>0.55 seconds)
   c. Symptoms at presentation (syncope, seizure, cardiac arrest)
   d. Young age at presentation (<1 month)
   e. Documented torsades de pointes or ventricular fibrillation
   f. T wave alternation (major changes in T wave morphology); this is a relative risk factor
2. General measures
   a. Physicians should avoid prescribing medications that prolong the QT interval (see Box 5-1 and updated Internet sources [www.torsades.org or www.qtdrugs.org]).
   b. No competitive sport is allowed. Swimming is not advised.
3. Treatment of congenital LQTS
   a. β-blockers. β-blockers are the current treatment of choice. They reduce both syncope and sudden cardiac death, but cardiac events continue to occur while on β-blocker therapy. There is a consensus that all symptomatic children with long QT syndrome should be treated with propranolol or other β-blockers (e.g., atenolol, metoprolol).
      (1) Whether to start asymptomatic children with QTc prolongation on beta blockers has been controversial. Any patients who score 4 or greater on the Schwartz diagnostic criteria should be treated regardless of symptoms. However, it may be prudent to follow those asymptomatic children whose QTc intervals are borderline (0.46 to 0.47 seconds). Symptoms are more likely to occur in patients with QTc intervals >0.48 seconds. In addition, treatment with beta blockers may be dangerous to some patients with the syndrome because treatment tends to produce bradycardia, a known risk factor for sudden death.
      (2) Schwartz (1997) has recommended definite treatment in the following circumstances: newborns and infants, patients with sensorineuronal hearing loss, affected siblings with LQTS and sudden cardiac death, extremely long QTc (>0.60 seconds) or T wave alternans, and to prevent family or patient anxiety.
   b. The ICD appears to be the most effective therapy for high-risk patients, defined as those with aborted cardiac arrests or recurrent cardiac events despite conventional therapy (with β-blockers), and those with extremely prolonged QTc intervals (e.g., >0.60 seconds). Patients with ICD should be kept on β-blockers.
   c. Left cardiac sympathetic denervation. Because of the availability of other options, such as pacing and ICD, this procedure is rarely performed.

d. Targeted pharmacologic therapy. Sodium channel blocker mexiletine was used in patients with mutation in the sodium channel gene *SCN5A (LQT3)* with significant shortening of the QTc.

4. Treatment of acquired long QT syndrome. The management of acquired LQTS involves acute treatment of arrhythmias (with intravenous magnesium), discontinuation of any precipitating drug (Table 5-1), and correction of any metabolic abnormalities (such as hypokalemia or hypomagnesemia).

PROGNOSIS. The prognosis is very poor in untreated patients, with annual mortality as high as 20% and 10-year mortality of 50%. β-blockers may reduce mortality to some extent, but they do not completely protect patients from sudden death. ICD appears promising in improving prognosis.

F. SHORT QT SYNDROME

Short QT syndrome is characterized by a very short QTc (≤300 ms), symptoms of palpitation, dizziness or syncope, and family history of sudden death. The cause of death is believed to be ventricular fibrillation. This syndrome is transmitted in an autosomal dominant manner. Treatment plans similar to those described for long QT syndrome should apply.

G. BRUGADA SYNDROME

This rare condition is more common among young men in Southeast Asia. Mutations in the sodium channel appear to be the cause of the condition. The patient may present with complaints of blackout or palpitations. Cardiac examination is usually normal. There is no demonstrable structural abnormality of the heart. The ECG typically shows RBBB with J point elevation and concave ST elevation best seen in V1. There may be a family history of sudden death. Diagnosis is suspected on the basis of the ECG appearance, which may not always be present, however. No antiarrhythmic drug, including β-blockers, appears to reduce the risk of death in these patients. The current standard practice, therefore, is to use an ICD to protect most patients.

II. ATRIOVENTRICULAR CONDUCTION DISTURBANCES

AV block is a disturbance in conduction between the normal sinus impulse and the eventual ventricular response. The block is assigned to one of three classes, according to the severity of the conduction disturbance. First-degree AV block is a simple prolongation of the PR interval, but all P waves are conducted to the ventricle. In second-degree AV block some atrial impulses are not conducted into the ventricle. In third-degree AV block (or complete heart block) none of the atrial impulses is conducted into the ventricle (Fig. 5-7).

A. FIRST-DEGREE AV BLOCK

1. **Description:** There is a prolongation of the PR interval beyond the upper limits of normal (see Table 1-11) due to an abnormal delay in conduction through the AV node (Fig. 5-7).

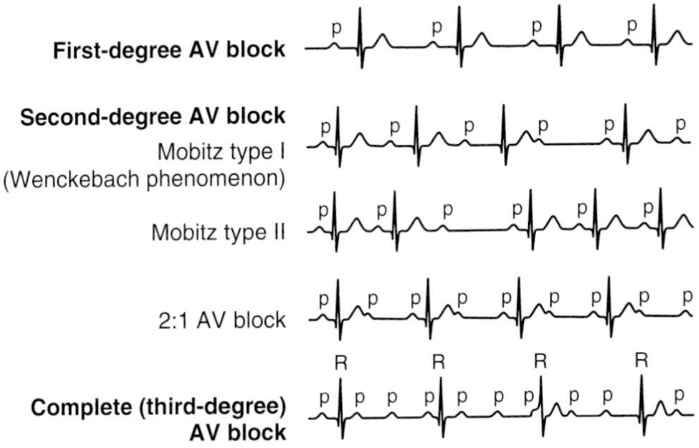

FIG. 5-7

AV block. *(From Park MK, Guntheroth WG:* How to read pediatric ECGs, *ed 4, Philadelphia, 2006, Mosby.)*

2. **Causes:** In otherwise healthy children and young adults, particularly athletes, infectious disease, inflammatory conditions (including acute rheumatic fever), cardiomyopathies, CHDs (e.g., ASD, Ebstein anomaly, endocardial cushion defect [ECD]), cardiac surgery, and certain drugs (digitalis toxicity, calcium channel blockers).

3. **Significance:** Usually no hemodynamic disturbance results. Sometimes it may progress to a more advanced AV block.

4. **Treatment:** No treatment is indicated except in digitalis toxicity.

B.   SECOND-DEGREE AV BLOCK

Some but not all P waves are followed by QRS complexes (dropped beats). There are several types.

MOBITZ TYPE I (WENCKEBACH PHENOMENON)

1. **Description:** The PR interval becomes progressively prolonged until one QRS complex is dropped completely (Fig. 5-7).

2. **Causes:** In otherwise healthy children, myocarditis, cardiomyopathy, myocardial infarction, CHD, cardiac surgery, and digitalis toxicity.

3. **Significance:** The block is at the level of the AV node. It usually does not progress to complete heart block. It occurs in individuals with vagal dominance.

4. **Treatment:** The underlying cause is treated.

MOBITZ TYPE II

1. **Description:** The AV conduction is "all or none." AV conduction is either normal or completely blocked (Fig. 5-7).

2. **Causes:** Same as for Mobitz type I.

3. **Significance:** The block is at the level of the bundle of His. It is more serious than type I block because it may progress to complete heart block, resulting in Stokes-Adams attacks.

4. **Treatment:** The underlying cause is treated. Prophylactic pacemaker therapy may be indicated.

TWO-TO-ONE (OR HIGHER) AV BLOCK

1. **Description:** A QRS complex follows every second (third or fourth) P wave, resulting in 2:1 (3:1 or 4:1, respectively) AV block (Fig. 5-7).

2. **Causes:** Similar to those of other second-degree AV blocks.

3. **Significance:** The block is usually at the bundle of His, alone or in combination with the AV nodal block. It may occasionally progress to complete heart block.

4. **Treatment:** The underlying cause is treated. Electrophysiologic studies may be necessary to determine the level of the block. Pacemaker therapy is occasionally necessary.

C. THIRD-DEGREE AV BLOCK (COMPLETE HEART BLOCK)

1. **Description:** In third-degree AV block, the atrial and ventricular activities are entirely independent of each other (Fig. 5-7). The P waves are regular (with regular PP interval) with a rate comparable with the heart rate of the patient's age. The QRS complexes are also quite regular (with regular RR interval), with a rate much slower than the P rate.

a. In *congenital* complete heart block the duration of the QRS complex is normal because the pacemaker for the QRS complex is at a level higher than the bifurcation of the bundle of His. The ventricular rate is faster (50 to 80 beats/min) than in the acquired type.

b. In surgically induced or *acquired* (from postmyocardial infarction) complete heart block the QRS duration is prolonged, and the ventricular rate is in the range of 40 to 50 beats/min (idioventricular rhythm). The pacemaker for the wide QRS complex is at a level below the bifurcation of the bundle of His.

2. **Causes**

a. The congenital type may be an isolated anomaly (without associated CHD). Maternal lupus erythematosus or mixed connective tissue disease or CHD such as L-TGA may be the cause of complete heart block.

b. The acquired type is usually a complication of cardiac surgery in children. Rarely, severe myocarditis, Lyme carditis, acute rheumatic fever, mumps, diphtheria, cardiomyopathies, tumors in the conduction system, or overdose of certain drugs causes it. It may also follow myocardial infarction. These causes produce either temporary or permanent heart block.

3. **Significance**

a. CHF may develop in infancy, particularly when there are associated CHDs.

b. Patients with isolated congenital heart block are usually asymptomatic during childhood and achieve normal growth and development.

c. Syncopal attacks (Stokes-Adams attack) or sudden death may occur
with the heart rate below 40 to 45 beats/min.

4. **Treatment**

a. Atropine or isoproterenol is indicated in symptomatic children and
adults until temporary ventricular pacing is secured.

b. No treatment is required for asymptomatic children with congenital
complete heart block with acceptable heart rate, narrow QRS complex, and normal ventricular function.

c. Pacemaker therapy is indicated in patients with congenital heart block
in the following cases.

   (1) The patient is symptomatic or develops CHF.

   (2) Dizziness or light-headedness may be an early warning sign of the
   need for a pacemaker.

   (3) An infant has a ventricular rate <50 to 55 beats/min or the infant
   has a CHD with a ventricular rate <70 beats/min.

   (4) The patient has a wide QRS escape rhythm, complex ventricular
   ectopy, or ventricular dysfunction.

d. A permanent artificial ventricular pacemaker is indicated in patients
with surgically induced heart block that is not expected to resolve or
persists at least 7 days after cardiac surgery.

III. PACEMAKERS AND IMPLANTABLE CARDIOVERTER-DEFIBRILLATORS IN CHILDREN

A. PACEMAKERS IN CHILDREN

A pacemaker is a device that delivers battery-supplied electrical stimuli over
leads to electrodes in contact with the heart. The electrical leads are inserted either directly over the epicardium or transvenously; the latter is the
method of choice. Electronic circuitry regulates the timing and characteristics of the stimuli. The power source usually is a lithium-iodine battery.
Battery life varies from 3 to 15 years depending on the type of the device,
which determines the amount of battery use. New pacemakers (physiologic
pacemakers) are capable of closely mimicking normal cardiac rhythm, and
most of them are small enough to be implanted in an infant.

Physicians encounter an increasing number of children with either temporary or permanent pacemakers. Basic knowledge about the pacemaker
and the pacemaker rhythm strip is essential in taking care of these children. This section presents examples of ECG rhythm strips from children
with various types of pacemakers and elementary information regarding
pacemaker and ICD therapy in children.

ECGS OF ARTIFICIAL CARDIAC PACEMAKERS

The need to recognize rhythm strips of artificial pacemakers has increased
in recent years, especially in intensive care and emergency department
settings. The position and number of the pacemaker spikes on the ECG
rhythm strip are used to recognize different types of pacemakers.

1. When the pacemaker stimulates the atrium, a P wave follows an
electronic spike. The resulting P wave demonstrates an abnormal P axis.

2. When the pacemaker stimulates the ventricle, a wide QRS complex appears after the electronic spike. The ventricle that is stimulated (or the ventricle on which the pacemaker electrode is placed) can be identified by the morphology of the QRS complexes. With the pacing electrode on the RV, the QRS complex resembles a LBBB pattern; with the pacemaker placed on the LV, a RBBB pattern results.

3. Three examples of pacemaker ECGs are shown in Figure 5-8.

a. Ventricular pacemaker (ventricular sensing and pacing). This mode of pacing is recognized by vertical pacemaker spikes that initiate ventricular depolarization with wide QRS complexes (Fig. 5-8, *A*). The electronic spike has no fixed relationship with atrial activity (P wave). The pacemaker rate may be fixed as in the figure, or it may be on a demand (or standby) mode in which the pacemaker fires only after a long pause between the patient's own ventricular beats.

b. Atrial pacemaker (atrial sensing and pacing). The atrial pacemaker is recognized by a pacemaker spike followed by an atrial complex. When AV conduction is normal, a QRS complex of normal duration follows (Fig. 5-8, *B*). This type of pacemaker is indicated in patients with sinus node dysfunction with bradycardia. When the patient has high-degree or complete AV block in addition to sinus node dysfunction, an additional ventricular pacemaker may be required (AV sequential pacemaker, not illustrated in the figure). The AV sequential pacemaker is recognized by two sets of electronic spikes—one before the P wave and another before the wide QRS complex.

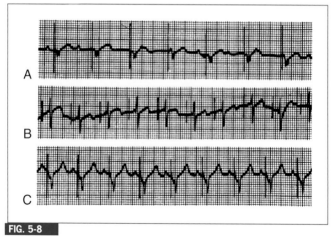

FIG. 5-8

Examples of some artificial pacemaker rhythm strips. **A,** Fixed-rate ventricular pacemaker. **B,** Atrial pacemaker. **C,** P wave–triggered pacemaker in a child with surgically induced complete heart block.

c. P wave–triggered ventricular pacemaker (atrial sensing, ventricular pacing). This pacemaker may be recognized by pacemaker spikes that follow the patient's own P waves at regular PR intervals and with wide QRS complexes (Fig. 5-8, *C*). The patient's own P waves are sensed and trigger a ventricular pacemaker after an electronically pre-set PR interval. This type of pacemaker is the most physiologic and is indicated when the patient has advanced AV block but a normal sinus mechanism. Advantages of this type of pacemaker are that the heart rate varies with physiologic need and the atrial contraction contributes to ventricular filling and improves cardiac output.

INDICATIONS

In general, pediatric conditions that require pacemaker implantation fit into one of four categories: (1) symptomatic bradycardia (with symptoms of syncope, dizziness, exercise intolerance, or congestive heart failure), (2) congenital AV block, (3) surgical or acquired advanced second- or third-degree AV block, and (4) recurrent bradycardia-tachycardia.

Bradycardia is the most common and noncontroversial indication for permanent pacemaker therapy in both children and adults. In children, sig-nificant bradycardia with syncope or near syncope results most commonly from extensive surgery involving the atria (such as the Fontan operation). Another noncontroversial indication is surgically acquired heart block that lasts more than 7 days after surgery.

Temporary pacing is indicated for (1) patients with advanced second-degree or complete heart block secondary to overdose of certain drugs, myocarditis, or myocardial infarction and (2) certain patients immediately after cardiac surgery.

TYPES OF PACING DEVICES

The North American Society of Pacing and Electrophysiology (NASPE) and the British Pacing and Electrophysiology Group (BPEG) devised a generic letter code to describe the types and functions of pacemakers (Table 5-2). The letter in the first position identifies the chamber paced (A, atrium; V, ventricle; D, dual) and the second is the chamber sensed (A, atrium; V, ventricle; D, dual; O, none). The third letter corresponds to the response of the pacemaker to an intrinsic cardiac event (I, inhibited; T, triggered; D, dual). For example:

1. A VOO device provides ventricular pacing, no sensing, and no re-sponse. This type of pacemaker is commonly used for emergency pacing.
2. A VVI device is ventricle stimulated and ventricle sensed; it inhibits paced output if endogenous ventricular activity occurs (thus preventing competition with native QRS activity). This type is commonly used for ep-isodic AV block or bradycardia in small infants.
3. An AAI device paces and senses the atrium and is inhibited by atrial activity. This type is commonly used in patients with sinus node dysfunc-tion with intact AV conduction.
4. A DDD device is a dual-chamber pacemaker that is capable of pacing either chamber, sensing activity in either chamber, and either triggering

TABLE 5-2
REVISED NASPE/BPEG GENERIC CODE FOR ANTIBRADYCARDIA PACING

I: CHAMBER(S) PACED	II: CHAMBER(S) SENSED	III: RESPONSE TO SENSING	IV: PROGRAMMABILITY, RATE MODULATION	V: ANTIARRHYTHMIA FUNCTION
O, None	O, None	O, None	O, None	O, None
A, Atrium	A, Atrium	T, Triggered	R, Rate modulation	A, Atrium
V, Ventricle	V, Ventricle	I, Inhibited		V, Ventricle
D, Dual (A+V)	D, Dual (A+V)	D, Dual (T+I)		D, Dual (A+V)

Adapted from Bernstein AD, Daubert AC, Fletcher RD et al and the NASPE/BPEG: The revised NASPE/BPEG generic code for antibradycardia, adaptive-rate, and multisite pacing, *Pacing Clin Electrophysiol* 25:260-264, 2002.

NASPE, North American Society of Pacing and Electrophysiology; BPEG, British Pacing and Electrophysiology Group.

or inhibiting paced output (with resulting AV synchrony). This type is used in AV block where AV synchrony is important.

5. The pacemaker choice is based on several factors, including the presence or absence of underlying cardiac disease, the size of the patient, and the relevant hemodynamic factors (including the need for atrial contribution in cardiac output).

B.   IMPLANTABLE CARDIOVERTER-DEFIBRILLATOR THERAPY

An ICD is used in patients at risk for recurrent, sustained ventricular tachycardia or fibrillation. The efficacy of ICD therapy in saving lives of patients at high risk of sudden death has been shown convincingly. All ICDs also have a built-in pacemaker. The ICD automatically detects, recognizes, and treats tachyarrhythmias and bradyarrhythmias using tiered therapy (i.e., bradycardia pacing, overdrive tachycardia pacing, low-energy cardioversion, high-energy shock defibrillation). ICDs can discharge voltages ranging from less than 1 V for pacing to 750 V for defibrillation. The ICD is implanted beneath the skin over the left chest (for right-handed persons) pectoralis muscle and the leads are connected to the ICD. Virtually all ICD systems are implanted transvenously. The longevity of the ICD depends on the frequency of shock delivery, the degree of pacemaker dependency, and other programmable options, but most are expected to last from 5 to 10 years. The most common problem with the ICD is inappropriate shocks, which are usually the result of detection of a supraventricular tachycardia, most commonly atrial fibrillation.

INDICATIONS

1. Two most common indications for ICD implantation in children are hypertrophic cardiomyopathy and long QT syndrome.

2. Other potential indications include idiopathic dilated cardiomyopathy, Brugada syndrome, and arrhythmogenic RV dysplasia.

3. A family history of sudden death may influence the decision to use an ICD in a pediatric patient.

C.   LIVING WITH A PACEMAKER OR ICD

Electromagnetic interference (EMI) can cause malfunction of the pacemaker or ICD by rate alteration, sensing abnormalities, reprogramming, and other functions, which may result in malfunction of the device or even damage to the pulse generator. Patients should be educated to avoid situations that may cause malfunction or damage to the device. EMI can occur within or outside the hospital. Patients with pacemakers should wear a medical identification bracelet or necklace in case of an emergency to show that they have the pacemaker or ICD.

Following are some common situations that may or may not affect pacemakers or ICDs.

1. Most home appliances in the following list will *not* interfere with the pacemaker signal.

a. Kitchen appliances (microwave ovens, blenders, toaster ovens, electric knives)

b. Televisions, stereos, FM and AM radios, ham radios, and CB radios

c. Electric blankets, heating pads

d. Electric shavers, hair dryers, curling irons

e. Garage door openers, gardening electric trimmers

f. Computers, copiers, and fax machines

g. Properly grounded shop tools (except power generators or arc welding equipment)

2. The patient must use caution in the following situations.

a. Security detectors at airports and government buildings such as court-houses. The patient should not stay near the electronic article surveillance system longer than is necessary or lean against the system.

b. Cellular phones. The patient should not carry a cell phone in the breast pocket when the ICD is implanted in the left upper chest. Keep the cell phone at least 6 inches away from the ICD. When talking on the cell phone, hold it on the opposite side of the body from the ICD.

c. Avoid working with, holding, or carrying magnets near the pacemaker.

d. Turn off large motors such as those in cars or boats when working on them. Do not use a chain saw.

e. Avoid industrial welding equipment. Most welding equipment used for "hobby" welding should not cause any significant problem.

f. Avoid high-tension wires, radar installations, smelting furnaces, electric steel furnaces, and other high-current industrial equipment.

g. Abstain from diathermy (the use of heat to treat muscles).

h. Contact sports are not recommended for children with a pacemaker or ICD.

3. Hospital sources of potentially significant EMI are as follows:

a. Electrocautery during surgical procedures. Notify the surgeon or dentist so that electrocautery will not be used to control bleeding. ICD therapy should be deactivated before surgery and reinitiated after surgery by a qualified professional. Alternatively, a magnet can be placed over the pacemaker throughout the procedure.

b. For cardioversion or defibrillation. Paddles should be placed in the anteroposterior position, keeping the paddles at least 4 inches from the pulse generator. A qualified pacemaker programmer should be available.

c. Magnetic resonance imaging (MRI) is considered a relative contraindication in patients with a pacemaker or ICD.

D. FOLLOW-UP FOR PACEMAKER AND ICD

Patients with pacemakers and ICDs must be followed on a regular schedule. Many of the same considerations are relevant to both pacemaker and ICD follow-up. Some physicians prefer regular office assessment, others prefer transtelephonic follow-up, and still others prefer a combination of the two techniques. The frequency of clinic follow-up and pacemaker interrogation by the pacemaker manufacturer vary between 3 and 12 months. A monthly transtelephonic evaluation system is simple, convenient, and inexpensive.

Special Problems

I. CONGESTIVE HEART FAILURE

Congestive heart failure (CHF) is a clinical syndrome in which the heart is unable to pump enough blood to the body to meet its needs, to dispose of systemic or pulmonary venous return adequately, or a combination of the two.

A. CAUSES

6

The heart failure syndrome may arise from diverse causes. Common causes of CHF are volume and/or pressure overload caused by either congenital or acquired heart disease, as well as myocardial diseases. By far the most common causes of CHF in infancy are congenital heart diseases (CHDs). Beyond infancy, myocardial dysfunction of various etiologies is an important cause of CHF. Tachyarrhythmias and heart block can also cause heart failure at any age.

1. **Congenital heart disease.** Volume overload lesions such as ventricular septal defect (VSD), patent ductus arteriosus (PDA), and endocardial cushion defect (ECD) are the most common causes of CHF in the first 6 months of life. In infancy the time of the onset of CHF varies predictably with the type of defect. Table 6-1 lists common defects according to the age at which CHF develops. Large left-to-right shunt (L-R shunt) lesions, such as VSD and PDA, do not cause CHF before 6 to 8 weeks of age because the pulmonary vascular resistance (PVR) does not fall low enough to cause a large shunt until this age. CHF may occur earlier in premature infants (within the first month) because of an earlier fall in the PVR. Note that children with tetralogy of Fallot (TOF) do not develop CHF and that children with atrial septal defect (ASD) rarely develop CHF in the pediatric age group, although ASD causes CHF in adulthood.

2. **Acquired heart disease.** Acquired heart disease of various etiologies can lead to CHF. Common entities (with the approximate time of onset of CHF) are as follows:

a. Viral myocarditis (in toddlers, occasionally in neonates with fulminating course)

b. Myocarditis associated with Kawasaki disease (1 to 4 years of age)

c. Acute rheumatic carditis (school-age children)

d. Rheumatic valvular heart diseases, such as mitral regurgitation (MR) or aortic regurgitation (AR) (older children and adults)

e. Idiopathic dilated cardiomyopathy (any age during childhood and adolescence)

f. Doxorubicin cardiomyopathy (months to years after chemotherapy)

g. Cardiomyopathies associated with muscular dystrophy and Friedreich ataxia (older children and adolescents)

257

TABLE 6-1

CAUSES OF CONGESTIVE HEART FAILURE DUE TO CONGENITAL HEART DISEASE ACCORDING TO THE TIME OF OCCURRENCE

TIME OF OCCURRENCE	CAUSES
At birth	Hypoplastic left heart syndrome (HLHS)
	Volume overload lesions (e.g., severe TR or PR, large systemic AV fistula)
First week	Transposition of the great arteries (TGA)
	PDA in small premature infants
	HLHS (with more favorable anatomy)
	TAPVR, particularly those with pulmonary venous obstruction
	Critical AS or PS
	Others: systemic AV fistula
1-4 weeks	COA (with associated anomalies)
	Critical AS
	Large L-R shunt lesion (e.g., VSD, PDA) in premature infants
	All other lesions listed above
4-6 weeks	Some L-R shunt lesions, such as ECD
6 weeks-4 months	Large VSD
	Large PDA
	Others: anomalous left coronary artery from the PA

ECD, endocardial cushion defect.

3. Miscellaneous causes
a. Metabolic abnormalities (severe hypoxia, acidosis, hypoglycemia, hypocalcemia) (newborns)
b. Hyperthyroidism (any age)
c. Supraventricular tachycardia (SVT) (early infancy)
d. Complete heart block associated with CHDs (the newborn period or early infancy)
e. Severe anemia (any age), hydrops fetalis (neonates), and sicklemia (childhood and adolescence)
f. Bronchopulmonary dysplasia (BPD) with right-sided failure (the first few months of life)
g. Primary carnitine deficiency (2 to 4 years)
h. Acute cor pulmonary caused by acute airway obstruction (early childhood)
i. Acute systemic hypertension with glomerulonephritis (school-age children)

B. CLINICAL MANIFESTATIONS

The diagnosis of CHF relies on several sources of clinical findings, including history, physical examination, and chest x-ray (CXR) films. Cardiomegaly is almost always present on CXR films. Echo studies are the most helpful non-invasive studies, confirming the diagnosis, cause, and severity of CHF.

Plasma levels of natriuretic peptides, atrial natriuretic peptide (ANP), and B-type natriuretic peptide (BNP) are increased in most adult patients with dyspnea from heart failure but not in dyspnea caused by pulmonary disease. Plasma levels of these peptides are normally elevated in the first weeks of life. Although increased levels of BNT and the N-terminal segment of its pro-hormone (NT-ProBNT) have been reported in most children with CHF, the usefulness of data on the levels of these peptides appears limited because an appropriate reference range has not been established. The levels of these peptides are different depending on the commercial testing kits used.

1. Poor feeding of recent onset, tachypnea, poor weight gain, and cold sweat on the forehead suggest CHF in infants. In older children, short-ness of breath, especially with activities; easy fatigability; puffy eyelids; or swollen feet may be presenting complaints.
2. Physical findings can be divided by pathophysiologic subgroups.
a. Compensatory responses to impaired cardiac function
   (1) Tachycardia, gallop rhythm, weak and thready pulse, and cardio-megaly on CXR films
   (2) Signs of increased sympathetic discharges (growth failure, perspi-ration, and cold wet skin)
b. Signs of pulmonary venous congestion (left-sided failure) include tachy-pnea, dyspnea on exertion (or poor feeding in small infants), orthopnea in older children, and rarely wheezing and pulmonary crackles.
c. Signs of systemic venous congestion (right-sided failure) include hepa-tomegaly and puffy eyelids. Distended neck veins and ankle edema are not seen in infants.
3. Cardiomegaly on CXR films is almost always present, except when the pulmonary venous return is obstructed; in that case pulmonary edema or venous congestion will be present.
4. The ECG is not helpful in deciding whether one is in CHF, although it may be helpful in determining the cause.
5. Echo studies confirm the presence of chamber enlargement or im-paired left ventricle (LV) function and help determine the cause of CHF.

C. MANAGEMENT
The treatment of CHF consists of (1) elimination of the underlying causes or correction of precipitating or contributing causes (e.g., infection, anemia, arrhythmias, fever, hypertension); (2) general supportive measures; and (3) control of heart failure state by inotropic agents, diuretics, or afterload-reducing agents.
1. Treatment of underlying causes or contributing factors
a. When surgically feasible, treatment of underlying CHDs or valvular heart disease is the best approach for complete cure.
b. Antihypertensive treatment for hypertension.
c. Antiarrhythmic agents or cardiac pacemaker therapy for arrhythmias or heart block.
d. Treatment of hyperthyroidism if it is the cause of CHF.

e. Antipyretics for fever.

f. Antibiotics for a concomitant infection.

g. Packed cell transfusion for anemia (to raise the hematocrit to ≥35%).

2. **General measures.** Nutritional supports are important. Infants in CHF need significantly higher caloric intakes than recommended for average children. The required calorie intake may be as high as 150 to 160 kcal/kg/day for infants in CHF.

a. Increasing caloric density of feeding may be required, and it may be accomplished with fortification of feeding (Box 6-1).

b. Frequent small feedings are better tolerated than large feedings in infants.

c. If oral feedings are not well tolerated, intermittent or continuous nasogastric (NG) feeding is indicated. To promote normal development of oral-motor function, infants may be allowed to take calorie-dense oral feeds throughout the day and then be given continuous NG feeds overnight.

d. In older children, salt restriction (<0.5 g/day) and avoidance of salty snacks (chips, pretzels) and table salt are recommended. Bed rest remains an important component of management. The availability of a television screen and computer games for entertainment ensures bed rest in older children.

3. **Drug therapy.** Three major classes of drugs are commonly used in the treatment of CHF in children: diuretics, inotropic agents, and afterload-reducing agents.

a. Diuretics

(1) Diuretics remain the principal therapeutic agent to control pulmonary and systemic venous congestion. Diuretics only reduce

---

BOX 6-1

METHODS OF INCREASING CALORIC DENSITY OF FEEDINGS

1. Human milk fortifier (Enfamil, Mead Johnson), 1 packet per 25 mL of breast milk ≡ 24 kcal/oz
2. Formula concentration to 24 kcal/oz by:
    a. 1 cup powdered formula + 3 cups water or
    b. 4 oz ready-to-feed + ½ scoop powdered formula
3. Supplementation of formula to 26-30 kcal/oz is accomplished in the following manner.
    a. Fat modular products
        (1) Medium chain triglycerides (MCT) oil (Mead Johnson), 8 kcal/mL
        (2) Microlipid (safflower oil emulsion, Mead Johnson), 4.5 kcal/mL
    b. Low-osmolality polymers
        (1) Polycose (Ross), 23 kcal/tablespoon
        (2) Moducal (Mead Johnson), 30 kcal/tablespoon
4. Pediasure (Ross), 30 kcal/oz ready-to-feed (for children over 1 year of age)

From Wright GE, Rochini AP: Primary and general care of the child with congenital heart disease, *ACC Current Journal Review* 89-93, March/April 2002.

preload and improve congestive symptoms; they do not
improve cardiac output or myocardial contractility (Fig. 6-1).
There are three main classes of diuretics that are commercially
available.

(a) Thiazide diuretics (e.g., chlorothiazide, hydrochlorothiazide),
which act at the proximal and distal tubules, are no longer
popular.

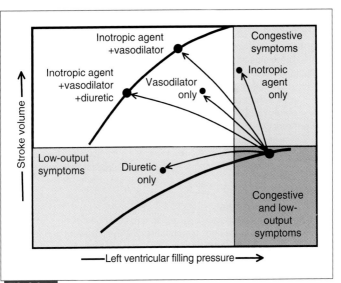

FIG. 6-1

Effects of anticongestive medications on the Frank-Starling relationship for ventricular
function. In normal persons with a normal heart, cardiac output increases as a function of ventricular filling pressure (*upper curve*). In patients with heart failure the normal relationship between the cardiac output (stroke volume) and filling pressure (preload) is shifted lower and to the right such that a low-output state and congestive
symptoms may coincide. Congestive symptoms (dyspnea, tachypnea) may appear
even in a normal heart if the filling pressure reaches a certain point. At one extreme
the addition of a pure inotropic agent, such as digoxin, primarily increases the stroke
volume with minimal impact on filling pressure (so that the patient may still have congestive symptoms). Conversely, the addition of a diuretic primarily decreases the filling
pressure (with improved congestive symptoms) but without improving cardiac output.
Clinically, it is common to use multiple classes of agents (usually a combination of inotropic agents, diuretics, and vasodilators) to produce both increased cardiac output
and decreased filling pressure. *(Adapted from Cohn JN, Franciosa JS: Vasodilator
therapy of cardiac failure [first of two parts].* N Engl J Med *297:27-31, 1977.)*

(b) Rapid-acting diuretics (e.g., furosemide, ethacrynic acid) are the drugs of choice. They act primarily at the loop of Henle ("loop diuretics").

(c) Aldosterone antagonist (e.g., spironolactone) acts on the distal tubule to inhibit sodium-potassium exchange. This drug has value in preventing hypokalemia produced by other diuretics and thus is used in conjunction with a loop diuretic. However, when angiotensin-converting enzyme (ACE) inhibitors are used, spironolactone should be discontinued to avoid hyperkalemia.

(2) Table 6-2 shows dosages of commonly available diuretic preparations. Side effects of diuretic therapy include hypokalemia (except when used with spironolactone) and hypochloremic alkalosis. These side effects predispose to digitalis toxicity.

b. Rapidly acting inotropic agents

(1) In critically ill infants with CHF, rapidly acting catecholamines with a short duration of action are preferable to digoxin. Dosages of this class of inotropic agents are suggested in Table 6-3.

(2) Amrinone is a noncatecholamine agent that exerts its inotropic effect and vasodilator effects by inhibiting phosphodiesterase (see Appendix E for dosage). Thrombocytopenia is a side effect; the drug should be discontinued if the platelet count falls below $150,000/mm^3$.

c. Digitalis glycosides

(1) Dosage of digoxin

(a) Digoxin increases the cardiac output (or contractile state of the myocardium), thereby resulting in an upward and leftward shift of the ventricular function curve relating cardiac output

TABLE 6-2		
DIURETIC AGENTS AND DOSAGES		
PREPARATION	**ROUTE**	**DOSAGE**
Thiazide Diuretics		
Chlorothiazide (Diuril)	Oral	20-40 mg/kg/day in two divided doses
Hydrochlorothiazide (HydroDIURIL)	Oral	2-4 mg/kg/day in two divided doses
Loop Diuretics		
Furosemide (Lasix)	IV	1 mg/kg/dose
	Oral	2-3 mg/kg/day in two or three divided doses
Ethacrynic acid (Edecrin)	IV	1 mg/kg/dose
	Oral	2-3 mg/kg/day in two or three divided doses
Aldosterone Antagonists		
Spironolactone (Aldactone)	Oral	3 mg/kg/day in two or three divided doses

TABLE 6-3

SUGGESTED DOSAGES OF RAPID-ACTING CATECHOLAMINES

DRUG	ROUTE AND DOSAGE	SIDE EFFECTS
Epinephrine (Adrenalin)	IV 0.1-1 μg/kg/min	Hypertension, arrhythmias
Isoproterenol (Isuprel)	IV 0.1-0.5 μg/kg/min	Peripheral and pulmonary vasodilation
Dobutamine (Dobutrex)	IV 5-8 μg/kg/min	Little tachycardia and vasodilation, arrhythmias
Dopamine (Inotropin)	IV 5-10 μg/kg/min	Tachycardia, arrhythmias, hypertension, or hypotension Dose-related cardiovascular effects of dopamine (μg/kg/min): Renal vasodilation (2-5) Cardiac (5-15) Vasoconstriction (15-20)

to filling volume of pressure (Fig. 6-1). Use of digoxin in infants with large L-R shunt lesions (e.g., large VSD) is controversial because ventricular contractility is normal in this situation. However, studies have shown that digoxin improves symptoms in these infants, perhaps because of other actions of digoxin, such as parasympathomimetic action and diuretic action.

(b) The total digitalizing dose (TDD) and maintenance dosage of digoxin by oral and intravenous routes are shown in Table 6-4. A high dose may be needed in treating SVT, in which the goal of treatment is to delay atrioventricular (AV) conduction. The maintenance dose is more closely related to the serum digoxin level than is the digitalizing dose, which is given to build a sufficient body store of the drug and to shorten the time required to reach the pharmacokinetic steady state.

TABLE 6-4

ORAL DIGOXIN DOSAGE FOR CONGESTIVE HEART FAILURE

PATIENT	TDD* (μG/KG)	MAINTENANCE*† (μG/KG/DAY)
Premature babies	20	5
Neonates	30	8
Less than 2 years	40-50	10-12
More than 2 years	30-40	8-10

From Park MK: The use of digoxin in infants and children with specific emphasis on dosage, *J Pediatr* 108:871-877, 1986.
*IV dose is 75% of the oral dose.
†Maintenance dose is 25% of the TDD in two divided doses.
TDD, total digitalizing dose.

(2) How to digitalize. One half of the total digitalizing doses are followed by one fourth and then the final one fourth of the total digitalizing dose at 6- to 8-hour intervals. The maintenance dose is given 12 hours after the final total digitalizing dose. An ECG strip before starting the maintenance dose is advised. This results in a pharmacokinetic steady state in 3 to 5 days. When an infant is in mild heart failure, the maintenance dose may be administered orally without loading doses; this results in a steady state in 5 to 8 days. A baseline ECG (rhythm and PR interval) and serum electrolytes are recommended. Hypokalemia and hypercalcemia predispose to digitalis toxicity.

(3) Monitoring for digitalis toxicity by ECG. With the relatively low dosage recommended in Table 6-4, digitalis toxicity is unlikely unless there are predisposing factors for the toxicity (Box 6-2). Serum digoxin levels obtained during the first 3 to 5 days after digitalization tend to be higher than those obtained when the pharmacokinetic steady state is reached. Therefore, detection of digitalis toxicity is best accomplished by monitoring with ECGs, not by serum digoxin levels during this period. Box 6-3 lists ECG signs of digitalis effects and toxicity. In general the digitalis effect is confined to *ventricular repolarization*, whereas toxicity involves disturbances in the *formation and conduction of the impulse.*

(4) Serum digoxin levels. Therapeutic ranges of serum digoxin levels for treating CHF are 0.8 to 2 ng/mL. Blood for serum digoxin levels should be drawn just before a scheduled dose or at least 6 hours after the last dose; samples obtained earlier than 6 hours after the last dose will give a falsely elevated level.

(5) Digitalis toxicity. The diagnosis of digitalis toxicity is based on the following clinical and laboratory findings.

BOX 6-2
FACTORS THAT MAY PREDISPOSE TO DIGITALIS TOXICITY
HIGH SERUM DIGOXIN LEVEL
High-dose requirement, as in treatment of certain arrhythmias
Decreased renal excretion (premature infants, renal disease)
Hypothyroidism
Drug interaction (e.g., quinidine, verapamil, amiodarone)
INCREASED SENSITIVITY OF MYOCARDIUM (WITHOUT HIGH SERUM DIGOXIN LEVEL)
Status of myocardium (myocardial ischemia, rheumatic *or* viral myocarditis)
Systemic changes (electrolytes [↓K, ↑Ca], hypoxia, alkalosis)
Catecholamines
Immediate postoperative period after heart surgery under cardiopulmonary bypass

---

BOX 6-3

ECG CHANGES ASSOCIATED WITH DIGITALIS

EFFECTS

Shortening of QTc is the earliest sign of digitalis effect

Sagging ST segment and diminished amplitude of T wave (T vector does not change)

Slowing of heart rate

TOXICITY

Prolongation of PR interval

Some normal children have a prolonged PR interval, making it mandatory to obtain a baseline ECG; may progress to advanced AV block

Profound sinus bradycardia or sinoatrial block

Supraventricular arrhythmias (atrial or nodal ectopic beats and tachycardias), particularly if accompanied by AV block, are more common than ventricular arrhythmias in children

Ventricular arrhythmias (such as ventricular bigeminy or trigeminy) are extremely rare in children, although common in adults with digitalis toxicity; isolated PVCs are not uncommon in children as a sign of toxicity

---

    (a) A history of accidental ingestion
    (b) Noncardiac symptoms in digitalized children: anorexia, nausea, vomiting, diarrhea, restlessness, drowsiness, fatigue, and visual disturbances in older children
    (c) Heart failure not improving or worsening
    (d) ECG signs of toxicity (Box 6-3)
    (e) An elevated serum level of digoxin (>2 ng/mL) in the presence of clinical findings suggestive of digitalis toxicity

d. Afterload-reducing agents
  (1) Reducing afterload tends to augment the stroke volume without a great change in the inotropic state of the heart and therefore without increasing myocardial oxygen consumption. Combined use of an inotropic agent, a vasodilator, and a diuretic produces most improvement in both inotropic state and congestive symptoms (Fig. 6-1).
  (2) Afterload-reducing agents may be used not only in infants with a large-shunt VSD, AV canal, or PDA but also in patients with dilated cardiomyopathies, myocardial ischemia, postoperative cardiac status, severe MR or AR, and systemic hypertension. Dosages and the site of action of the afterload-reducing agents are presented in Table 6-5.

e. Other drugs
  (1) β-Adrenergic blockers
    (a) As reported in adults, β-adrenergic blockers have been shown to be beneficial in some pediatric patients with chronic CHF who were treated with standard anticongestive drugs. Adrenergic overstimulation, often seen in patients with chronic CHF,

TABLE 6-5
DOSAGES OF VASODILATORS

DRUG	ROUTE AND DOSAGE	COMMENTS
Arteriolar Vasodilators		
Hydralazine (Apresoline)	IV: 0.15-0.2 mg/kg/dose, every 4-6 hr (maximum 20 mg/dose)	May cause tachycardia; may be used with propranolol
	Oral: 0.75-3 mg/kg/day, in 2-4 doses (maximum 200 mg/day)	May cause gastrointestinal symptoms, neutropenia, and lupuslike syndrome
Venodilators		
Nitroglycerin	IV: 0.5-1 µg/kg/min (maximum 6 µg/kg/min)	Start with small dose and titrate based on effects
Mixed Vasodilators		
Captopril (Capoten)	Oral:	May cause hypotension, dizziness, neutropenia, and proteinuria
	Newborn: 0.1-0.4 mg/kg, TID-QID	
	Infant: Initially 0.15-0.3 mg/kg, QD-QID; titrate upward if needed; max dose 6 mg/kg/24 hr	Dose should be reduced in patients with impaired renal function
	Child: Initially 0.3-0.5 mg/kg, BID-TID; titrate upward if needed; max 6 mg/kg/24 hr	
	Adolescents and adults: Initially 12.5-25 mg, BID-TID; increase weekly if needed by 25 mg/dose to max dose 450 mg/24 hr	
Enalapril (Vasotec)	Oral: 0.1 mg/kg, once or twice daily	Patient may develop hypotension, dizziness, or syncope
Nitroprusside (Nipride)	IV: 0.3-0.5 µg/kg/min; titrate to effects (max dose 10 µg/kg/min)	May cause thiocyanate or cyanide toxicity (e.g., fatigue, nausea, disorientation), hepatic dysfunction, or light sensitivity

may have detrimental effects on the failing heart by inducing myocyte injury and necrosis. However, β-adrenergic blockers should not be given to those with decompensated heart failure.

(b) When added to standard medical therapy for CHF, carvedilol, a nonselective β-adrenergic blocker with additional α1-antagonist activities, has been shown to be beneficial in children with idiopathic dilated cardiomyopathy, chemotherapy-induced cardiomyopathy, postmyocarditis myopathy, muscular dystrophy, and postsurgical heart failure (e.g., Fontan operation). Metoprolol was also beneficial in dilated cardiomyopathy. See Appendix E for the dosages and side effects of carvedilol and metoprolol. Propranolol added to conventional treatment for CHF was also beneficial in a small number of infants with large L-R shunts at the dose of 1.6 mg/kg per day.

(2) Carnitine, which is an essential cofactor for transport of long-chain fatty acids into mitochondria for oxidation, has been shown to be beneficial in some cases of dilated cardiomyopathy. The dosage of L-carnitine used was 50 to 100 mg/kg/day, given BID or TID orally (maximum daily dose 3 g).

4. **Surgical management.** If medical treatment as outlined previously does not improve CHF caused by CHD within a few weeks to months, one should consider either palliative or corrective cardiac surgery for the underlying cardiac defect when technically feasible. Cardiac transplantation is an option for a patient with progressively deteriorating cardiomyopathy despite maximal medical treatment.

II. CHILD WITH CHEST PAIN

Although chest pain does not indicate serious disease of the heart or other systems in most pediatric patients, in a society with a high prevalence of atherosclerotic cardiovascular disease it can be alarming to the child and parents. Physicians should be aware of the differential diagnosis of chest pain in children and should make every effort to find a specific cause before making a referral to a specialist or reassuring the child and the parents of the benign nature of the complaint.

A. CAUSE AND PREVALENCE

Table 6-6 lists the frequency of the causes of chest pain in children according to organ systems. The three most common causes of chest pain in children are costochondritis, trauma to or muscle strain of the chest wall, and respiratory diseases, especially those associated with coughing. These three conditions account for 45% to 65% of cases of chest pain in children.

TABLE 6-6

FREQUENCY OF CAUSES OF CHEST PAIN IN CHILDREN

CAUSE	INCIDENCE (%)
Idiopathic	12-45
Costochondritis	9-22
Musculoskeletal trauma	21
Cough, asthma, pneumonia	15-21
Psychogenic	5-9
Gastrointestinal system	4-7
Cardiac disorder	0-4
Sickle cell crisis	2
Miscellaneous	9-21

Chest pain of cardiac origin occurs in only 0% to 4% of children with complaint of chest pain. Box 6-4 is a partial list of possible causes of non-cardiac and cardiac chest pain in children. Psychogenic causes are less likely found in children younger than 12 years old; such causes are more likely to be found in females older than 12 years of age.

B.   CLINICAL MANIFESTATIONS

1. **Idiopathic chest pain.** No cause can be found in 12% to 45% of patients, even after a moderately extensive investigation. In children with chronic chest pain a cardiac cause is less likely to be found.

2. **Noncardiac causes of chest pain.** Identifiable noncardiac causes of chest pain are found in 56% to 86% of reported cases, most often in the thorax and respiratory system (Table 6-6).

a. Costochondritis
   (1) Costochondritis is found in 9% to 22% of children with chest pain. It is more common in girls than boys and may persist for several months. It is characterized by mild to moderate anterior chest pain, usually unilateral but occasionally bilateral. The pain may radiate to the remainder of the chest and back and may be exaggerated by breathing or physical activities. Physical examination is diagnostic; the clinician finds a reproducible tenderness on palpation over the chondrosternal or costochondral junctions. It is a benign condition.
   (2) *Tietze syndrome* is a rare form of costochondritis characterized by a large, tender, fusiform (spindle-shaped), and nonsuppurative swelling at the chondrosternal junction. It usually affects the second and third costochondral junctions.

b. Musculoskeletal. A history of vigorous exercise, weight lifting, or direct trauma to the chest and the presence of tenderness of the chest wall or muscles clearly indicate muscle strain or trauma.

c. Respiratory
   (1) Respiratory causes (10% to 20% of cases) may result from lung pathology, pleural irritation, or pneumothorax. A history of severe cough, tenderness of intercostal or abdominal muscles, and crackles or wheezing on examination suggests a respiratory cause of chest pain.
   (2) Exercise-induced asthma. The response of the asthmatic patient to exercise is quite characteristic. Strenuous exercise for 3 to 8 minutes causes bronchoconstriction in virtually all asthmatic subjects, especially when the heart rate rises to 180 beats per minute. Symptoms may include coughing, wheezing, dyspnea, and/or pain. Patients also complain of limited endurance during exercise. Exercise-induced bronchospasm provocation test is diagnostic.

d. Gastrointestinal. Gastroesophageal reflux (GER) may produce burning substernal pain that worsens with a reclining posture or abdominal pressure. In young children, ingested foreign bodies (such as coins or

BOX 6-4

CAUSES OF CHEST PAIN IN CHILDREN AND ADOLESCENTS

NONCARDIAC CAUSES

THORACIC CAGE

Costochondritis

Trauma or muscle strain

Abnormalities of rib cage or thoracic spine

Breast tenderness (mastalgia)

RESPIRATORY SYSTEM

Severe cough or bronchitis

Pleural effusion

Lobar pneumonia

Exercise-induced asthma

Spontaneous pneumothorax or pneumomediastinum

GASTROINTESTINAL SYSTEM

Gastroesophageal reflux (GER)

Gastritis

Peptic ulcer disease

Foreign body

Cholecystitis

PSYCHOGENIC ORIGINS

Hyperventilation

Conversion symptoms

Somatization disorder

Depression

MISCELLANEOUS ORIGINS

Texidor's twinge

Herpes zoster

Pleurododynia

CARDIAC CAUSES

ISCHEMIC VENTRICULAR DYSFUNCTION

Structural abnormalities of heart (severe AS or PS, HOCM, Eisenmenger syndrome)

Mitral valve prolapse

Coronary artery abnormalities (old Kawasaki, congenital anomaly, coronary heart disease, hypertension, sickle cell disease)

Cocaine (drug abuse)

Aortic dissection and aortic aneurysm (Turner, Marfan, or Noonan syndrome)

INFLAMMATION

Pericarditis (viral, bacterial, or rheumatic)

Postpericardiotomy syndrome

Myocarditis, acute or chronic

Kawasaki disease

ARRHYTHMIAS (WITH PALPITATION)

Supraventricular tachycardia

Frequent PVCs or ventricular tachycardia ($\pm$)

caustic substances) may cause chest pain. Cholecystitis presents with postprandial pain referred to the right upper quadrant of the abdomen and part of the chest.
e. Psychogenic. Psychogenic causes of chest pain are more likely seen in female adolescents. Often a recent stressful situation parallels the onset of the chest pain: a death or separation in the family, a serious illness, a disability, a recent move, failure in school, or sexual molestation. However, a psychological cause of chest pain should not be lightly assigned without a thorough history taking and a follow-up evaluation. Psychological or psychiatric consultation may be indicated.
f. Miscellaneous
 (1) The precordial catch (Texidor's twinge or stitch in the side), a one-sided chest pain, lasts a few seconds or minutes and is associated with bending or slouching.
 (2) Slipping rib syndrome (resulting from excess mobility of the eighth to tenth ribs, which do not directly insert into the sternum).
 (3) Mastalgia in some male and female adolescents.
 (4) Pleurodynia (devil's grip) is an unusual cause of chest pain caused by coxsackievirus infection.
 (5) Herpes zoster is another unusual cause of chest pain.
 (6) Spontaneous pneumothorax and pneumomediastinum are rare respiratory causes of acute chest pain. Children with asthma, cystic fibrosis, or Marfan syndrome are at risk. Inhalation of cocaine can provoke pneumomediastinum and pneumothorax.
 (7) Hyperventilation can produce chest discomfort and is often associated with paresthesia and light-headedness.
3. **Cardiac causes of chest pain.** Cardiac chest pain may be caused by ischemic ventricular dysfunction, pericardial or myocardial inflammatory processes, or arrhythmias, and these cardiac causes occur in 0% to 4% of cases (Box 6-4). Table 6-7 summarizes important clinical findings of cardiac causes of chest pain in children.
a. Ischemic myocardial dysfunction
 (1) Congenital heart defects. Severe aortic stenosis (AS), subaortic stenosis, severe pulmonary stenosis (PS), and pulmonary hypertension (Eisenmenger syndrome) may cause ischemic chest pain. The pain is usually associated with exercise and is a typical anginal pain.
 (2) Mitral valve prolapse. Chest pain associated with mitral valve prolapse (MVP) is usually a vague, nonexertional pain of short duration, located at the apex, without a constant relationship to effort or emotion. Occasionally, supraventricular or ventricular arrhythmias may result in cardiac symptoms, including chest discomfort. Nearly all patients with Marfan syndrome have MVP. A midsystolic click with or without a late systolic murmur is the hallmark of the condition.
 (3) Cardiomyopathy. Hypertrophic and dilated cardiomyopathy can cause chest pain from ischemia, with or without exercise, or from rhythm disturbances.

TABLE 6-7
IMPORTANT CLINICAL FINDINGS OF CARDIAC CAUSES OF CHEST PAIN

CONDITION	HISTORY	PHYSICAL EXAMINATION	ECG	CXR FILM
Severe AS	CHD (+)	Loud (≥ grade 3/6) systolic ejection murmur at URSB with radiation to the neck	LVH with or without strain	Prominent ascending aorta and aortic knob
Severe PS	CHD (+)	Loud (≥ grade 3/6) systolic ejection murmur at ULSB	RVH with or without strain	Prominent MPA segment
HOCM	FH (+) in 33% of cases	Variable heart murmurs; brisk brachial pulses (±)	LVH, deep Q/small R or QS pattern in LPLs	Mild cardiomegaly with globular heart
MVP	Positive FH (±)	Midsystolic click with or without late systolic murmur; thin body build; thoracic skeletal anomalies (80%)	Inverted T waves in aVF (±)	Normal heart size; straight back (±); narrow AP diameter (±)
Eisenmenger syndrome	CHD (+)	Cyanosis or clubbing; RV impulse; loud and single S2, soft or no heart murmur	RVH	Markedly prominent MPA with normal heart size
Anomalous origin of left coronary artery	Symptomatic in early infancy, with recurrent episodes of distress	Soft or no heart murmur	MI, anterolateral	Moderate to marked cardiomegaly
Sequelae of Kawasaki or other coronary artery disease	Kawasaki disease (±); typical exercise-related anginal pain	Usually normal; continuous murmur in coronary fistula	ST segment elevation (±); old MI pattern (±)	May be normal or mild cardiomegaly
Cocaine abuse	Substance abuse (±)	Hypertension; nonspecific heart murmur (±)	ST segment elevation (±)	May be normal in acute cases

cont'd

TABLE 6-7—cont'd
IMPORTANT CLINICAL FINDINGS OF CARDIAC CAUSES OF CHEST PAIN

CONDITION	HISTORY	PHYSICAL EXAMINATION	ECG	CXR FILM
Pericarditis, myocarditis	URI (±); sharp chest pain	Friction rub; muffled heart sounds; nonspecific heart murmur (±)	Low QRS voltages; ST segment shift; arrhythmias (±)	Cardiomegaly of varying degrees
Postpericardiotomy syndrome	Recent heart surgery; sharp pain, dyspnea	Muffled heart sounds (±); friction rub	Persistent ST segment elevation	Cardiomegaly of varying degrees
Arrhythmias (+ palpitation)	WPW (±); FH of long QT syndrome (±)	May be normal; irregular rhythm (±)	Arrhythmias (±); WPW preexcitation (±); long QTc (>0.46 sec)	Normal

FH, family history; MI, myocardial infarction; MPA, main pulmonary artery; ULSB, upper left sternal border; URI, upper respiratory infection; URSB, upper right sternal border.

(4) Coronary artery disease. Coronary artery anomalies, either congenital (aberrant or single coronary artery, coronary artery fistula) or acquired (aneurysm or stenosis of the coronary arteries as a result of Kawasaki disease, or as a result of previous cardiac surgery involving the coronary arteries) can rarely cause chest pain.

(5) Cocaine abuse. Cocaine blocks the reuptake of norepinephrine with an increase in circulating levels of catecholamines causing coronary vasoconstriction. Cocaine also induces the activation of platelets, increases endothelin production, and decreases nitric oxide production. These effects collectively produce anginal pain, infarction, arrhythmias, or sudden death.

b. Pericardial or myocardial disease

(1) Pericarditis. Older children with pericarditis may complain of a sharp, stabbing precordial pain that worsens when they lie down and improves after they sit and lean forward. Echo examination is usually diagnostic.

(2) Myocarditis. Acute myocarditis often involves the pericardium to a certain extent and can cause chest pain.

c. Arrhythmias. Chest pain may result from a variety of arrhythmias, especially with sustained tachycardia resulting in myocardial ischemia. Even without ischemia, children may consider palpitation or forceful heartbeats as chest pain. In this situation, chest pain may be associated with dizziness and palpitation.

C. DIAGNOSTIC APPROACH

A careful history taking and physical examination will suffice to rule out cardiac causes of chest pain in most cases and often find a specific noncardiac cause of the pain. Even if physicians cannot find a specific cause of chest pain, it is relatively easy to rule out cardiac causes of chest pain.

1. **History of present illness.** The initial history is directed at determining whether the pain is likely of cardiac origin. One asks about the nature of the pain, in terms of its association with exertion or physical activities, the intensity, character, frequency, duration, and points of radiation. A typical *anginal pain is* located in the precordial or substernal area and radiates to the neck, jaw, either or both arms, back, or abdomen. Exercise, heavy physical activities, or emotional stress typically precipitate the pain. It is not a sharp pain. The patient describes the pain as a deep, heavy pressure; the feeling of choking; or a squeezing sensation. Nonexertional sharp pain of short duration is usually not of cardiac origin. Associated symptoms such as syncope, dizziness, or palpitation with chest pain suggest potential cardiac origin of the pain. Pain that changes with position of the body may suggest pleural pain. The following are some examples of questions used in determining the nature of chest pain.

a. What seems to bring on the pain (e.g., exercise, eating, trauma, emotional stress)?

b. Do you get the same type of pain while you watch TV or sit in class?

c. What is the pain like (e.g., sharp, pressure sensation, squeezing)?

d. What are the location (e.g., specific point, localized, or diffuse), severity, radiation, and duration (seconds, minutes) of the pain?

e. Does the pain get worse with deep breathing? (If so, the pain may be caused by pleural irritation or chest wall pathology.) Does the pain improve with certain body positions? (This is sometimes seen with pericarditis.)

f. Does the pain have any relationship with your meals?

g. How often and how long have you had similar pain (frequency and chronicity)?

h. Have you been hurt while playing, or have you used your arms excessively for any reason?

i. Are there any associated symptoms, such as presyncope, syncope, dizziness, palpitation?

j. Have you been coughing a lot lately?

2. **Past and family histories**

a. Past history of congenital or acquired heart disease, cardiac surgery, infection, asthma, or Kawasaki disease

b. Medications, such as asthma medicines or birth control pills

c. Family history of recent chest pain or a cardiac death

d. Family history of long QT syndrome, cardiomyopathies, or unexpected sudden death

e. History of exposure to drugs (cocaine) or cigarettes

3. **Physical examination**

a. The chest should be carefully inspected for trauma or asymmetry. The chest wall should be palpated for signs of tenderness or subcutaneous air. Special attention should be paid to the possibility of costochondritis as the cause of chest pain. Physicians should use the soft part of the terminal phalanx of a middle finger to palpate each costochondral and chondrosternal junction, not the palm of a hand. Pectoralis muscles and shoulder muscles should be examined for tenderness.

b. The skin and extremities should be examined for trauma or chronic disease.

c. The abdomen should be carefully examined because it may be the source of pain referred to the chest.

d. The heart and lungs should be auscultated for arrhythmias, heart murmurs, rubs, muffled heart sounds, gallop rhythm, crackles, wheezes, or decreased breath sounds. One must be careful not to interpret commonly occurring innocent murmurs as pathologic.

4. **Other investigations.** CXR films (for pulmonary pathology, cardiac size and silhouette, and pulmonary vascularity) and an ECG (for arrhythmias, hypertrophy, conduction disturbances, Wolff-Parkinson-White [WPW] pre-excitation, and prolonged QT intervals) may be obtained. Drug screening is ordered when cocaine-induced chest pain is suspected. Clinical findings of cardiac causes of chest pain are summarized in Table 6-7.

5. **Tentative diagnosis of noncardiac chest pain**
a. The chest pain is likely of noncardiac origin if the following are true.
   (1) It is nonexertional, occurring while watching TV or sitting in class; sharp pain; or of chronic nature (many cases of costochondritis have a chronic history of pain, having been there for weeks or months).
   (2) The family history is negative for hereditary heart disease (such as long QT syndrome, cardiomyopathies, unexpected sudden death).
   (3) The past history is negative for heart disease or Kawasaki disease.
   (4) The cardiac examination is unremarkable.
   (5) The ECG and CXR films are normal.
b. At this point, the clinician can reassure the patient and family of the probable benign nature of the chest pain. Simple follow-up may clarify the cause or the pain may subside without recurrence. The physician should then consider a condition in other systems, such as gastrointestinal, respiratory systems, or psychogenic origin. Drug screening for cocaine may be worthwhile in adolescents who have acute, severe chest pain and distress with an unclear cause. Appropriate referral to a specialist may be considered at this time.

6. **Referral to cardiologists.** The following are some indications for referral to a cardiologist for cardiac evaluation of chest pain.
a. When chest pain is triggered or worsened by physical activities or chest pain is accompanied by other symptoms such as palpitation, dizziness, or syncope
b. When there are abnormal findings in the cardiac examination or when abnormalities occur in the CXR films or ECG
c. When there is a family history of cardiomyopathy, long QT syndrome, sudden unexpected death, or other hereditary diseases commonly associated with cardiac abnormalities
d. When there are high levels of anxiety in the family and patient and the pain is of a chronic, recurring nature

D. TREATMENT

When a specific cause of chest pain is identified, treatment is directed at correcting or alleviating the cause.

1. Costochondritis can be treated by reassurance and occasionally by nonsteroidal antiinflammatory agents (such as ibuprofen) or acetaminophen. Ibuprofen is a better choice because it is an antiinflammatory as well as analgesic agent.

2. Most musculoskeletal and nonorganic causes of chest pain can be treated with rest, acetaminophen, or nonsteroidal antiinflammatory agents.

3. Exercise-induced asthma is most effectively prevented by inhalation of a $\beta2$-agonist immediately before exercise. Inhaled albuterol usually affords protection for 4 hours.

4. If gastritis, gastroesophageal reflux, or peptic ulcer disease is suspected, trials of antacids, hydrogen ion blockers, or prokinetic agents

(such as metoclopramide [Reglan]) are helpful therapeutically (as well as diagnostically).

5. If organic causes of chest pain are not found and psychogenic etiology is suspected, psychological consultation may be considered.

6. The correct therapy for acute cocaine toxicity has not been established. Calcium channel blockers (nifedipine, nitrendipine), β-adrenergic blockers, nitrates, and thrombolytic agents have resulted in varying levels of success. The use of β-blockers is controversial; they may worsen coronary blood flow.

III. SYNCOPE

A. PREVALENCE

As many as 15% of children and adolescents are estimated to have a syncopal event between the ages of 8 and 18 years.

B. DEFINITION

Syncope is a transient loss of consciousness and muscle tone that results from inadequate cerebral perfusion. Presyncope is the feeling that one is about to pass out while remaining conscious with a transient loss of postural tone. The most common prodromal symptom is dizziness.

C. CAUSES

The normal function of the brain depends on a constant supply of oxygen and glucose. Significant alterations in the supply of oxygen and glucose may result in a transient loss or near loss of consciousness. Syncope may be due to noncardiac causes (usually autonomic dysfunction), cardiac conditions, neuropsychiatric, and metabolic disorders. Box 6-5 lists possible causes of syncope.

In adults, most cases of syncope are caused by cardiac problems. In children and adolescents, however, most incidents of syncope are benign, resulting from vasovagal episodes (probably the most common cause), other orthostatic intolerance entities, hyperventilation, and breath holding. Before age 6 years, syncope is likely caused by a seizure disorder, breath holding, or cardiac arrhythmias. Only circulatory causes of syncope will be discussed in some detail.

1. Noncardiac causes of syncope
a. Orthostatic intolerance. Three easily definable entities of orthostatic intolerance are vasovagal syncope, orthostatic hypotension, and postural orthostatic tachycardia syndrome (POTS).
   (1) Vasovagal syncope
      (a) Vasovagal syncope (also called simple fainting or neurocardiogenic syncope) is the most common type of syncope in otherwise healthy children and adolescents. This syncope is uncommon before 10 to 12 years of age but quite prevalent in adolescents, especially girls. It is characterized by a prodrome lasting a few seconds to a minute; the prodrome may include

BOX 6-5

CAUSES OF SYNCOPE

AUTONOMIC (NONCARDIAC)

Orthostatic intolerance group

Vasovagal syncope (also known as simple, neurocardiogenic, or neurally mediated syncope)

Orthostatic (postural) hypotension (dysautonomia)

Postural orthostatic tachycardia syndrome (POTS)

Exercise-related syncope (see further discussion in text)

Situational syncope

Breath holding; cough, micturition; defecation, etc.

Carotid sinus hypersensitivity

Excess vagal tone

CARDIAC

Arrhythmias

Tachycardias: SVT, atrial flutter/fibrillation, ventricular tachycardia (seen with long QT syndrome, arrhythmogenic RV dysplasia)

Bradycardias: sinus bradycardia, asystole, complete heart block, pacemaker malfunction

Obstructive lesions

Outflow obstruction: AS, PS, hypertrophic cardiomyopathy, pulmonary hypertension;

Inflow obstruction: MS, tamponade, constrictive pericarditis, atrial myxoma

Myocardial: coronary artery anomalies, hypertrophic cardiomyopathy, dilated cardiomyopathy, MVP, arrhythmogenic RV dysplasia

NEUROPSYCHIATRIC

Hyperventilation

Seizure

Migraine

Tumors

Hysteria

METABOLIC

Hypoglycemia

Electrolyte disorders

Anorexia nervosa

Drugs/toxins

---

dizziness, nausea, pallor, diaphoresis, palpitation, blurred vision, headache, and/or hyperventilation. The prodrome is followed by the loss of consciousness and muscle tone with a fall. The unconsciousness does not last more than a minute. The syncope may occur after rising in the morning or in association with prolonged standing, anxiety or fright, pain, blood drawing or the sight of blood, fasting, hot and humid conditions, or crowded places.

(b) The normal responses to the assumption of an upright posture are a reduced cardiac output, an increase in heart rate, and an unchanged or slightly diminished systolic pressure (Fig. 6-2) with about 6% decrease in cerebral blood flow. Pathophysiology of vasovagal syncope is not completely understood, but one theory is as follows: In susceptible individuals, a sudden decrease in venous return to the ventricle produces a large increase in the force of ventricular contraction, which causes activation of the left ventricular mechanoreceptors. A sudden increase in neural traffic to the brainstem somehow mimics the conditions seen in hypertension and thereby produces a paradoxical withdrawal of sympathetic activity, resulting in a peripheral vasodilation, hypotension, bradycardia, and subsequent decrease in cerebral perfusion (Fig. 6-2).

(c) History is most important in establishing the diagnosis of vasovagal syncope. Tilt testing of various protocols is useful in diagnosing vasovagal syncope, but its specificity and reproducibility are questionable.

(2) Orthostatic hypotension (dysautonomia)

(a) The normal response to standing is reflex arterial and venous constriction and a slight increase in heart rate. In orthostatic hypotension the normal adrenergic vasoconstriction of the

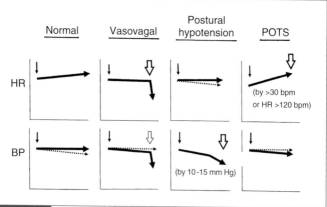

FIG. 6-2

Schematic drawing of changes in heart rate (HR) and systolic blood pressure (BP) observed during the head-up tilt test. Thin arrows mark the start of orthostatic stress. Large unfilled arrows indicate appearance of symptoms with changes seen in HR and BP. POTS, postural orthostatic tachycardia syndrome. *(From Park MK: Pediatric cardiology for practitioners, ed 5, Philadelphia, 2008, Mosby.)*

arterioles and veins in the upright position is absent or inadequate, resulting in hypotension without a reflex increase in heart rate (Fig. 6-2). Unlike the prodrome seen with vasovagal syncope, in orthostatic hypotension, patients experience only light-headedness. They do not display the autonomic nervous system signs seen with vasovagal syncope, such as pallor, diaphoresis, and hyperventilation. Prolonged bed rest, prolonged standing, dehydration, drugs that interfere with the sympathetic vasomotor response (e.g., calcium channel blockers, antihypertensive drugs, vasodilators, phenothiazines), and diuretics may exacerbate orthostatic hypotension.

(b) In patients suspected of having orthostatic hypotension, blood pressure (BP) should be measured in the supine and standing positions. A fall in systolic/diastolic pressure of more than 20/10 mm Hg within 3 minutes of assuming the upright position without moving the arms or legs, with no increase in the heart rate but without fainting, suggests the diagnosis.

(3) Postural orthostatic tachycardia syndrome (POTS)

(a) This new syndrome, most often observed in young women, is a form of an autonomic neuropathy that predominantly affects the lower extremities. Venous pooling associated with assuming a standing position leads to a reduced venous return and a resulting increase in sympathetic discharge with a significant degree of tachycardia. Affected patients often complain of chronic fatigue, exercise intolerance, palpitation, light-headedness, nausea, and recurrent near syncope (and sometimes syncope). These symptoms may be related to *chronic fatigue syndrome* and may be misdiagnosed as having panic attacks or chronic anxiety. Occasionally patients develop swelling of the lower extremities with purplish discoloration of the dorsum of the foot and ankle.

(b) For the diagnosis of POTS, heart rate and blood pressure are measured in the supine, sitting, and standing positions. POTS is defined as the development of orthostatic symptoms that are associated with at least a 30-beat per minute increase in heart rate (or a heart rate of ≥ 120 beats per minute) that occurs within the first 10 minutes of standing or upright tilt, with occurrence of symptoms described previously (Fig. 6-2).

b. Exercise-related syncope. Athletic adolescents may experience syncope or presyncope during or after strenuous physical activities. This may signal serious cardiac problems, but in most cases it occurs because of a combination of venous pooling in vasodilated leg muscles, inadequate hydration, and high ambient temperature. To prevent venous pooling, athletes should keep moving after running competitions. Secondary hyperventilation from exercise activities with resulting hypocapnia may also contribute to this form of syncope. Tingling or numbness of extremities may occur with hypocapnia.

c. Situational syncope

    (1) Micturition syncope is a rare form of orthostatic hypotension. In this condition, rapid bladder decompression results in decreased total peripheral vascular resistance with splanchnic stasis and reduced venous return to the heart, resulting in postural hypotension.

    (2) Cough syncope follows paroxysmal nocturnal coughing in asthmatic children. Paroxysmal coughing produces a marked increase in intrapleural pressure with a reduced venous return and reduced cardiac output, resulting in altered cerebral blood flow and loss of consciousness.

2. **Cardiac causes of syncope.** Cardiac causes of syncope may include obstructive lesions; myocardial dysfunction; and arrhythmias, including long QT syndrome.

a. Obstructive lesions. Patients with severe AS, PS, or hypertrophic obstructive cardiomyopathy (HOCM), as well as those with pulmonary hypertension, may have syncope. Exercise often precipitates syncope associated with these conditions. These patients may also complain of chest pain, dyspnea, and palpitation.

b. Myocardial dysfunction. Although rare, myocardial ischemia or infarction secondary to congenital anomalies of the coronary arteries or acquired disease of the coronary arteries (such as Kawasaki disease or atherosclerotic heart disease) may cause syncope.

c. Arrhythmias. Either extreme tachycardia or bradycardia can cause syncope. Commonly encountered rhythm disturbances include SVT, ventricular tachycardia, sick sinus syndrome, and complete heart block.

    (1) No identifiable structural defects. Syncope from arrhythmias in children with structurally normal hearts may be seen in long QT syndrome, WPW syndrome, right ventricular (RV) dysplasia, and Brugada syndrome.

    (2) Structural heart defects. The following congenital and acquired heart conditions, unoperated or operated, may cause syncope resulting from arrhythmias.

        (a) Preoperative CHDs (such as Ebstein anomaly, mitral stenosis [MS] or MR, and L-TGA) may cause arrhythmias.

        (b) Postoperative CHDs (such as TOF, transposition of the great arteries [TGA], after Fontan operation) may have sinus node dysfunction, SVT, ventricular tachycardia, or complete heart block.

        (c) Dilated cardiomyopathy can cause sinus bradycardia, SVT, or ventricular tachycardia.

        (d) Hypertrophic cardiomyopathy is a rare cause of ventricular tachycardia and syncope.

D. EVALUATION OF A CHILD WITH SYNCOPE

The goal of the evaluation of a patient with syncope is to identify high-risk patients with underlying cardiac disease, which may recur or result in sudden death. The evaluation should extend to other family members when a genetic condition is suspected or identified.

1. **History.** Accurate history taking is most important in determining cost-effective diagnostic strategies.

a. About the syncopal event

   (1) The time of the day. Syncope occurring after rising in the morning suggests vasovagal syncope. Hypoglycemia is a very rare cause of syncope.

   (2) The patient's position. Syncope while sitting or recumbent suggests arrhythmias or seizures. Syncope after standing for some time suggests vasovagal syncope or other orthostatic intolerance group.

   (3) Relationship to exercise

      (a) Syncope occurring during exercise suggests arrhythmias.

      (b) Syncope occurring immediately after cessation of strenuous physical activities (such as football practice or a game) may be caused by venous pooling in the leg and is rarely caused by arrhythmias. Vigorousness and duration of the activity, relative hydration status, and ambient temperature are important.

   (4) Associated symptoms

      (a) Palpitation or racing heart rate suggests arrhythmia or tachycardia.

      (b) Chest pain suggests possible myocardial ischemia (due to obstructive lesions, cardiomyopathy, carditis, etc.).

      (c) Shortness of breath or tingling or numbness of extremities suggests hyperventilation.

      (d) Nausea, epigastric discomfort, and diaphoresis suggest vasovagal syncope.

      (e) Headache or visual changes also suggest vasovagal syncope.

   (5) The duration of syncope

      (a) Syncopal duration of less than 1 minute suggests vasovagal syncope, hyperventilation, or syncope due to another orthostatic mechanism.

      (b) A longer duration of syncope suggests convulsive disorders, migraine, or cardiac arrhythmias.

   (6) The patient's appearance during and immediately following the episode

      (a) Pallor indicates hypotension.

      (b) Abnormal movement or posturing, confusion, focal neurologic signs, amnesia, or muscle soreness suggests the possibility of seizure.

b. Past history of cardiac, endocrine, neurologic, or psychological disorders may suggest a disorder in that system.

   c. Medications, including prescribed, over-the-counter, and recreational drugs, should be checked.

   d. Family history should include the following data:

      (1) Myocardial infarction (MI) in family members younger than 30 years of age.

      (2) Cardiac arrhythmia, CHD, cardiomyopathies, long QT syndrome, seizures, metabolic and psychological disorders.

      (3) Positive family history of fainting is common in patients with vasovagal syncope.

   e. Social history is important in assessing whether there is a possibility of substance abuse, pregnancy, or factors leading to a conversion reaction.

2. Physical examination. Although physical examination is usually normal, it should always be performed, focusing on the cardiac and neurologic systems.

   a. Careful auscultation includes heart murmurs or abnormally loud second heart sounds.

   b. If orthostatic intolerance group is suspected, the heart rate and BP should be measured repeatedly while the patient is supine and after standing without moving for up to 10 minutes.

   c. Neurologic examination should include a fundoscopic examination, test for Romberg sign, gait evaluation, deep tendon reflexes, and cerebellar function.

3. Diagnostic studies. History and physical examinations guide practitioners in choosing the diagnostic tests that apply to a given syncopal patient.

   a. Data on serum glucose and electrolyte levels are of limited value because patients are seen hours or days after the episode.

   b. When an arrhythmia is suspected as the cause of syncope

      (1) the ECG should be inspected for heart rate (bradycardia), arrhythmias, WPW preexcitation, heart block, long QTc interval, as well as abnormalities suggestive of cardiomyopathies and myocarditis.

      (2) ambulatory ECG monitoring should be performed (24-hour Holter monitor or event recorder).

   c. Echo studies are performed to rule out CHDs, pulmonary hypertension, and cardiomyopathies, and to check on the status of postoperative CHDs.

   d. An exercise stress test is indicated if the syncopal event is associated with exercise.

   e. Rarely, cardiac catheterization and an electrophysiologic study may be indicated in some equivocal cases.

   f. Head-up tilt table test. If patients with positional syncope have autonomic symptoms (such as pallor, diaphoresis, or hyperventilation), a tilt table test is sometimes performed by some centers.

      (1) The goal of the test is to provoke patients' symptoms during an orthostatic stress while closely monitoring cardiac rhythm, heart

rate, and BP responses associated with symptoms. Orthostatic stress is created by a tilting table with the patient placed in an upright position for a certain period of time. Various protocols are available.

(2) Positive responses commonly include light-headedness, dizziness, nausea, visual changes, and frank syncope. Sinus bradycardia, junctional bradycardia, and asystole for as long as 30 seconds are common. Hypotension generally is manifested by systolic blood pressures of less than 70 mm Hg. Returning these patients to the supine position produces resolution of symptoms rapidly, usually with a reactive tachycardia. There are, however, serious questions about the sensitivity, specificity, diagnostic yield, and day-to-day reproducibility of the tilt test. In adults the overall reproducibility of syncope by the tilt test is disappointingly low (62%). About 25% of adolescents with no prior fainting history fainted during the tilt test. Moreover, among habitual fainters 25% to 30% did not faint during the test on a given day.

(3) Besides the specificity and reproducibility issues, several distinct abnormal patterns have been identified following the head-up tilt table tests (Fig. 6-2).

   (a) Vasovagal: an abrupt decrease in BP usually with bradycardia leading to syncope
   (b) Dysautonomia (or postural hypotension): a gradual decrease in BP without an increase in heart rate, leading to syncope
   (c) POTS: an excessive increase in heart rate to maintain an adequate BP to prevent syncope

g. Neurologic consultation. Patients exhibiting prolonged loss of consciousness, seizure activity, and a postictal phase with lethargy or confusion should be referred for neurologic consultation.

E. TREATMENT

1. Orthostatic intolerance group. Regardless of the type, the same preventive measures are used for all orthostatic intolerance groups. Beginning the therapy empirically without performing a head-up tilt table test is not unreasonable.

a. The patient is advised to avoid extreme heat and dehydration and to increase salt and fluid intake.

b. Fludrocortisone (Florinef), a mineralocortisone, 0.1 mg PO, QD or BID for children, 0.2 mg/day for adults, with increased salt intake or a salt tablet (1 g daily) may be tried. Average children commonly gain 1 kg or 2 kg water weight into their circulating volume within 2 or 3 weeks.

c. β-Blocker therapy is used commonly, especially in adolescents and young adults, to modify the feedback loop. Atenolol (1 to 1.2 mg/kg/day PO QD, maximum dose 2 mg/kg/day) or metoprolol (1.5 mg/kg/day given PO in two or three doses) is most commonly used.

d. β-Agonist therapy using pseudoephedrine (60 mg, PO, BID) or an ephedrine-theophylline combination (Marax) stimulates the heart rate and increases the peripheral vascular tone, preventing reflex bradycardia and vasodilation.

2. Cardiac arrhythmias presenting as syncopal events require antiarrhythmic therapy (see treatment for specific arrhythmias in Chapter 5). Long QT syndrome is treated with β-blockers, pacemakers, or an implantable cardioverter-defibrillator (ICD). Occasionally catheter ablation may be indicated in patients with WPW syndrome causing frequent SVT.

F. DIFFERENTIAL DIAGNOSIS OF SYNCOPE

1. Epilepsy. Patients with epilepsy may have incontinence, marked confusion in the postictal state, and abnormal electroencephalograms (EEGs). Patients are rigid rather than limp and may have sustained injuries. Patients do not experience the prodromal symptoms of syncope (e.g., dizziness, pallor, palpitation, and diaphoresis). The duration of unconsciousness is longer than that typically seen with syncope (<1 minute).

2. Hypoglycemia. Hypoglycemic attacks differ from syncope in that the onset and recovery occur more gradually; they do not occur during or shortly after meals.

3. Hyperventilation. Hyperventilation produces hypocapnia, which in turn produces intense cerebral vasoconstriction, causing syncope. It may also have a psychological component. The patient often experiences air hunger, shortness of breath, chest tightness, abdominal discomfort, palpitations, dizziness, numbness or tingling of the face and extremities, and rarely loss of consciousness. The syncopal episode can be reproduced in the office when the patient hyperventilates.

4. Hysteria. Syncope resulting from hysteria is not associated with injury and occurs only in the presence of an audience. During these attacks the patient does not experience the pallor and hypotension that characterize true syncope. The attacks may last longer (up to an hour) than a brief syncopal spell. Episodes usually occur in an emotionally charged setting and are rare before 10 years of age.

IV. PALPITATION

A. DEFINITION AND DESCRIPTION

The term *palpitation* is used loosely to describe an unpleasant subjective awareness of one's own heartbeats. This usually occurs as a sensation in the chest of rapid, irregular, or unusually strong heartbeats. Rarely, slow heart rates may cause palpitation.

B. CAUSES

Box 6-6 lists causes of palpitation. A high percentage of patients with palpitation have no etiology that can be established. Certain drugs and stimulants, such as caffeine, can be identified as a cause of palpitation. Caffeine is found in many foods and drinks, such as coffee, tea, hot cocoa, soda,

BOX 6-6

CAUSES OF PALPITATION

Normal physiologic event: exercise, excitement, fever

Psychogenic or psychiatric: fear, anger, stress, anxiety disorders, panic attack or panic disorder

Certain drugs and substances

Stimulants: caffeine (coffee, tea, soda, chocolate), some energy drinks, smoking

Over-the-counter drugs: decongestants, diet pills, etc.

Drugs that cause tachycardia: catecholamines, theophylline, hydralazine, minoxidil, cocaine

Drugs that cause bradycardia: β-blockers, antihypertensive drugs, calcium channel blockers

Drugs that cause arrhythmias: tricyclic antidepressants, phenothiazine, antiarrhythmics (some of which are proarrhythmic)

Certain medical conditions: anemia, hyperthyroidism, hypoglycemia, hyperventilation, poor physical condition

Heart diseases

Certain CHDs

Following surgeries for CHD: Fontan connection

Mitral valve prolapse

Cardiomyopathy (hypertrophic or dilated)

Cardiac tumors or infiltrative diseases

Cardiac arrhythmias

Tachycardia: sinus tachycardia, SVT, and VT

Bradycardia, including sick sinus syndrome

Ectopic beats (PACs, PVCs)

Atrial fibrillation

chocolate, and some medicines. Most energy drinks (such as Venom, Whoopass, Red Bull, Adrenalin Rush) contain large doses of caffeine and other legal stimulants, including ephedrine, guarana, taurine, and ginseng. Some medical conditions, such as hyperthyroidism, anemia, and hypoglycemia, may be the cause of palpitation. Rarely, cardiac arrhythmias should be looked into as a cause of palpitation, although most arrhythmias are not perceived and reported as palpitations. Some patients report palpitation while having sinus tachycardia. Occasionally a psychogenic or psychiatric cause for their symptoms can be suspected. Some adult patients with palpitations have panic disorder or panic attack.

C. EVALUATION

1. **History**
a. The nature and onset of palpitation may suggest causes.
   (1) Isolated "jumps" or "skips" suggest premature beats.
   (2) Sudden start and stop of rapid heartbeat or a pounding of the chest suggests SVT. Some children will appear sweaty or pale with SVT.

(3) A gradual onset and cessation of palpitation suggest sinus tachycardia or anxiety state.

(4) Palpitation characterized by slow heart rate may be due to AV block or sinus node dysfunction.

b. Relationship to exertion

(1) A history of palpitation during strenuous physical activity may be a normal phenomenon (due to sinus tachycardia), although it could be due to exercise-induced arrhythmias.

(2) Nonexertional palpitation may suggest atrial flutter/fibrillation, febrile state, thyrotoxicosis, hypoglycemia, or anxiety state.

(3) Palpitation on standing suggests postural hypotension.

c. Associated symptoms

(1) Symptoms of dizziness or fainting associated with palpitation may indicate ventricular tachycardia.

(2) The presence of other symptoms, such as chest pain, sweating, nausea, or shortness of breath, may increase the likelihood of identifiable causes of palpitation.

d. Personal and family history

(1) Caffeine-containing drinks (such as coffee, tea, hot cocoa, chocolate drinks, and energy drinks)

(2) Prescription and over-the-counter medications

(3) Family history of syncope, sudden death, or arrhythmias

2. **Physical examination**

a. Most children with palpitation have normal physical examinations, except for those with hyperthyroidism.

b. Cardiac examination may reveal findings of MVP, obstructive lesions, or possibly cardiomyopathy.

3. **Recording of ECG rhythm**

a. Routine ECG may show prolonged QTc interval, WPW preexcitation, or AV block.

b. Depending on the frequency of the complaint, a 24-hour Holter monitoring (for daily occurrence), event recorder (for occasional complaints, up to 30 days), or an implantable loop recorder (for very rare occurrences) may be indicated.

c. If the symptoms occur during exercise, an exercise stress test may be helpful in making the diagnosis.

4. **Laboratory studies.** Full blood count (for anemia), electrolytes, blood glucose, and thyroid function testing may be indicated.

D. MANAGEMENT

1. Stimulant-containing drinks (coffee, tea, hot cocoa, chocolate drinks, sodas, and energy drinks) should be reduced or eliminated.

2. Treat medical causes of palpitation (such as hypothyroidism), if present.

3. Examination of all medications that the patient is taking may be helpful in the diagnosis and in modifying the dosage or schedule or changing it to other medications.

4. If the rhythm recorded on an ECG monitor shows sinus tachycardia during the complaint of palpitation, all one has to do is to reassure the parents and child of the normal, benign nature of palpitation.

5. For isolated premature atrial contractions (PACs) or premature ventricular contractions (PVCs), nothing needs to be done except avoidance of the stimulants listed previously.

6. If a significant cardiac arrhythmia or an AV conduction disturbance is found, appropriate therapy should be given for the conditions found.

7. If palpitation is associated with symptoms, such as fainting, dizziness, chest pain, pallor, or diaphoresis, further evaluation is guided as described under Syncope or Child with Chest Pain in this chapter.

V. SYSTEMIC HYPERTENSION

A. DEFINITION

For adults a BP level of 120/80 mm Hg, previously considered normal, is now classified as prehypertension, and levels lower than 120/80 are now considered normal. Hypertension is further classified as stage 1 and stage 2 depending on the level of abnormalities (Table 6-8).

For children, hypertension is defined as systolic and/or diastolic pressure levels that are greater than the 95th percentile for age and gender or ≥120/80 mm Hg as in an adult on at least three occasions. Prehypertension is defined as an average systolic and/or diastolic pressure between the 90th and 95th percentiles for age and gender. Hypertension is further classified into stages 1 and 2 as follows: Stage 1 hypertension is present when BP readings are between the 95th and 99th percentiles and stage 2 hypertension is present when BP readings are 5 mm Hg or more above the 99th percentile values (Table 6-8). "White coat hypertension" is present when BP readings in health care facilities are in hypertensive ranges but are normotensive outside a clinical setting.

TABLE 6-8
CLASSIFICATION OF BLOOD PRESSURE FOR ADULTS AND CHILDREN

BP CLASSIFICATION	ADULTS		CHILDREN AND ADOLESCENTS*
	SYSTOLIC BP	DIASTOLIC BP	
Normal	<120	<80	<90th percentile
Prehypertension	120-139	80-89	90th-95th percentile
Stage 1 hypertension	140-159	90-99	95th-99th percentile
Stage 2 hypertension	≥160	≥100	≥5 mm Hg + 99th percentile value

Adapted from Chobanian AV, Bakris GL, Black HR et al: The seventh report of the Joint National Committee on Prevention, Detection, Evaluation, and Treatment of High Blood Pressure: the JNC 7 report, *JAMA* 21:2560-2572, 2003.
*Pediatric classification is according to the Fourth Report on the Diagnosis, Evaluation, and Treatment of High Blood Pressure in Children and Adolescents, *Pediatrics* 111:555-576, 2004.

A prerequisite for the pediatric definition of hypertension is the availability of reliable normative BP standards. However, the BP tables provided by the Working Group of the National High Blood Pressure Education Program (NHBPEP) are not acceptable standards because they are obtained by a methodology discordant from the Group's own recommendations, are statistically unsound, and are impractical for practitioners (as discussed in Chapter 2). Normative BP standards from the San Antonio Children's Blood Pressure Study are the only reliable sets available at this time. (The auscultatory BP standards for children 5 to 17 years old are shown in Tables B-3 and B-4, Appendix B). BP readings obtained by Dinamap monitor model 8100, a popular oscillometric device, are not interchangeable with those obtained by the auscultatory method. Dinamap readings are on average 10 mm Hg higher for the systolic pressure and 5 mm Hg higher for the diastolic pressure than the auscultatory method. (Normative oscillometric BP standards for children 5 to 17 years old from the same study are presented in Tables B-5 and B-6, Appendix B). Oscillometric BP standards for neonates and small children up to 5 years of age are presented in Table 1-3.

B. CAUSES

Although the incidence of essential hypertension in children and adolescents is not known, more than 90% of secondary hypertension in nonobese children is caused by three conditions: renal parenchymal disease, renal artery disease, and coarctation of the aorta (COA) (Box 6-7). With the

---

BOX 6-7

CAUSES OF SECONDARY HYPERTENSION

RENAL

Renal parenchymal disease

   Glomerulonephritis, acute and chronic

   Pyelonephritis, acute and chronic

   Congenital anomalies (polycystic or dysplastic kidneys)

   Obstructive uropathies (hydronephrosis)

   Hemolytic-uremic syndrome

   Collagen disease (periarteritis, lupus)

   Renal damage from nephrotoxic medications, trauma, or radiation

Renovascular disease

   Renal artery disorders (e.g., stenosis, polyarteritis, thrombosis)

   Renal vein thrombosis

CARDIOVASCULAR

Coarctation of the aorta

Conditions with large stroke volume (patent ductus arteriosus, aortic insufficiency, systemic arteriovenous fistula, complete heart block) (these conditions cause only systolic hypertension)

BOX 6-7—cont'd

ENDOCRINE

Hyperthyroidism (systolic hypertension)

Excessive catecholamine levels

   Pheochromocytoma

   Neuroblastoma

Adrenal dysfunction

   Congenital adrenal hyperplasia

      11-b-hydroxylase deficiency

      17-hydroxylase deficiency

   Cushing syndrome

   Hyperaldosteronism

      Primary: Conn's syndrome, idiopathic nodular hyperplasia, dexamethasone-suppressible hyperaldosteronism

      Secondary: renovascular hypertension, renin-producing tumor (juxtaglomerular cell tumor)

Hyperparathyroidism (and hypercalcemia)

NEUROGENIC

Increased intracranial pressure (any cause, especially tumors, infections, trauma)

Poliomyelitis

Guillain-Barré syndrome

Dysautonomia (Riley-Day syndrome)

DRUGS AND CHEMICALS

Sympathomimetic drugs (nose drops, cough medications, cold preparations, theophylline)

Amphetamines

Steroids

Nonsteroidal antiinflammatory drugs

Oral contraceptives

Heavy-metal poisoning (mercury, lead)

Cocaine, acute or chronic use

Cyclosporine

Large amount of licorice (hypokalemia and hypertension)

MISCELLANEOUS

Hypervolemia and hypernatremia

Stevens-Johnson syndrome

Bronchopulmonary dysplasia (newborns)

increasing prevalence of obesity in recent decades, overweight and obesity may be the most common cause of pediatric hypertension. In general the younger the child and the more severe the hypertension, the more likely an underlying cause can be identified. Primary hypertension is rare in children younger than 10 years of age.

C. DIAGNOSIS AND WORKUP

Diagnosis of hypertension relies on accurate BP measurement and comparing the reading with reliable BP standards. The diagnosis of hypertension should not be made until one confirms *persistently* elevated BP levels on at least three consecutive examinations. This is because "white coat hypertension" is quite common at the initial visit to the doctor's office. Careful history, physical examination, and laboratory tests should direct physicians to a correct cause of hypertension.

1. History
a. Neonatal: use of umbilical artery catheters or bronchopulmonary dysplasia.
b. History of palpitation, headache, and excessive sweating (signs of excessive catecholamine levels).
c. Renal: history of obstructive uropathies; urinary tract infection; and radiation, trauma, or surgery to the kidney area.
d. Cardiovascular: history of COA or surgery for it.
e. Endocrine: weakness and muscle cramps (hypokalemia seen with hyperaldosteronism).
f. Medications: corticosteroids, amphetamines, antiasthmatic drugs, cold medications, oral contraceptives, nephrotoxic antibiotics, cyclosporine, or cocaine use.
g. Family history of essential hypertension, atherosclerotic heart disease, and stroke.
h. Familial or hereditary renal disease (polycystic kidney, cystinuria, familial nephritis).
i. Most children with mild hypertension are asymptomatic. Only those children with acute severe hypertension may be symptomatic (with headache, dizziness, nausea and vomiting, irritability, personality changes). Rarely, severe hypertension may present with neurologic signs, CHF, renal dysfunction, or stroke.
2. Physical examination
a. Accurate measurement of BP is essential.
b. Physical examination should focus on delayed growth (renal disease), bounding peripheral pulse (PDA or AR), weak or absent femoral pulses or BP differential between the arms and legs (COA), abdominal bruits (renovascular), and tenderness over the kidney (renal infection).
c. Children's weight and body mass index (BMI) percentile (obesity-related hypertension).
d. In general children younger than 10 years of age with sustained hypertension require extensive evaluation because identifiable and potentially curable causes are more likely to be found. Adolescents with mild hypertension and a positive family history of essential hypertension are more likely to have essential hypertension, and extensive studies are not indicated.
3. Laboratory tests

a. Initial laboratory tests should be directed toward detecting renal parenchymal disease, renovascular disease, and COA and therefore should include urinalysis; urine culture; serum electrolyte, blood urea nitrogen, creatinine, and uric acid levels; ECG; CXR films; and possibly echo (Table 6-9).

b. When overweight is the likely cause of hypertension, metabolic aspects of risk factors should be checked.

TABLE 6-9

ROUTINE AND SPECIAL LABORATORY TESTS AND THEIR SIGNIFICANCE

LABORATORY TEST	SIGNIFICANCE
Urinalysis, urine culture, blood urea nitrogen, creatinine, uric acid	Renal parenchymal disease
Serum electrolytes (hypokalemia)	Hyperaldosteronism (primary or secondary)
	Adrenogenital syndrome
	Renin-producing tumors
ECG, chest x-ray studies, and possibly echocardiography	Cardiac cause of hypertension; also baseline function
Intravenous pyelogram (or ultrasonography, radionuclide studies, computed tomography, or magnetic resonance imaging of the kidneys)	Renal parenchymal disease
	Renovascular hypertension
	Tumors (neuroblastoma, Wilms tumor)
Plasma renin activity (peripheral)	High-renin hypertension (renovascular hypertension, renin-producing tumors, some Cushing syndrome, some essential hypertension)
	Low-renin hypertension (adrenogenital syndrome, primary hyperaldosteronism)
24-hour urine collection for 17-ketosteroid and 17-hydroxycorticosteroids	Cushing syndrome
	Adrenogenital syndrome
24-hour urine collection for catecholamine levels and vanillylmandelic acid	Pheochromocytoma
	Neuroblastoma
Aldosterone	Hyperaldosteronism (primary or secondary)
	Renovascular hypertension
	Renin-producing tumors
Renal vein plasma renin activity	Unilateral renal parenchymal disease
	Renovascular hypertension
Abdominal aortogram	Renovascular hypertension
	Abdominal coarctation of the aorta
	Unilateral renal parenchymal disease
	Pheochromocytoma
Intraarterial digital subtraction angiography	Renovascular hypertension

c. More specialized studies may be indicated for the detection of rare causes of secondary hypertension (Table 6-9).

D. MANAGEMENT

1. **Essential hypertension**

a. **Nonpharmacologic intervention.** Nonpharmacologic intervention should be started as an initial treatment, which includes counseling on weight reduction, if indicated; low-salt (and potassium-rich) foods; regular aerobic exercise; and avoidance of smoking and oral contraceptives.

b. **Pharmacologic intervention.** Drugs are used when a nonpharmacologic approach is not effective. Although there are no clear guidelines for identifying those who should be treated with antihypertensive drugs, the following are generally considered indications for initiating drug therapy in hypertensive children.

   (1) Severe symptomatic hypertension (with intravenous antihypertensive medications)

   (2) Significant secondary hypertension (e.g., renovascular and renoparenchymal diseases)

   (3) Target-organ damage (such as LV hypertrophy by echo studies)

   (4) Family history of early complications of hypertension

   (5) Diabetes (types 1 and 2)

   (6) Child who has dyslipidemia and other coronary artery risk factors

   (7) Persistent hypertension despite nonpharmacologic measures

c. **The choice of drug** for initial antihypertensive therapy rests on the preference of the responsible physician.

   (1) One approach is to initiate therapy with a small dose of a thiazide diuretic and proceed to a full dose. If it is not effective, a second drug such as an ACE inhibitor may be added to it, starting with a small dose and proceeding to a full dose. The efficacy of β-blockers appears disappointing and their popularity has declined, at least in adults.

   (2) A combination therapy is gaining popularity. In adults a combination of a thiazide diuretic and an ACE inhibitor (or angiotensin-receptor blocker [ARB]) is quite popular. Similarly, a calcium channel blocker (without diuretics) appears to be safe and equally effective. The same approach may be reasonable in children and adolescents. β-blockers appear not as effective as once thought. Table 6-10 shows the dosages of commonly used antihypertensive drugs for children. Specific classes of antihypertensive drugs should be used preferentially in patients with specific underlying or concurrent medical conditions (Table 6-11).

   (3) If the BP still remains elevated with the combination of two drugs, a third drug could be added to the regimen. At this point, however, the possibility of secondary hypertension should be reconsidered.

TABLE 6-10

ORAL DOSAGES OF SELECTED ANTIHYPERTENSIVE DRUGS FOR CHILDREN

DRUGS	INITIAL DOSE	TIMES/DAY
Diuretics		
Hydrochlorothiazide (HydroDIURIL)	1 mg/kg/day (max 3 mg/kg/day up to 50 mg/day)	1
Chlorthalidone	0.3 mg/kg/day (max 2 mg/kg/day up to 50 mg/day)	1
Furosemide (Lasix)	0.5-2 mg/kg/dose (max 6 mg/kg/day)	1-2
Spironolactone (Aldactone)	1 mg/kg/day (max 3.3 mg/kg/day up to 100 mg/day)	1-2
Triamtrene (Dyrenium)	1-2 mg/kg/day (max 3-4 mg/kg/day up to 300 mg/day)	2
Adrenergic Inhibitors		
Propranolol (Inderal)	1-2 mg/kg/day (max 4 mg/kg/day up to 640 mg/day)	2-3
Metoprolol (Lopressor)	1-2 mg/kg/day (max 6 mg/kg/day up to 200 mg/day)	2
Atenolol (Tenormin)	0.5-1 mg/kg/day (max 2 mg/kg/day up to 100 mg/day)	1-2
Angiotensin-Converting Enzyme Inhibitors		
Captopril (Capoten)	0.3-0.5 mg/kg/dose (max 6 mg/kg/day)	3
Enalapril (Vasotec)	0.08 mg/kg/day up to 5 mg/day (max 0.6 mg/kg/day up to 40 mg/day)	1-2
Lisinopril (Zestril, Prinivil)	0.07 mg/kg/day up to 5 mg/day (max 0.6 mg/kg/day up to 40 mg/day)	1
Angiotensin-Receptor Blocker		
Losartan (Cozaar)	0.7 mg/kg/day up to 50 mg/day (max 1.4 mg/kg/day up to 100 mg/day)	1
Calcium Channel Blockers		
Amlopidine (Norvasc)	6-17 yr: 2.5-5 mg/day	1
Extended-release nifedipine (Adalat, Procardia)	0.25-0.5 mg/kg/day (max 3 mg/kg/day up to 120 mg/day)	1-2
Direct-Acting Vasodilator		
Hydralazine (Apresoline)	0.75 mg/kg/day (max 7.5 mg/kg/day up to 200 mg/day)	4

Adapted from the Fourth Report on the Diagnosis, Evaluation, and Treatment of High Blood Pressure in Children and Adolescents, *Pediatrics* 114:555-576, 2004.

TABLE 6-11

PREFERENCES AND CONTRAINDICATIONS FOR THE USE OF
ANTIHYPERTENSIVE DRUGS

CLASS OF DRUGS	PREFERRED (INDICATIONS)	CONTRAINDICATED
Diuretics	Diabetes	Gout
	Asthmatics	
	Blacks?	
β-Adrenergic blockers	Migraine	Diabetes
	Hyperdynamic hypertension (with rapid pulse rates)	Asthmatics
	Hyperthyroidism	
	Non-blacks?	
ACE inhibitors or angiotensin-receptor blockers	Diabetes	Pregnancy
	Other nephropathy or pro-teinuria	Bilateral renal artery stenosis
	Non-blacks?	Hyperkalemia
Calcium channel blockers	Migraine	Heart block
	Blacks?	

d. **The goal of the treatment** is reduction of BP to <95th percentile for
   children with uncomplicated primary hypertension without hypertensive end-organ damage. For children with chronic renal disease, diabetes, or hypertensive target organ damage, the goal is reduction of
   BP to <90th percentile.
e. Classes of antihypertensive drugs
   (1) **Diuretics** are the cornerstone of antihypertensive drug therapy,
       except in patients with renal failure. Their action is related to a
       decrease in extracellular and plasma volume initially and later it is
       related to a decline in the peripheral resistance. The thiazide di-
       uretics (hydrochlorothiazide and chlorthalidone) are most com-
       monly used. An important side effect of diuretic therapy in chil-
       dren is hypokalemia, occasionally requiring potassium
       supplementation in the diet or as potassium salt. Diuretics may
       increase glucose, insulin, and cholesterol levels. Potassium-
       sparing diuretics (spironolactone, triamterene) may cause hyperka-
       lemia, especially if given with ACE inhibitors or ARBs.
   (2) **Adrenergic inhibitors.** Propranolol (Inderal), a β-adrenergic
       blocker, acts at three important locations: on the juxtaglomerular
       apparatus of the kidney to suppress the renin-angiotensin system,
       on the central vasomotor center to decrease systemic vascular
       resistance, and on the myocardium to suppress contractility.
       β-Adrenergic blockers should not be used in insulin-dependent
       diabetics. Propranolol is contraindicated in patients with asthma.
   (3) **ACE inhibitors.** Captopril and new long-acting agents (enalapril
       and lisinopril) are effective in pediatric hypertension. A diuretic

clearly enhances the effectiveness of ACE inhibitors. Side effects of ACE inhibitors include rash, loss of taste, and leukopenia. Occasional side effects include cough and angioedema. If cough appears, an ARB may be used. ACE inhibitors are contraindicated in pregnancy. Serum electrolytes and creatinine should be checked for hyperkalemia and azotemia.

(4) **ARBs** are a new class of antihypertensive agents that act by displacing angiotensin II from its receptor, antagonizing all of angiotensin's known effects with a resulting decrease in peripheral resistance. Cough is not a side effect of losartan, although angioedema can occur. ARBs are contraindicated in pregnancy.

(5) **Calcium channel blockers** are being used increasingly in the treatment of adult hypertension. Nifedipine has the greatest peripheral vasodilatory action, with little effect on cardiac automaticity, conduction, or contractility. Concomitant dietary sodium restriction or the use of a diuretic agent may not be necessary because calcium antagonists cause natriuresis by producing renal vasodilation. Amlopidine (Norvasc) is safe and effective in children with various forms of hypertension. Occasional side effects include headache, flushing, and local ankle edema.

(6) **Direct-acting vasodilators.** Hydralazine (Apresoline) produces side effects related to increased cardiac output (flushing, headache, tachycardia, palpitation) and salt retention, and therefore, the concomitant use of a β-adrenergic blocker and a diuretic is recommended. Hydralazine can cause a lupuslike syndrome. Minoxidil can cause hypertrichosis when used on a chronic basis.

2. **Secondary hypertension.** Treatment of secondary hypertension should be aimed at removing the cause of hypertension whenever possible.

a. **Cardiovascular causes.** Surgical or catheter interventional correction is indicated for coarctation of the aorta.

b. **Renal parenchymal disease.** The same therapy as discussed for essential hypertension is given. Salt restriction, avoidance of excessive fluid intake, and antihypertensive drug therapy can control hypertension caused by most renal parenchymal diseases. If hypertension is difficult to control and the disease is unilateral, unilateral nephrectomy may be considered.

c. **Surgical treatment.** Renovascular disease may be cured by successful surgery, such as reconstruction of a stenotic renal artery, autotransplantation, or unilateral nephrectomy. Hypertension caused by tumors that secrete vasoactive substances, such as pheochromocytoma, neuroblastoma, and juxtaglomerular cell tumor, are treated primarily by surgery.

3. **Hypertensive crisis**

a. In hypertensive crisis, blood pressure is rapidly rising or a high BP level is associated with neurologic manifestations, heart failure, or pulmonary edema. It may be loosely divided into the following subgroups.

(1) Hypertensive urgency is a situation in which reduction of BP is needed within hours, usually with oral agents.

(2) Hypertensive emergency is a situation in which immediate reduction of BP (within minutes) is needed, usually with parenteral therapy.

(3) Accelerated malignant hypertension is a situation in which papilledema, hemorrhage, and exudate are associated with a markedly elevated BP; the diastolic pressure is usually >140 mm Hg.

(4) Hypertensive encephalopathy is a situation in which markedly elevated BP is associated with severe headache and various alterations in consciousness. This may be seen in a previously normotensive patient who suddenly becomes hypertensive, such as children with acute glomerulonephritis or young women with eclampsia.

b. Aggressive parenteral administration of antihypertensive drugs is indicated to lower BP in most situations.

(1) Labetalol (α- and β-blocker), 0.2 to 2 mg/kg/hour IV drip; diazoxide (Hyperstat), 3 to 5 mg/kg as an intravenous bolus; or nitroprusside (Nipride), 1 to 3 μg/kg per minute as an intravenous drip, are the treatments of choice.

(2) If hypertension is less severe, hydralazine (Apresoline), 0.15 mg/kg intravenously or intramuscularly, may be used. The dose may be repeated at 4- to 6-hour intervals. Nifedipine, 0.2 to 0.5 mg/kg (maximum, 10 mg), may be given orally every 4 to 6 hours.

(3) A rapid-acting diuretic, such as furosemide (1 mg/kg), is given intravenously to initiate diuresis.

(4) Seizures may be treated with slow IV infusion of diazepam (Valium), 0.2 mg/kg, or another anticonvulsant medication.

(5) Fluid balance must be controlled carefully, so intake is limited to urine output plus insensible loss.

(6) When a hypertensive crisis is under control, oral medications replace the parenteral medications (see Table 6-10 for oral dosages).

VI. PULMONARY HYPERTENSION

A. DEFINITION

In the cardiac cath lab, the normal pulmonary artery (PA) systolic pressure in children and adults is ≤30 mm Hg (with the PA mean pressure ≤25 mm Hg) at sea level. Noninvasive Doppler method, however, often overestimates the PA pressure. Using tricuspid regurgitation (TR) jet velocity and the Bernoulli equation, with an assumed right atrial (RA) pressure of 10 mm Hg, the upper limit of normal PA systolic pressure is around 37 mm Hg (with ranges of 36 to 40 mm Hg). (The 37 mm Hg value will result from a TR jet velocity of 2.6 m/sec in the absence of PS.) Pulmonary hypertension (PH) is present when the PA pressure is higher than the upper limit of normal for each method.

B. CAUSES

PH is a group of conditions with multiple causes rather than a single one.
The causes of pulmonary hypertension can be grouped into the following
five (Box 6-8).

1. Increased pulmonary blood flow (as seen with large L-R shunt
lesions)
2. Alveolar hypoxia
3. Increased pulmonary venous pressure
4. Primary pulmonary vascular disease

BOX 6-8

CAUSES OF PULMONARY HYPERTENSION

1. Large left-to-right shunt lesions (hyperkinetic pulmonary hypertension): VSD,
   PDA, ECD
2. Alveolar hypoxia
   a. Pulmonary parenchymal disease
      (1) Extensive pneumonia
      (2) Hypoplasia of lungs (primary or secondary, such as that seen in
          diaphragmatic hernia)
      (3) Bronchopulmonary dysplasia
      (4) Interstitial lung disease (Hamman-Rich syndrome)
      (5) Wilson-Mikity syndrome
   b. Airway obstruction
      (1) Upper airway obstruction (large tonsils, macroglossia, micrognathia,
          laryngotracheomalacia, sleep-disordered breathing)
      (2) Lower airway obstruction (bronchial asthma, cystic fibrosis)
   c. Inadequate ventilatory drive (central nervous system diseases, obesity
      hypoventilation syndrome)
   d. Disorders of chest wall or respiratory muscles
      (1) Kyphoscoliosis
      (2) Weakening or paralysis of skeletal muscle
   e. High altitude (in certain hyperreactors)
3. Pulmonary venous hypertension: MS, cor triatriatum, TAPVR with obstruction,
   chronic left heart failure
4. Primary pulmonary vascular disease
   a. Persistent pulmonary hypertension of the newborn
   b. Primary pulmonary hypertension
5. Other diseases that involve pulmonary parenchyma or pulmonary vasculature
   a. Thromboembolism: ventriculoatrial shunt for hydrocephalus, sickle cell
      anemia, thrombophlebitis
   b. Connective tissue disease: scleroderma, systemic lupus erythematosus,
      mixed connective tissue disease, dermatomyositis, rheumatoid arthritis
   c. Disorders directly affecting the pulmonary vasculature: schistosomiasis,
      sarcoidosis, histiocytosis X

5. Other diseases that involve pulmonary parenchyma or pulmonary vasculature

C. PATHOPHYSIOLOGY

1. The endothelial cells and lung tissues normally synthesize and/or activate some vasoactive hormones and inactivate others. Balance among the vasoactive substances maintains vascular tone in normal and pathologic situations.

a. Normally, balanced release of nitric oxide (NO, a vasodilator) and endothelin (a potent vasoconstrictor) by endothelial cells is a key factor in the regulation of the pulmonary vascular tone.

b. Prostaglandin (PG) I_2 and PGE_1 are vasodilators, whereas $PGF_{2\alpha}$ and PGA_2 are vasoconstrictors.

c. Stimulation of α-adrenoceptors and β-adrenoceptors produces vasoconstriction and vasodilation, respectively.

d. Serotonin is a vasoconstrictor that promotes smooth muscle cell hypertrophy.

e. Angiotensin II, a potent vasoconstrictor, is activated from angiotensin I in the lungs by ACE.

2. Reduced alveolar oxygen tension (*alveolar hypoxia*) induces vasoconstriction (by reducing NO production and increasing endothelin production). Acidosis significantly increases PVR, acting synergistically with hypoxia. High altitude (with low alveolar oxygen tension) is associated with pulmonary vasoconstriction (and pulmonary hypertension), for which a large species and individual variations exist.

3. Pressure (P) is related to both flow (F) and vascular resistance (R), as shown in the following formula.

$$P \equiv F \times R$$

An increase in pulmonary blood flow, pulmonary vascular resistance, or both can result in PH. Regardless of its cause, PH eventually involves constriction of the pulmonary arterioles, resulting in an increase in PVR and hypertrophy of the RV.

4. The normally thin RV cannot sustain a sudden increase in PA pressure greater than 40 to 50 mm Hg, and such an increase results in RV failure. However, if PH develops slowly, the RV hypertrophies and it can tolerate higher pressures, which can reach systemic pressure.

5. Normal PVR is 1 Wood unit (or 67 ± 23 [SD] dyne-sec/cm^2), which is about 10% of systemic vascular resistance.

D. PATHOGENESIS

Pathogenesis differs among different subgroups of PH.

1. **Hyperkinetic pulmonary hypertension**

a. PH associated with large L-R shunt lesions (e.g., VSD, PDA) is called *hyperkinetic pulmonary hypertension.* It is the result of an increase in pulmonary blood flow, a direct transmission of the systemic pressure to the PA, and compensatory pulmonary vasoconstriction. Endothelial cell dysfunction with overproduction of endothelin and reduced NO production results. Hyperkinetic PH is usually reversible if the cause is eliminated before permanent changes occur in the pulmonary arterioles (see later section).

b. If large L-R shunt lesions are left untreated, irreversible changes take place in the pulmonary vascular bed, with severe PH and cyanosis due to a reversal of the L-R shunt. This stage is called Eisenmenger syndrome or pulmonary vascular obstructive disease (PVOD). Surgical correction is not possible at this stage. The time of development of PVOD varies. Many patients with TGA begin to develop PVOD within the first year of life. Children with Down syndrome with large L-R shunt lesions tend to develop PVOD much earlier than normal children with similar lesions.

2. **Alveolar hypoxia.** An acute or chronic reduction in the oxygen tension (Po_2) in the alveolar capillary region (alveolar hypoxia) elicits a strong pulmonary vasoconstrictor response, which may be augmented by acidosis. Although the exact mechanisms of the pulmonary vasoconstrictor response to alveolar hypoxia are not completely understood, endothelin and nitric oxide (NO) are the strongest candidates responsible for the response. Alveolar hypoxia may be an important basic mechanism of many forms of PH, including that seen in pulmonary parenchymal disease, airway obstruction, inadequate ventilatory drive (central nervous system diseases), disorders of chest wall or respiratory muscles, and high altitude.

3. **Pulmonary venous hypertension.** Increased pressure in the pulmonary veins produces reflex vasoconstriction of the pulmonary arterioles and raises the PA pressure to maintain a high enough pressure gradient between the PA and the pulmonary vein. The mechanism for the vasoconstriction is not entirely clear, but a neuronal component may be present. Moreover, an elevated pulmonary venous pressure may also narrow or close small airways, resulting in alveolar hypoxia, which may contribute to the vasoconstriction. Mitral stenosis, total anomalous pulmonary venous return (TAPVR) with obstruction (of pulmonary venous return to the left atrium [LA]), and chronic left-sided heart failure are examples of this entity. PH with increased pulmonary venous pressure is usually reversible when the cause is eliminated, with the exception of congenital pulmonary vein stenosis, for which no curative surgery is available.

4. **Primary pulmonary vascular disease.** Primary pulmonary hypertension is characterized by progressive, irreversible vascular changes similar to those seen in Eisenmenger syndrome but without intracardiac lesions. The pathogenesis of primary pulmonary hypertension is not fully understood, but endothelial dysfunction of the pulmonary vascular bed (with overproduction of endothelin) and enhanced platelet activities may be important factors. Overproduction of endothelin is associated with not only vasoconstriction but also cell proliferation, inflammation, medial hypertrophy, and fibrosis. This condition is rare in pediatric patients; it is a

condition of adulthood and is more prevalent in women. It has a poor prognosis.

5. **Other disease states.** Pulmonary hypertension associated with other disease states has a pathogenesis similar to that described in the preceding four categories, singly or in combination.

E. PATHOLOGY

1. Heath and Edwards classified the changes into six grades. Grade 1 consists of hypertrophy of the medial wall of the small muscular arteries; grade 2, hyperplasia of the intima; and grade 3, hyperplasia and fibrosis of the intima with narrowing of the vascular lumen. Changes up to grade 3 are considered reversible if the cause is eliminated. In grades 4 to 6, dilation and plexiform lesions, angiomatous and cavernous lesions, hyalinization of intimal fibrosis, and necrotizing arteritis are seen. Changes seen in grades 4 through 6 are considered irreversible and preclude surgical repair of CHDs.

2. The progressive vascular changes that occur in primary PH are identical to those that occur with CHDs.

3. With pulmonary venous hypertension the pulmonary arteries may show severe medial hypertrophy and intimal fibrosis. However, the changes are limited to grades 1 through 3 of the Heath and Edwards classification, and they are often reversible when the cause is eliminated.

F. CLINICAL MANIFESTATIONS

1. With significant PH, exertional dyspnea and fatigue may manifest. Some patients complain of headache. Syncope, presyncope, or chest pain also occurs on exertion.

2. Cyanosis with or without clubbing may be present. The neck veins are distended and a right ventricular lift or tap occurs on palpation.

3. The S2 is loud and single. An ejection click and an early diastolic decrescendo murmur of pulmonary regurgitation (PR) are usually present along the mid-left sternal border (MLSB). A holosystolic murmur of TR may be audible at the lower left sternal border (LLSB). Signs of right-sided heart failure (e.g., hepatomegaly, ankle edema) may be present.

4. The ECG shows right axis deviation (RAD) and right ventricular hypertrophy (RVH) with or without "strain." Right atrial hypertrophy (RAH) is frequently seen late. Arrhythmias occur in the late stage.

5. CXR films show either a normal or slightly enlarged heart. A prominent PA segment and dilated hilar vessels with clear lung fields are characteristic.

6. Echo studies usually demonstrate the following:

a. The right atrium (RA) and RV are enlarged; LV dimensions are normal or small.

b. With an elevated RV pressure, the interventricular septum shifts toward the LV and appears flattened at the end of systole.

c. PA pressure can be estimated by a Doppler study (see Chapter 2 for a detailed discussion).

   (1) Using the peak TR velocity, the RV systolic pressure can be estimated by the simplified Bernoulli equation ($\Delta P \equiv 4V^2$) and adding assumed RA pressure of 10 mm Hg.

   (2) With a shunt lesion, such as VSD or PDA, the peak systolic velocity across the shunt is used to estimate the RV pressure.

   (3) The end-diastolic (not early diastolic) velocity of PR is used to estimate the *diastolic* pressure in the PA.

7. Natural history and prognosis

a. PH secondary to the upper airway obstruction is usually reversible when the cause is eliminated.

b. Chronic pulmonary conditions that produce alveolar hypoxia have a relatively poor prognosis.

c. PH associated with large L-R shunt lesions or with pulmonary venous hypertension improves or disappears after surgical removal of the cause, if performed early.

d. Primary PH is progressive and has a fatal outcome, usually 2 to 3 years after the onset of symptoms.

e. PH associated with Eisenmenger syndrome, collagen disease, and chronic thromboembolism is usually irreversible and has a poor prognosis but may be stable for 2 to 3 decades.

f. Right-sided heart failure and cardiac arrhythmias occur in the late stage. Chest pain, hemoptysis, and syncope are ominous signs.

G.   DIAGNOSIS

1. Noninvasive tools (ECG, CXR films, and echo) are used to detect and estimate the severity of PH. Collectively, they are reasonably accurate in assessing severity.

2. Cardiac catheterization is performed to confirm the diagnosis and severity of PH. It will also determine whether the elevated pulmonary vascular resistance is due to active vasoconstriction ("responders") or to permanent changes in the pulmonary arterioles ("nonresponders"). Tolazoline (Priscoline, α-adrenoceptor blocker), oxygen administration, intravenous adenosine or epoprostenol (prostacyclin), or inhaled nitric oxide can be used to test the responsiveness of the pulmonary vascular bed.

3. Lung biopsies have been used in an attempt to evaluate the "operability" of patients with PH and CHD. Unfortunately, pulmonary vascular changes are not uniformly distributed and the biopsy findings correlated poorly with the natural history of the disease or the operability.

H.   MANAGEMENT

1. Measures to remove or treat the underlying cause should be the primary emphasis whenever possible.

a. Timely corrective surgery for CHDs (such as large-shunt VSD, ECD, or PDA)

b. Tonsillectomy and adenoidectomy when the cause of PH is the upper airway obstruction

c. Treatment of underlying diseases, such as cystic fibrosis, asthma, pneumonia, or bronchopulmonary dysplasia

2. General measures are aimed at preventing further elevation of PA pressure or treating its complications.

a. Avoidance or limitation of strenuous exertion, isometric activities (weight lifting).

b. Avoidance of trips to high altitudes.

c. Oxygen supplementation is provided as needed.

d. Patients should be strongly advised to avoid pregnancy. Pregnancy may increase the risk of pulmonary embolism from deep vein thrombosis or amniotic fluid and may cause syncope and cardiac arrest.

e. Oral contraceptives worsen pulmonary hypertension (surgical contraception is preferred).

f. Avoidance of vasoconstrictor drugs, including decongestants with α-adrenergic properties.

g. CHF is treated with digoxin and diuretics and a low-salt diet.

h. Cardiac arrhythmias are treated.

i. Partial erythropheresis is performed for polycythemia and headache.

j. Annual flu shots are recommended.

3. Anticoagulation and antiplatelet agent

a. Anticoagulation with warfarin (with the INR of 2.0 to 2.5) is widely recommended in patients with thromboembolic disease. It may be beneficial in patients with PH from other causes.

b. Some recommend antiplatelet drugs (aspirin) instead of warfarin to prevent microembolism in the pulmonary circulation.

4. For "responders." Vasodilators are used after testing vascular responsiveness in the catheterization laboratory. Most of the experiences are based on adult trials. Some vasodilators may lower the systemic vascular resistance more than the pulmonary vascular resistance and thus are not suitable.

a. Nifedipine, a calcium channel blocking agent (0.2 mg/kg PO every 8 hours), is one of the oldest drugs used, with beneficial effects seen in 40% of children with primary PH. Hypotension is a side effect of the medication.

b. Prostacyclines. Continuous intravenous infusion of epoprostenol (PGI_2) has been shown to improve quality of life and survival in patients with primary PH, Eisenmenger syndrome, or chronic lung disease. The starting dose of epoprostenol was 2 ng/kg/min, with increments of 2 ng/kg/min every 15 minutes, until desired effects appeared; the average final dose was 9 to 11 ng/kg/min.

c. Endothelin receptor antagonists bosentan and sitaxsentan are new therapeutic agents that have been used in both primary pulmonary hypertension and Eisenmenger syndrome.

(1) In children with primary pulmonary hypertension or Eisenmenger syndrome, oral bosentan, a nonselective endothelin receptor blocker, in the dose of 31.25 mg BID for children <20 kg, 62.5 mg BID for children 20 to 40 kg, and 125 mg BID for children >40 kg (with or without concomitant IV prostacycline therapy) for a median duration of 14 months resulted in a significant functional improvement in about 50% of the cases. A rare side effect of the drug is increased liver enzyme.

(2) Sitaxsentan, a selective endothelin-A (ETA) receptor antagonist, given orally once daily at a dose of 100 mg (for mostly adult patients and children older than 12 years) resulted in improved exercise capacity after 18 weeks of treatment. Elevation of aspartate aminotransferase (AST) and alanine aminotransferase (ALT) was a rare side effect.

d. Sidenafil, a phosphodiesterase inhibitor, 0.25 to 1 mg/kg, 4 times daily for 12 months' duration given orally, has resulted in improvement in hemodynamics and exercise capacity.

e. Nitric oxide inhalation is effective in lowering PA pressure in primary pulmonary hypertension and persistent pulmonary hypertension of the newborn.

f. In addition to the vasodilators just mentioned, inotropic agents (e.g., digoxin, dopamine) are often helpful in lowering PA pressure.

5. For "nonresponders," the following measures can be used.

a. Nitric oxide inhalation and continuous intravenous or possibly nebulized prostacycline (prostaglandin I_2) may provide selective pulmonary vasodilation.

b. Atrial septectomy (either by catheter or surgery) improves survival rates and abolishes syncope by providing a right-to-left (R-L) atrial shunt and thereby helping to maintain cardiac output.

c. Lung transplantation. Bilateral lung transplantation is preferred at most centers, but some centers prefer single lung transplantation.

VII. ATHLETES WITH CARDIAC PROBLEMS

Many physicians are involved in medical clearance for participation in school sports activities. To help reduce or prevent sudden death or other serious events occurring during athletic competitions, physicians should be aware of cardiac conditions that may cause problems during athletic activities. Physicians should also have general understanding of the eligibility guidelines for the participation in sports activities for patients with specific cardiovascular conditions.

The topics discussed include causes of sudden death, preparticipation screening of athletes, classification of sports, participation eligibility for athletes with congenital and acquired heart disease, athletes with cardiac arrhythmias, and athletes with hypertension. The following are summarized from the recent recommendations from the American College of Cardiology and the American Heart Association (AHA).

A. CAUSES OF SUDDEN UNEXPECTED DEATH IN YOUNG ATHLETES

Sudden unexpected death in young athletes is estimated to occur in about 1 per 200,000 high school sports participants per academic year. Among a variety of causes of sudden death during athletic competition, hypertrophic cardiomyopathy (HCM) is the single most common cause of sudden death in young athletes (up to 40%) (Table 6-12). Congenital anomalies and acquired diseases of the coronary arteries are the next important group, accounting for about 30% of sudden unexpected deaths. Less common abnormalities associated with sudden cardiac death in athletes include myocarditis, mitral valve prolapse, and cardiac arrhythmias. Sudden death is far more common in boys than girls. In the United States, football and basketball are the sports more frequently associated with sudden cardiac death.

B. PREPARTICIPATION SCREENING

Customary screening for U.S. high school and college athletes is confined to history taking and physical examination, which is known to be limited in its power to consistently identify important cardiovascular abnormalities. The AHA panel has recently recommended a 12-element screening strategy

TABLE 6-12

CARDIOVASCULAR ANOMALIES IN 134 YOUNG COMPETITIVE ATHLETES WITH SUDDEN DEATH

PRIMARY CARDIOVASCULAR LESIONS	PERCENT
Hypertrophic cardiomyopathy	36.0
Unexplained increase in cardiac mass (possible hypertrophic cardiomyopathy)	10.0
Aberrant coronary arteries	13.0
Other coronary anomalies	6.0
Ruptured aortic aneurysm	5.0
Tunneled left anterior descending coronary artery (myocardial "bridges")	5.0
Aortic valve stenosis	4.0
Myocarditis	3.0
Idiopathic myocardial scarring	3.0
Idiopathic dilated cardiomyopathy	3.0
Arrhythmogenic right ventricular dysplasia	3.0
Mitral valve prolapse	2.0
Atherosclerotic coronary artery disease	2.0
Other congenital heart disease	1.5
Long QT syndrome	0.5
Sarcoidosis	0.5
Sickle cell trait	0.5
Normal heart	2.0

From Maron BJ, Shirani J, Poline LC et al: Sudden death in young competitive athletes: clinical, demographic and pathological profiles, *JAMA* 276:199-208, 1996.

that includes gathering of medical and family histories and a physical examination (Box 6-9). A positive finding on any of these 12 items would result in referral for cardiovascular evaluation based on the discretion of the examiner. Some European countries require the use of routine 12-lead ECG in addition to the history and physical examination in screening athletes, but the AHA panel does not recommend routine use of ECG in the preparticipation screening because of its low specificity, high rate of false positives, and high cost. Medical clearance for sports does not necessarily imply the absence of cardiovascular disease or complete protection from sudden death. Even with the use of specialized tools available to cardiologists, complete prevention of such death is nearly impossible, given the rarity of some of the causes of sudden expected death.

The AHA panel recommends a complete screening for high school athletes before participation in organized sports and again after 2 years.

BOX 6-9

THE 12 ELEMENTS: AHA RECOMMENDATIONS FOR PREPARTICIPATION CARDIOVASCULAR SCREENING OF COMPETITIVE ATHLETES

PERSONAL HISTORY*

1. Exertional chest pain/discomfort
2. Unexplained syncope or near syncope[†]
3. Excessive exertional and unexplained dyspnea/fatigue, associated with exercise
4. Prior recognition of a heart murmur
5. Elevated systolic blood pressure

FAMILY HISTORY*

6. Premature death (sudden and unexpected, or otherwise) before age 50 years due to heart disease, in at least one relative
7. Disability from heart disease in a close relative <50 years of age
8. Specific knowledge of certain cardiac conditions in family members: hypertrophic or dilated cardiomyopathy, long QT syndrome or other ion channelopathies, Marfan syndrome, or clinically important arrhythmias

PHYSICAL EXAMINATION

9. Heart murmur[‡]
10. Femoral pulses to exclude aortic coarctation
11. Physical stigmata of Marfan syndrome
12. Brachial artery blood pressure (sitting position)[§]

From Maron BJ, Thompson PD, Ackermann MJ et al: Recommendations and considerations related to preparticipation screening of cardiovascular abnormalities in competitive athletes, *Circulation* 115:1643-1655, 2007.
*Parental verification is recommended for high school and middle school athletes.
[†]Judged not to be neurocardiogenic (vagal); of particular concern when related to exertion.
[‡]Auscultation should be performed in both supine and standing positions (or with Valsalva maneuver), specifically to identify murmurs of dynamic left ventricular outflow tract obstruction.
[§]Preferably taken in both arms.

College athletes should be evaluated before training and competition and annually for the next 3 years.

Cardiologists use 2D echo to reliably diagnose HCM. The diastolic LV wall thickness ≥15 mm (or on occasion, 13 or 14 mm), usually with LV dimension <45 mm, is accepted for the clinical diagnosis of HCM in adults. For children, a z-score of 2 or more relative to body surface area is theoretically compatible with the diagnosis. Some highly trained athletes may show hypertrophy of the LV wall, but an LV wall thickness of 13 mm and greater is very uncommon in highly trained athletes and is always associated with an enlarged LV cavity (with LV diastolic dimension greater than 54 mm).

C. CLASSIFICATION OF SPORTS

For the purpose of making recommendation on athletes' participation eligibility, Task Force 8 of the 36th Bethesda Conference (Mitchell JH, et al. J Am Coll Cardiol 2005) has presented the following classification of sports (Fig. 6-3). In this method, sports are classified into dynamic and

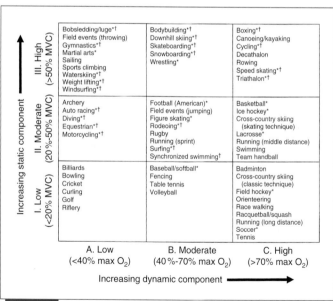

FIG. 6-3

Classification of sports. Max O_2, maximal oxygen uptake; MVC, maximal voluntary contraction. *Danger of bodily collision. †Increased risk if syncope occurs. (*Modified from Mitchell JH, Haskell W, Snell P et al: Task Force 8: classification of sports,* J Am Coll Cardiol 45:1364-1367, 2005.)

static exercises, and each sport is categorized by the level of intensity (low, medium, high).

There are two broad types of exercise: dynamic and static. Dynamic exercise causes a marked increase in cardiac output, heart rate, stroke volume, and systolic BP and a decrease in diastolic pressure and systemic vascular resistance. Static exercise, in contrast, causes a small increase in cardiac output and heart rate and a marked increase in systolic, diastolic, and mean arterial pressures but no appreciable change in total peripheral resistance. Thus, dynamic exercise primarily causes a volume load on the left ventricle, whereas static exercise causes a pressure load.

D. ELIGIBILITY DETERMINATION OF ATHLETES WITH CARDIOVASCULAR DISEASE

Most of the following recommendations are summarized from the 36th Bethesda Conference. These recommendations apply to athletes in high school and college. For further details on a specific condition, readers are encouraged to refer to the original article.

It should be noted that β-blockers used to treat certain heart conditions and arrhythmias are expressly banned in sports like riflery (class IA) and archery (class IIA) in which the athlete would benefit from a slow heart rate. Therefore, β-blockers should not be prescribed for athletes in these sports because it would put them at risk of having a positive drug test.

1. **Acyanotic congenital heart defects.** Participation eligibility of athletes with acyanotic heart diseases (e.g., L-R shunt lesions and obstructive lesions) is primarily determined by the level of PA systolic pressure and the status of left ventricular (LV) systolic function.
   a. Pulmonary artery systolic pressure (PA SP)
      (1) When PA SP is ≤30 mm Hg in the cardiac catheterization laboratory (or Doppler-estimated PA systolic pressure <36 to 40 mm Hg), full participation in all competitive sports is allowed.
      (2) When PA SP >30 mm Hg (or Doppler-estimated PA systolic pressure >36 to 40 mm Hg), a full evaluation will determine limitations in participation eligibility. With mild PH, low-intensity sports (class IA) are permitted. With PVOD, no competitive sports are allowed.
   b. LV systolic function
      (1) When LV ejection fraction (EF) is ≥50%, full participation is allowed.
      (2) With mild LV dysfunction (EF 40% to 50%), low-intensity static sports (class IA, IB, and IC) are allowed.
      (3) With moderate to severe LV dysfunction (EF <40%), no competitive sports are allowed.
2. **Cyanotic congenital heart defects.** In patients with arterial oxygen desaturation from cyanotic CHD, moderate to severe restriction in sports participation is recommended.

a. Patients with cyanotic CHDs, which are unoperated or for which palliative procedures have been done, can participate only in low-intensity competitive sports, such as class IA.

b. Most patients with cyanotic CHD for which surgical repair has been done can participate only in low-intensity sports.

c. Patients who have received an excellent result from the surgical repair of TOF or arterial switch operation for TGA may participate in all competitive sports.

3. **Coronary artery abnormalities.** For most patients with congenital abnormalities of the coronary arteries or following Kawasaki disease, moderate to severe restriction in sports participation is recommended. Those children who had no coronary artery involvement during the acute phase of Kawasaki disease may participate in all sports 6 to 8 weeks after the illness. Stress testing is often required before prescribing participation eligibility.

4. **Valvular heart diseases.** The severity of the valvular lesion determines eligibility of participation in competitive sports.

a. For patients with mild valvular lesions (such as MS, MR, AS, and AR), participation in all competitive sports is allowed.

b. For patients with moderate valvular lesions, participation is limited to low-intensity to moderate-intensity sports.

c. For patients with severe obstructive lesions such as severe AS, participation in competitive sports is not permitted.

d. For patients with valvular lesions that produce significant pulmonary hypertension, no participation in competitive sports is permitted.

e. For those patients with a prosthetic valve and who are taking warfarin, no sports involving the risk of bodily contact are allowed.

5. **Cardiomyopathy, pericarditis, and other myocardial diseases**

a. Athletes who have either a confirmed or probable diagnosis of HCM or arrhythmogenic RV dysplasia are excluded from most competitive sports, with the possible exception of class IA sports.

b. Athletes with myocarditis or pericarditis of any etiology should be excluded from all competitive sports during the acute phase. After complete recovery from these illnesses, they may gradually participate in sports.

c. Athletes with Marfan syndrome can participate only in class IA or IB sports.

d. Athletes with mitral valve prolapse who have any symptoms or abnormalities in ECG, LV function, or arrhythmias are permitted to participate only in low-intensity sports.

E. CARDIAC ARRHYTHMIAS AND SPORTS

1. The presence of a symptomatic cardiac arrhythmia requires exclusion from physical activity until this problem can be adequately evaluated and controlled by a cardiologist.

2. Patients with PACs can participate in all competitive sports.

3. Asymptomatic athletes with atrial flutter or fibrillation and a structurally normal heart may participate in competitive sports when the arrhythmias are fully under control either by medication or ablation.

4. Athletes with SVT and a structurally normal heart may participate in all competitive sports when the SVT is in full control with medication or following successful ablation.

5. For athletes with a structurally normal heart who have PVCs or more complex arrhythmias, an exercise stress test is a useful technique. If the PVCs disappear when the heart rate reaches 140 to 150 beats per minute, the PVCs are benign and full participation may be permitted.

6. Athletes with ventricular tachycardia (VT) who had successful treatment to prevent recurrence of the arrhythmias may participate in sports, provided that VT is not inducible by exercise-stress test or electrophysiologic study.

7. Asymptomatic adult athletes with WPW preexcitation with no history of SVT may participate in all competitive sports, but children with the same diagnosis require in-depth evaluation.

8. Athletes with long QT syndrome can participate only in class IA sports.

9. Athletes who had a successful ablation for any of the arrhythmias may participate in all competitive sports after verification of the success by appropriate tests.

10. Athletes with structural heart disease and an arrhythmia can participate in sports within the limits determined by the structural defect, usually class IA sports.

11. Athletes who have a pacemaker implanted and those who are on anticoagulants should not be permitted to engage in activities with danger of bodily collision. Participation in class IA sports is usually permitted.

12. Athletes with first-degree AV block or Mobitz type 1 second-degree AV block can participate in all sports provided the block does not worsen with exercise.

13. Athletes with Mobitz type 2 second-degree AV block or complete heart block usually require pacemaker implantation before being permitted to participate in any sports.

14. Asymptomatic athletes with right bundle branch block (RBBB) or left bundle branch block (LBBB) who do not have ventricular arrhythmias or develop AV block during exercise can participate in all sports. However, patients with LBBB who have an abnormal prolongation of HV interval on an electrophysiologic study should receive a pacemaker.

F. ATHLETES WITH SYSTEMIC HYPERTENSION

Reports of cerebrovascular accident during maximal exercise have raised concerns that the rise in BP accompanying strenuous activity may cause harm. Task Force 5: Systemic Hypertension, 36th Bethesda Conference on Eligibility Recommendation for competitive sports has recommended the following (summarized from Kaplan NM, et al. *J Am Coll Cardiol* 2005;1346-1348):

1. Athletes with prehypertension
a. These athletes may participate in physical activity but should be encouraged to modify lifestyle (such as weight control).
b. If prehypertension persists, echo studies are done to see if there is left ventricular hypertrophy (LVH) (beyond that seen with "athletes' heart").
c. If LVH is present, athletic participation is limited until BP is normalized by appropriate drug therapy.
2. Athletes with stage 1 hypertension
a. These athletes may participate in any competitive sport, in the absence of target organ damage, including LVH or concomitant heart disease. However, hypertension should be checked every 2 to 4 months (or more frequently) to monitor the impact of exercise.
b. If LVH is present, athletic participation is limited until BP is normalized by appropriate drug therapy.
3. Athletes with stage 2 (severe) hypertension: Even in the absence of target organ damage (such as LVH), athletic participation should be restricted, particularly from high static sports (class IIIA, IIIB, and IIIC), until their hypertension is controlled by either lifestyle modification or drug therapy.
a. All drugs being taken must be registered with appropriate governing bodies to obtain a therapeutic exemption. When hypertension coexists with another cardiovascular disease, eligibility for participation in competitive sports is usually based on the type and severity of the associated condition.
b. With respect to the treatment of hypertension, β-blockers are not banned for most sports, including football and basketball. However, β-blockers are banned for riflery or archery. In addition, athletes with essential hypertension do not tolerate β-blockers well because they reduce their maximum performance. One should, therefore, avoid treating hypertensive athletes with β-blockers. Instead, ACE inhibitors are preferred. One should be aware of potential teratogenic effects of ACE inhibitors if taken during pregnancy. Calcium channel blockers may also be used instead of β-blockers in treating hypertension.

VIII. DYSLIPIDEMIA

High levels of total cholesterol and low-density lipoprotein cholesterol (LDL-C) and low levels of high-density lipoprotein cholesterol (HDL-C) are all risk factors for coronary atherosclerosis. A link has been established between increased levels of triglycerides and coronary heart disease as well. Cholesterol reduction results in reduced angiographic progression of coronary artery disease and even modest regression in some cases. The National Cholesterol Education Program (NCEP) Expert Panel on Blood Cholesterol Levels in Children and Adolescents (1991) recommended strategies for the prevention and detection of hyperlipidemia in children in the hope of preventing or retarding the progress of atherosclerosis.

A. MEASUREMENT OF CHOLESTEROL AND LIPOPROTEINS

1. The child does not have to be fasting for the measurement of total cholesterol.

2. A lipoprotein analysis is obtained by measuring total cholesterol, HDL, and triglyceride levels after an overnight fast of 12 hours. The LDL level is usually estimated by the Friedewald formula.

$$LDL \equiv Total\ cholesterol - HDL - (Triglyceride/5)$$

a. This formula is not accurate if the child is not fasting, if the triglyceride level is >400 mg/100 mL, or if chylomicrons or dysbetalipoproteinemia (type III hyperlipoproteinemia) is present. Methods are currently available to measure LDL-C directly, which allow LDL-C determination on specimens with the triglyceride level >400 mg/dL. Direct LDL-C measurement does not require a fasting specimen.

b. Children and adolescents with total cholesterol >200 mg/dL, LDL-C >130 mg/dL, HDL-C <40 mg/dL, or triglycerides >200 mg/dL need to be evaluated for possible dyslipidemia. (For adults, the desirable level of triglycerides is <150 mg/dL.) Cholesterol levels are reasonably consistent after 2 years of age (with some small increment during adolescence). Table C-1, Appendix C, provides age-specific percentile values for total cholesterol, LDL-C, HDL-C, and triglycerides.

3. Other useful derivatives of lipid profile are as follows:

a. Total cholesterol-to-HDL ratio: The usual total cholesterol/HDL-C ratio in children is approximately 3 (based on total cholesterol of 150 mg/dL and an HDL-C of 50 mg/dL). The higher the ratio, the higher is the risk of developing cardiovascular disease.

b. Non-HDL-C: Serum non-HDL-C is obtained by subtracting HDL-C from total cholesterol. It consists of all classes of atherogenic (apoprotein B–containing) lipoproteins, including VLDL-C, intermediate density lipoproteins (IDL), LDL-C, and lipoprotein (a) (or Lp[a]). In children, normal non-HDL-C is higher than LDL-C by 13 to 17 mg/dL.

B. GENETIC LIPOPROTEIN DISORDERS

1. **Primary hypercholesterolemia.** Young patients with elevated LDL-C levels are more likely to have a familial disorder of LDL metabolism. Screening of all family members is recommended to determine whether the disorder is familial and to emphasize the need for all family members to change their eating patterns.

a. Familial hypercholesterolemia (FH). Familial hypercholesterolemia is caused by a lack of or a reduction in LDL receptors, which normally take up approximately 70% of circulating LDL.

HETEROZYGOUS FH

(1) This autosomal dominant disorder is fairly common, occurring in 1 of every 500 people, in which about a 50% reduction in LDL receptors is present. In this condition one parent and one out of

two siblings have severe elevation of total and LDL-C levels, but unaffected first-degree relatives have completely normal levels. Total cholesterol and LDL-C levels are 2 to 3 times higher than normal. Affected individuals' total cholesterol levels are most often >240 mg/100 mL (with an average value of 300 mg/100 mL) and their LDL-C levels are greater than 160 mg/100 mL (with an average value of 240 mg/100 mL). Triglycerides and HDL-C are usually in the normal ranges or only mildly abnormal.

(2) Physical examination is usually normal. Tendon xanthomas are rarely found before the age of 10 years. They are seen in the Achilles tendons and extensor tendons of the hands, in the second decade, in only 10% to 15% of patients. The presence of xanthomas in the parents of such children almost confirms the diagnosis. Angina pectoris may develop in the late teenage years. Secondary hypercholesterolemia should be ruled out by basic laboratory tests (hypothyroidism, liver disease, and renal disease).

(3) Treatment of heterozygotes includes a diet low in cholesterol and saturated fat and water-soluble fibers. Recent reports show that statins are safe, effective, and well tolerated (see later section). One should evaluate family members for the condition as well. Bile acid sequestrants are rarely used because of gritty texture and gastrointestinal complaints.

HOMOZYGOUS FH

(1) Homozygotes have little or no receptor activity. This rare condition occurs in about one in a million. The total cholesterol and LDL-C levels are 5 to 6 times greater than normal. Cholesterol levels average 700 mg/100 mL but may reach higher than 1000 mg/100 mL. Both parents must have severe elevations in LDL-C. Triglyceride levels are usually normal or mildly elevated and HDL-C levels are normal or slightly low.

(2) Clinical findings may include the following: Planar xanthomas (orange-colored skin lesions) may be present by the age of 5 years in the webbing of the hands and over the elbows and buttocks. Tendon xanthomas, especially on extensor tendons of the hands or Achilles tendon, occur by the age of 10, with articular symptoms such as tendinitis or arthralgia. Arcus corneae and clinically significant coronary artery disease (CAD) are often present in the first decade of life. The murmur of aortic stenosis may develop (due to the generalized atherosclerosis of the aortic valve).

(3) Children with homozygous FH respond somewhat to high doses of potent statins and to niacin. Cholesterol absorption inhibitors (CAI) also lower LDL to some extent, especially in combination with a more potent statin. However, most FH homozygotes will require LDL apheresis (with extracorporeal affinity LDL absorption column and plasma reinfusion) every 2 weeks to lower LDL-C to a range that is less atherogenic. The Liposorber system is an

example that selectively binds apo B–containing lipoproteins (LDL, Lp[a], and VLDL). Liver transplantation may be indicated in selected cases.

2. **Hypertriglyceridemia**

a. Familial combined hyperlipidemia (FCH)

   (1) In FCH, both the levels of cholesterol and triglycerides are increased. This autosomal dominant condition is more common than FH. It occurs in families of survivors of myocardial infarction, presenting with variable phenotypic expression: elevated LDL level alone (type IIa), elevated LDL-C with hypertriglyceridemia (type IIb), or normal LDL-C with hypertriglyceridemia (type IV). Clinically, it may be difficult to separate this entity from FH.

   (2) The diagnosis of FCH is suspected when a first-degree family member (often a parent or sibling) has a different lipoprotein phenotype than the proband. LDL-C levels fluctuate from time to time, with triglyceride levels fluctuating in the opposite direction. Plasma total cholesterol levels are usually between 190 and 220 mg/100 mL. The LDL-C level is usually normal or only mildly elevated. HDL-C levels are often decreased. The elevated triglyceride levels are generally due to an increase in VLDL. In FCH, most patients lack tendon xanthomas, and extreme hyperlipidemia is absent in childhood. Their phenotypes often have other characteristics such as hyperinsulinemia, glucose intolerance, hypertension, and visceral obesity. The combined expression of three or more of these traits constitutes the metabolic syndrome.

   (3) Treatment of FCH includes a low-fat diet, weight reduction, and regular aerobic exercise. Statins are the most effective in lowering LDL-C. Fibric acid and niacin, which are effective in adults, are not ordinarily used in pediatric patients. Metformin has been used to treat obese hyperinsulinemic adolescents with the metabolic syndrome. Metformin may enhance insulin sensitivity and reduce fasting blood glucose, insulin levels, plasma lipids, free fatty acids, and leptin.

b. Familial hyperchylomicronemia (type I hyperlipoproteinemia)

   (1) Hypertriglyceridemia results from markedly reduced or absent lipoprotein lipase (LPL) activity, with resulting increase in the level of chylomicrons and VLDL, especially after meals.

   (2) Fasting plasma triglyceride levels are markedly elevated (>1000 mg/dL) and rarely as high as 10,000 mg/dL. Recurrent bouts of pancreatitis are common, which occurs when triglyceride levels exceed 1000 mg/dL. Eruptive xanthomas and lipemia retinalis (a creamy appearance of the retinal veins and arteries due to a high concentration of lipids in the blood) can also be found. Plasma from these patients may be milky white, and a clear band of chylomicrons can be seen on top of the plasma.

    (3) Treatment of acute pancreatitis includes an intravenous hydration and avoidance of fat in the diet. Plasma filtration is required only rarely. Treatment of chronic pancreatitis includes avoidance of dietary fats and alcohol. Short-chain fatty acids (which are not incorporated in chylomicrons) can be used to supplement the diet.

  c. Familial hypertriglyceridemia (type IV hyperlipoproteinemia)

    (1) This disorder is caused by hepatic overproduction of VLDL-C. Lipolysis by LPL does not appear to be a rate-limiting factor.

    (2) This condition is not associated with clinical signs such as arcus corneae and xanthoms. Plasma triglyceride levels are moderately to markedly elevated (200 to 500 mg/dL). LDL-C and HDL-C levels are usually low. Total cholesterol is normal or elevated depending on VLDL-C levels. Hypercoagulable state may result.

    (3) Treatment is based on lifestyle modification, including a low-fat and low-calorie diet, limiting carbohydrate intake, weight control, limiting alcohol intake, and increasing exercise. Statins may be used if diet is ineffective and cardiovascular risk factors are present.

  d. Dysbetalipoproteinemia (type III hyperlipoproteinemia). This is a rare genetic disorder caused by a defect in apo E, which results in increased accumulation of chylomicron remnants and VLDL remnants. Patients with this disorder have increased cardiovascular risk. Palmar xanthomas may be present. Cholesterol and triglyceride levels are equally elevated to greater than 300 mg/dL, but this disorder is not usually seen in childhood. A low-fat diet, treatment of metabolic syndrome, and drug treatment (fibric acid or statin) are very effective.

3. Low levels of HDL-C: Familial hypoalphalipoproteinemia (low HDL syndrome)

  a. In this rare genetic form of low HDL-C, apo A-I and apo A-II concentrations are decreased and apo C-III is absent. Several variants have been identified, which include familial apo A-I deficiency, familial apo A-I structural mutations, familial LCAT deficiency, fish eye disease, Tangier disease, and familial hypoapo-lipoproteinemia. Frederickson classification does not include this group of conditions. In *Tangier disease* (first identified in the Chesapeake Bay Island of Tangier in the United States), HDL-C is nearly absent (with markedly enlarged yellow tonsils). LDL-C levels in affected individuals are low, which appears to have a protective effect.

  b. Secondary causes of low HDL-C are more common than the genetic form. The following are some examples of secondary causes of low HDL-C levels.

    (1) High triglyceride levels (which push down HDL-C levels)

    (2) Diets very high in carbohydrates (>60% of total calories) or polyunsaturated fats

    (3) Metabolic syndrome

    (4) Inactivity (obesity)

    (5) Others—cigarette smoking and hypertension

c. In general, familial forms present with much lower levels of HDL-C than the secondary forms (20 to 39 mg/dL).

d. There is no drug that specifically raises HDL-C levels. The primary target is to lower the LDL-C level to reduce cardiovascular risks. If, however, the triglyceride levels are very high (>500 mg/dL), hypertriglyceridemia should be addressed first. Although drugs are rarely used in cases of isolated low HDL-C, niacin is the most effective agent currently available. Lifestyle modification for weight loss and aerobic exercise are important. Fish oil capsules may be beneficial.

C. NONFAMILIAL AND SECONDARY DYSLIPIDEMIA

Nonfamilial (or polygenic) hypercholesterolemia is much more common than familial (or primary) hypercholesterolemia. Several disease states (hypothyroidism, renal disease, and liver disease) and drugs (progestins, anabolic steroids, glucocorticoids) are associated with the secondary form of hypercholesterolemia.

1. **Nonfamilial hypercholesterolemia**

a. Nonfamilial or polygenic hypercholesterolemia is the most common form of elevated serum cholesterol concentrations, occurring in 26% of American adults. This condition is caused by a susceptible genotype aggravated by excessive intake of saturated fat, trans–fatty acid, and cholesterol.

b. Some patients with mixed dyslipidemias probably have nonfamilial hypercholesterolemia that manifests as elevated LDL-C levels and insulin resistance. The latter manifests as low HDL-C levels, high triglyceride levels, or both. Cholesterol is moderately elevated (240 to 350 mg/dL), and serum triglyceride levels are in the normal range. Hypercholesterolemia does not produce symptoms. Tendon xanthomas are not present in nonfamilial hypercholesterolemia. (Their presence suggests familial hypercholesterolemia or familial defective apoprotein B-100.)

c. Treatment of mild to moderate hypercholesterolemia includes lifestyle modification with a low-fat diet and regular exercise. Although exercise has little effect on LDL-C concentration per se, aerobic exercise may improve insulin sensitivity, HDL-C concentrations, and triglyceride levels and thus may help reduce CAD risk. "Statins" are the most effective drugs in lowering LDL-C levels.

2. **Secondary dyslipoproteinemia**

a. Secondary dyslipoproteinemias result from other underlying disorders and increase predisposition to premature CAD and pancreatitis.

b. The following are causes of secondary dyslipidemia in children.

    (1) Disease states

        (a) Hypothyroidism

        (b) Metabolic (diabetes, metabolic syndrome)

        (c) Hepatic disease (biliary cirrhosis)

        (d) Renal (chronic renal failure, nephrotic syndrome, and glomerulonephritis)

    (2) Lifestyle: obesity, physical inactivity, diets rich in fat and saturated fat, alcohol intake

    (3) Medications: thiazide diuretics, β-adrenergic blockers, glucocorticoids, certain anticonvulsants, estrogens, testosterones, oral contraceptives, isotretinoin (Accutane), anabolic steroids, immunosuppressive agents (cyclosporine).

c. All children with LDL-C levels ≥130 mg/dL or triglyceride levels ≥150 mg/dL need to be evaluated for possible secondary dyslipoproteinemia. In addition to a careful history and physical examination (including weight status), determination of blood glucose levels and appropriate tests of liver, kidney, and thyroid function may be indicated. Lipoprotein patterns may differ according to the causes of dyslipidemia (Table 6-13).

d. Treatment of the underlying condition when possible or discontinuation of the offending drugs usually leads to an improvement in the hyperlipidemia. Specific lipid-lowering therapy may be required in certain circumstances.

D. CHOLESTEROL-LOWERING STRATEGIES

The NCEP Expert Panel has recommended two complementary approaches: a population approach and an individualized approach.

1. **Population approach.** For children older than 2 years of age, the following are recommended.

a. Nutritional adequacy should be achieved by eating a wide variety of foods.

b. Adequate calories should be provided for normal growth and development.

c. The following pattern of nutrient intake is recommended (the same as a step-one diet of the AHA).

    (1) Saturated fatty acids less than 10% of total calories.

    (2) Total fat ≤30% of total calories.

    (3) Dietary cholesterol less than 300 mg/day.

TABLE 6-13

LIPOPROTEIN PATTERNS IN SECONDARY DYSLIPIDEMIA

LCL-C	TG	HDL-C	CONDITIONS
↑	↑		1. Hypothyroidism
			2. Glomerulonephritis, nephrosis
			3. Thiazide diuretics, retinoic acid
	↑	↓	1. Metabolic syndrome, diabetes, obesity
			2. β-blockers
			3. Corticosteroids and immunosuppressive agents (glucocorticoids and cyclosporine)
			4. Chronic renal failure
	↑	↑	Estrogen

2. **Individualized approach**
a. The NCEP Expert Panel recommends *selective* screening of children and adolescents who meet the following specific criteria.
   (1) Patients whose parents or grandparents, at ≤55 years of age for men and ≤65 years of age for women, had coronary atherosclerosis after angiography or underwent balloon angioplasty or coronary artery bypass surgery
   (2) Patients whose parents or grandparents, at ≤55 years of age for men and ≤65 years of age for women, had documented MI, angina pectoris, peripheral vascular disease, cerebrovascular disease, or sudden cardiac death
   (3) The offspring of a parent who had high total cholesterol levels (≥240 mg/100 mL)
   (4) Children and adolescents whose parental or grandparental history is unobtainable, particularly those with other risk factors
b. The Panel's recommendations for selective screening are controversial. Several studies published in the pediatric literature have indicated that more than 60% of children with high LDL levels will be missed if a positive family history of premature CAD is used as the sole screening criterion. Some authorities recommend general screening of preschool children. Given the current state of knowledge, optional cholesterol testing by the practicing physician may be appropriate in children judged to be at higher risk for CAD.
c. The Expert Panel's recommendations on the initial laboratory tests are as follows:
   (1) For high parental cholesterol levels, the initial step is measurement of total cholesterol.
   (2) For children who have positive family histories (as listed previously), a lipoprotein analysis is recommended.
d. The Panel further recommends follow-up plans according to the levels of cholesterol or LDL-C.
   (1) For those children who had total cholesterol levels measured, the levels are classified as acceptable (<170 mg/dL), borderline (170 to 199 mg/dL), and high (≥200 mg/dL), and the follow-up plans are summarized in Fig. 6-4.
   (2) For those children who had LDL levels measured, the levels are classified as acceptable (LDL-C <110 mg/dL), borderline (110 to 129 mg/dL), or high (≥130 mg/dL), and specific recommendations for each group of patients are shown in Fig. 6-5.

E. **MANAGEMENT**
1. **Hypercholesterolemia**
a. Diet therapy is prescribed in two steps that progressively reduce the intake of saturated fatty acids and cholesterol.

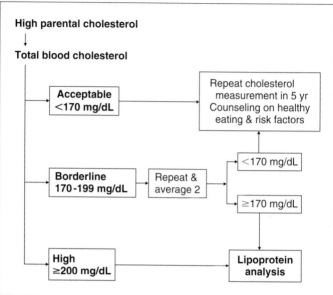

High parental cholesterol
↓
Total blood cholesterol

- **Acceptable** <170 mg/dL → Repeat cholesterol measurement in 5 yr Counseling on healthy eating & risk factors
- **Borderline** 170-199 mg/dL → Repeat & average 2 → <170 mg/dL / ≥170 mg/dL
- **High** ≥200 mg/dL → Lipoprotein analysis

FIG. 6-4

The Expert Panel's recommendations on the initial laboratory test and follow-up plans on children whose parents have high levels of cholesterol. *(Modified from Expert Panel on Blood Cholesterol Levels in Children and Adolescents: National Cholesterol Education Program, NIH Publication No. 91-2732, September 1991.)*

    (1) The step-one diet is recommended, which is the same nutrient intake as recommended in the population approach to lowering cholesterol levels (Table 6-14).

    (2) If the step-one diet fails to achieve the minimal goals of therapy in 3 months, the step-two diet is prescribed (Table 6-14). This diet further reduces the saturated fatty acid intake to less than 7% of calories and the cholesterol intake to less than 200 mg a day.

  b. Drug therapy

    (1) The NCEP Expert Panel recommends drug therapy in children age 10 years and older if an adequate trial of diet therapy (6 months to 1 year) fails to achieve the goal, specifically for the following groups of children.

      (a) Children with LDL-C level ≥190 mg/100 mL, with a negative or unobtainable family history of premature coronary cardiovascular disease

      (b) Children with LDL-C level ≥160 mg/100 mL *plus*

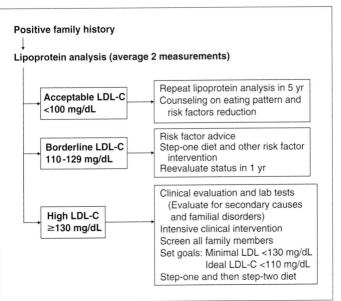

Positive family history

↓

Lipoprotein analysis (average 2 measurements)

Acceptable LDL-C <100 mg/dL	Repeat lipoprotein analysis in 5 yr Counseling on eating pattern and risk factors reduction
Borderline LDL-C 110-129 mg/dL	Risk factor advice Step-one diet and other risk factor intervention Reevaluate status in 1 yr

High LDL-C ≥130 mg/dL	Clinical evaluation and lab tests
	  (Evaluate for secondary causes
	  and familial disorders)
	Intensive clinical intervention
	Screen all family members
	Set goals: Minimal LDL <130 mg/dL
	        Ideal LDL-C <110 mg/dL
	Step-one and then step-two diet

FIG. 6-5

The Expert Panel's recommendations on the initial laboratory test and follow-up plans on children who have positive family history of coronary artery disease. *(Modified from Expert Panel on Blood Cholesterol Levels in Children and Adolescents: National Cholesterol Education Program, NIH Publication No. 91-2732, September 1991.)*

> (i) A positive family history of premature cardiovascular dis-
>   ease (before 55 years of age in men and before 65 years
>   in women), or
> (ii) Two or more other cardiovascular disease risk factors
>   (e.g., low HDL-C levels, cigarette smoking, high BP, obe-
>   sity, diabetes) (Box 6-10) or metabolic syndrome (see Box
>   6-12 for the definition) is present

(2) Two classes of pharmaceutical agents are currently used in children over 10 years with sufficiently elevated LDL-cholesterol levels. They are bile acid sequestrants (cholestyramine, colestipol)
and HMG-CoA reductase inhibitors (statins). Bile acid sequestrants are used only rarely because of their gritty texture and gastrointestinal complaints. The efficacy of Ezetimibe, a cholesterol
absorption inhibitor, in preventing CAD has recently been questioned, and it is not yet approved by the Food and Drug Administration (FDA) for use in children. Nicotinic acid and fibrates are
not routinely used in pediatrics.

TABLE 6-14

NUTRIENT COMPOSITION OF STEP-ONE AND STEP-TWO DIETS

NUTRIENT	STEP-ONE DIET	STEP-TWO DIET
Total fat (% total calories)	<30%	<30%
Saturated fatty acids	<10%	<7%
Polyunsaturated fatty acids	Up to 10%	Up to 10%
Monounsaturated fatty acids	10%-15%	10%-15%
Carbohydrates (% total calories)	50%-60%	50%-60%
Protein (% total calories)	10%-20%	10%-20%
Cholesterol (per day)	<300 mg	<200 mg
Total calories	To achieve and maintain desirable weight	To achieve and maintain desirable weight

(3) "Statins" (hydroxymethylglutaryl-coenzyme [HMG-CoA] reductase inhibitors) are widely used to lower total cholesterol and LDL-cholesterol in adults. Numerous studies have demonstrated the safety and efficacy of statins in adolescents with FH. Four statins—atorvastatin, lovastatin, pravastatin, and simvastatin—are currently approved by the FDA for use in adolescents. Statins lower LDL-C by inhibiting HMG-CoA reductase, the enzyme that regulates the rate-limiting step in cholesterol synthesis. The amount of the intermediate (i.e., mevalonate) is lowered, and, subsequently, cholesterol levels are reduced in hepatic cells. This, in turn, results in up-regulation of LDL receptors and increased hepatic uptake of LDL from the circulation. Periodic measurements of ALT, AST (preferred because it is also found in muscles), and creatine phosphokinase (CPK) should be taken to assess for possible adverse effects of the statins (when lipid levels are measured). Side effects of statins reported in adolescents include the following:
  (a) An increase in liver enzymes (up to 3 times the upper limits of normal) with high doses of statins
  (b) Instances of asymptomatic increases in CPK
  (c) Rarely muscle pain or weakness, myositis, rhabdomyolysis with renal failure
(4) Based on recently published clinical trials in children and adolescents, the following may be a reasonable pediatric dosage of the four statins that are approved for pediatric use. In pediatric trials, starting doses were usually half of the adult lower-range dose, increased by 10 mg every 4 to 8 weeks to a half dose or full dose of the upper-range adult dosage with periodic measurements of cholesterols. The final maintenance dosage of the drug is decided by periodic determinations of cholesterol levels.

(a) Atorvastatin (Lipitor): Starting dose of 10 mg is increased to 20 mg at 4 to 6 weeks, and further to 40 mg/day (maximum adult dose is 80 mg/day).

(b) Lovastatin (Mevacor): Starting dose is 10 mg/day for 6 to 8 weeks, with a 10-mg increase every 6 to 8 weeks, to a maximum 40 mg/day.

(c) Pravastatin (Pravachol): Starting dose of 10 mg/day is increased to 20 or 40 mg/day.

(d) Simvastatin (Zocor): Starting dose is 10 mg, increment of 10 mg every 6 to 8 weeks to maximum 40 mg/day.

2. **Hypertriglyceridemia**

a. A very low-fat diet (10% to 15% of calories) that can be supplemented by medium chain triglycerides (MCT). Portagen, a soybean-based formula enriched in MCT, is available for infants with LPL deficiency. Lipid-lowering drugs are ineffective in LPL deficiency.

b. The primary aim of therapy is to reach the LDL goal by the use of statins, intense weight management, and an increase in physical activity.

c. If triglycerides are ≥200 mg/dL when the LDL goal is reached, nicotinic acid or fibrate alone—or better, in combination with a statin—may be used to reduce the non-HDL-cholesterol level to the level of 30 mg/dL + LDL goal.

d. A prescription omega-3 fatty acid product (e.g., Omacor) 4 g/day and 8 g/day reduced triglyceride levels by 30% and 43%, respectively, from baseline values. (Most fish oil capsules have an omega-3 fatty acid content only a third of that contained in Omacor.) Omega-3 fatty acid plus a statin may be an effective alternative to a fibrate or niacin plus a statin.

3. **Low levels of HDL-cholesterol.** Statins that are effective in lowering LDL-cholesterol are not very effective in raising HDL-cholesterol. The following has been suggested for adults to raise low levels of HDL-cholesterol.

a. Regular exercise. Thirty minutes of brisk aerobic exercise every day or every other day is recommended.

b. Weight control. Every 3 kg of weight loss results in a 1 mg/dL increase in HDL.

c. Diet low in saturated fat and rich in polyunsaturated fatty acids. Examples are oils (olive, canola, soy, flaxseed), nuts (almonds, peanuts, walnuts, pecans), coldwater fish (salmon, mackerel), and shellfish.

d. Consumption of high glycemic index carbohydrates should be avoided.

e. Drugs

(1) Niacin is the most effective therapy for raising HDL-C (20% to 35% increase).

(2) Fibrate raises HDL-C 10% to 25%.

f. Fish oil capsules containing omega-3 fatty acids may be beneficial.

g. For adult patients, quitting smoking can raise HDL an average 4 mg/dL. Mild to moderate consumption of alcohol (one to two drinks a day) can raise 4 mg/dL of HDL_3 subfraction (but should not be recommended for those with liver disease or addiction problems).

IX. PREVENTIVE CARDIOLOGY

The primary mission of pediatrics has been prevention of disease and ensuring normal growth and development. It is natural for pediatricians to pay attention to early detection of children at risk of developing cardiovascular disease (and type 2 diabetes) and provide counseling, intervention, and/or treatment whenever possible.

A. CHILDHOOD ONSET OF ATHEROSCLEROSIS

Atherosclerotic cardiovascular disease is a major cause of morbidity and mortality and is responsible for more than 50% of all the deaths in the United States and other Western countries. Atherosclerotic lesions start to develop in early childhood and progress to irreversible lesions in adolescence and adulthood. The strongest evidence of childhood onset of coronary artery disease comes from the Bogalusa Heart Study and the Pathological Determinants of Atherosclerosis in Youth (PDAY) Research Group. Autopsy studies found that atherosclerosis originates in childhood, with a rapid increase in the prevalence of coronary pathology during adolescence and young adulthood. Fatty streak, the earliest lesion of atherosclerosis, occurred by 5 to 8 years of age and fibrous plaque, the advanced lesion, appeared in the coronary arteries in subjects in their late teens. Fibrous plaque was found in more than 30% of 16- to 20-year-old patients, and the prevalence of the lesion reached nearly 70% by age 26 to 39. These studies also confirmed that the extent of pathologic changes in the aorta and coronary arteries increased with age and that the number of known cardiovascular risk factors (Box 6-10) that the individual had at the time of death.

B. MAJOR CARDIOVASCULAR RISK FACTORS

The major risk factors for the development of coronary artery disease are listed in Box 6-10. A family history of premature CAD in first-degree relatives (parents and siblings) is the single best predictor of risk for adults. For children, however, family history includes the first- *and* second-degree relatives (including parents, siblings, grandparents, or blood-related aunts and uncles) who have or had CAD before age 55 for males and before age 65 for females. The reason that the second-degree relatives are included in family history for children is because some children's parents are too young to have developed clinical CAD when their children are examined.

C. DYSLIPIDEMIAS AS CAUSES OF CORONARY ATHEROSCLEROSIS

The pathogenesis of atherosclerosis and death from CAD has significant links to high levels of total cholesterol and LDL-C and low levels of HDL-C. Recently, a link has also been established between increased levels of

---

BOX 6-10

MAJOR RISK FACTORS FOR CORONARY HEART DISEASE

Family history of premature coronary heart disease, cerebrovascular or occlusive
    peripheral vascular disease (with onset before age 55 years for men and
    65 years for women in parents or grandparents)
Cigarette smoking
Hypercholesterolemia
Hypertension (BP >140/90 mm Hg or on antihypertensive medication)
Low levels of high-density lipoprotein (<40 mg/100 mL)
Diabetes mellitus (as a coronary heart disease risk equivalent)

Adapted from Summary of the Third Report of the National Cholesterol Education Program
(NCEP) Expert Panel on Detection, Education, and Treatment of High Blood Cholesterol in Adults
(Adult Treatment Panel III) final report, *Circulation* 106:3143-3421, 2002.

---

triglycerides and CAD. Cholesterol reduction results in reduced angiographic
progression and even modest regression of CAD in some cases.

D. OBESITY AND ITS COMORBIDITY AS CARDIOVASCULAR RISK FACTORS

Recent studies have shown that obesity is a risk factor for CAD independently of the standard risk factors, probably through the emerging risk factors. The emerging risk factors, which are commonly found in obese persons, include atherogenic dyslipidemia (also known as "lipid triad," which
consists of raised levels of triglycerides and small LDL particles and low
levels of HDL-C), insulin resistance (hyperinsulinemia), a proinflammatory
state (elevation of serum high-sensitivity C-reactive protein), and a prothrombotic state (increased amount of plasminogen activator inhibitor-1
[PAI-1]). The cluster of these risk factors occurring in one person is known
as "the metabolic syndrome." In metabolic syndrome, LDL-C levels may not
be elevated but apoprotein B (apo B) and small LDL particles are elevated;
the smallest particles in the LDL fraction are known to have the greatest
atherogenicity. This syndrome occurs more commonly in individuals with
abdominal (visceral) obesity, although there are exceptions, especially in individuals from Asia. With increasing adiposity, the lipid triad becomes more
pronounced. Hispanics and South Asians seem to be particularly susceptible to the syndrome. Black men have a lower frequency of the syndrome
than do white men.

Clinically identifiable components of the metabolic syndrome for
adults are listed in Box 6-11. The presence of at least three risk factors
is required to make the diagnosis of the metabolic syndrome in adults.
Evidence has supported that waist circumference (reflecting visceral
adiposity) is a better predictor of cardiovascular disease than body mass
index (BMI). Other components of metabolic syndrome, such as proinflammatory and prothrombotic states, are not routinely measured in

---

BOX 6-11

CLINICAL IDENTIFICATION OF THE METABOLIC SYNDROME IN ADULTS

The presence of at least three of these abnormalities constitutes metabolic syndrome.

1. Abdominal obesity: men, waist circumference ≥40 inches (102 cm); women, ≥35 inches (88 cm)
2. Elevated triglyceride ≥150 mg/dL
3. Reduced HDL-cholesterol: men <40 mg/dL; women <50 mg/dL
4. Hypertension ≥130/85 mm Hg
5. Elevated fasting glucose ≥100 mg/dL*

Adapted from Grundy SM, Hansen B, Smith SC, et al. Clinical management of metabolic syndrome. Report of the American Heart Association/National Heart, Lung, and Blood Institute/American Diabetes Association Conference on scientific issues related to management. *Circulation* 109:551-556, 2004.

*The American Diabetes Association (ADA) has recently established a cutpoint of ≥100 mg/dL, above which persons either have prediabetes (impaired fasting glucose) or diabetes. The original report of the conference recommended elevated fasting glucose level as ≥110 mg/dL.

---

clinical practice. C-reactive protein ≥3 mg/L may be significant in adults.

A direct association between obesity and insulin resistance also exists in children. Pediatric definition of the metabolic syndrome is shown in Box 6-12. As in adults, waist circumference is a better predictor of cardiovascular disease in children than body mass index. Fasting glucose level ≥100 mg/dL may be appropriate for children as well. The presence of at least three of the risk factors is required to make the diagnosis of the metabolic syndrome in children. The prevalence of the metabolic syndrome in overweight adolescents is about 30% to 50%.

There are significant differences in waist circumference (WC) according to ethnicity and gender (see Tables C-2, C-3, and C-4, Appendix C). In general, Mexican American (MA) boys and girls have higher WCs than counterparts of other ethnicities. Children with WCs at the 75th and 90th percentile are at an increased risk for cardiovascular and metabolic disorders (with significantly higher levels of total cholesterol, BP, and triglycerides and lower levels of HDL-cholesterol). BMI percentile curves are presented as Figures C-1 and C-2, Appendix C.

Prevention of the metabolic syndrome may prevent CAD. The mainstay of prevention is achieving optimum weight, normal BP, and normal lipid profile by dietary intervention and promotion of active lifestyle. Each component of the metabolic syndrome present should be treated aggressively to reduce cardiovascular risk factors and prevent diabetes. Pharmacologic intervention is usually not required in children, but drugs may be used on selected high-risk patients.

BOX 6-12

PROPOSED DEFINITION OF THE METABOLIC SYNDROME IN ADOLESCENTS

The presence of at least three of these abnormalities constitutes metabolic syndrome.

1. Triglycerides ≥110 mg/dL
2. HDL-cholesterol ≤40 mg/dL
3. Waist circumference ≥90th percentile (see Tables C-2, C-3, and C-4, Appendix C) or body mass index ≥95th percentile (see Figs. C-1 and C-2, Appendix C)
4. Fasting glucose ≥110 mg/dL
5. Systolic blood pressure ≥90th percentile for age and gender

From Cook S, Weitzman M, Auinger P et al: Prevalence of a metabolic syndrome phenotype in adolescents: findings from the third National Health and Nutrition Examination Survey, 1988-1994, *Arch Pediatr Adolesc Med* 157:821-827, 2003.

Weight reduction is of prime importance in managing the metabolic syndrome. All successful pediatric weight management programs include four components: (1) dietary component, (2) exercise, (3) behavior modification, and (4) family component. Among these, dietary intervention and regular exercise combined are the cornerstones of weight management. Only through behavior modification can long-term healthy eating and activity patterns be established; attempts at employing diet and exercise for quick weight loss usually fail. Without involvement of the parents and family, behavior modification in children and adolescents is difficult to achieve. Consultations with registered dietitians, psychologists, and/or exercise specialists may be sought or a referral to a multidisciplinary weight management program may become necessary.

E.   CIGARETTE SMOKING AS A CARDIOVASCULAR RISK FACTOR

Cigarette smoking is a powerful independent risk factor for myocardial infarction, sudden death, and peripheral vascular disease. Even passive exposure to smoke causes alterations in the risk factors in children.

The prevalence of cigarette smoking nationwide among high school students remains high. Current use of any tobacco product ranges from 13% among middle school students to 28% among high school students. Among college students, 33% are current users of tobacco products. There are usually smokers in the household of middle school and high school student smokers.

Physicians should assess the status of smoking, provide smoking prevention messages, and help counsel parents and children about smoking cessation. The following are some pathophysiologic effects of smoking on the cardiovascular system, which can be used in counseling patients to stop smoking. All of the pathophysiologic effects are involved in accelerating atherosclerosis in the coronary and peripheral arteries or increasing the probability of thrombosis (with potential for stroke).

1. Atherogenic dyslipidemia (increasing LDL and VLDL cholesterols and triglycerides and lowering HDL-C levels)
2. Prothrombotic predisposition: increasing levels of fibrinogen, factor VII, and other factors involved in the fibrin clotting cascade and decreasing the concentration of plasminogen; it also activates platelets, increasing their ability to adhere to the vessel wall
3. Increase in blood viscosity by increasing hemoglobin levels (through carbon monoxide–induced increase in carboxyhemoglobin) and by an elevation of plasma fibrinogen levels
4. Acceleration of the atherosclerotic process by increasing monocyte adhesion to endothelial cell (the initial step in atherogenesis), by decreasing nitric oxide synthesis (with resulting endothelial dysfunction), and by decreasing synthesis of prostacycline
5. Peripheral arterial disease through endothelial dysfunction
6. Increase in BP, heart rate, and myocardial oxygen consumption (by stimulation of sympathetic nervous system)

F. PRACTICE OF PREVENTIVE CARDIOLOGY

Atherosclerotic cardiovascular disease has its onset during childhood. The prevalence of obesity is increasing during childhood with its comorbidities (the metabolic syndrome) (Box 6-12). Intervention to reduce the cardiometabolic risk factors in childhood has been successful with low-calorie diets, smoking prevention, an increase in physical activities, and family-based weight control programs. This is due to the fact that some of the risk factors are detectable, modifiable, or treatable.

1. Family history of cardiovascular disease is very important in assessing a child's risk of developing CAD later in life. Although it is not modifiable, its presence is a marker for a high risk of heart disease. A history of premature CAD in first- or second-degree relatives (parents, siblings, grandparents, or blood-related aunts and uncles) before age 55 for males and before age 65 for females should prompt physicians to check on other risk factors.
2. Hypercholesterolemia is a major risk factor that is identifiable and treatable.
3. Hypertension is also an identifiable and treatable risk factor.
4. Other risk factors, such as smoking, consumption of atherogenic diets, and physical inactivity, are all modifiable by behavior changes.
5. Obesity is easily detectable. Although treatment of obesity can be frustrating to both patient and physician, patient education and behavior modification can be productive.
6. Inclusion of HbA_{1c} should be considered in the screening protocol to detect a diabetic or prediabetic state.
7. The American Heart Association has updated a guideline for the prevention of cardiovascular disease. Table 6-15 is a summary of goals and recommendations for reducing risks in children and adolescents identified as high risks for future cardiovascular disease.

TABLE 6-15

SUMMARY GUIDELINES FOR PREVENTIVE PEDIATRIC CARDIOLOGY

RISK IDENTIFICATION	TREATMENT GOALS	RECOMMENDATIONS
Blood cholesterol		
Total cholesterol:	Goals:	If LDL-C is above goals, initiate additional therapeutic lifestyle
>170 mg/dL is borderline	LDL-C <160 mg/dL (<130 mg/dL is even	changes, including diet (<7% of calories from saturated fat;
>200 mg/dL is elevated	better)	<200 mg cholesterol per day), in conjunction with a trained
LDL-C:	For patients with diabetes, LDL-C <100 mg/dL	dietitian.
>110 mg/dL is borderline		Consider LDL-lowering dietary options (increase soluble fiber by using
>130 mg/dL is elevated		age [in years] plus 5-10 g up to age 15, when the total remains at
		25 g per day) in conjunction with a trained dietitian.
		Emphasize weight management and increased physical activity.
		If LDL-C is persistently above goals, evaluate for secondary causes
		(thyroid-stimulating hormone, liver function tests, renal function
		tests, urinalysis).
		Consider pharmacologic therapy for individuals with LDL
		>190 mg/dL with no other risk factors for CVD, or >160 mg/dL
		with other risk factors present (blood pressure elevation, diabetes,
		obesity, strong family history of premature CVD).
		Pharmacologic intervention for dyslipidemia should be accomplished
		in collaboration with a physician experienced in treatment of disor-
		ders of cholesterol in pediatric patients.

cont'd

TABLE 6-15—cont'd

SUMMARY GUIDELINES FOR PREVENTIVE PEDIATRIC CARDIOLOGY

RISK IDENTIFICATION	TREATMENT GOALS	RECOMMENDATIONS
Other lipids and lipoprotein		
Triglycerides: >150 mg/dL	Goals: Fasting TG <150 mg/dL	Elevated fasting TG and reduced HDL-C are often seen in the context of overweight with insulin resistance. Therapeutic lifestyle change should include weight management with appropriate energy intake and expenditure. Decrease intake of simple sugars.
HDL-C: <40 mg/dL	HDL-C >40 mg/dL	If fasting TG are persistently elevated, evaluate for secondary causes such as diabetes, thyroid disease, renal disease, and alcohol abuse. No pharmacologic interventions are recommended in children for isolated elevation of fasting TG unless this is very marked (treatment may be initiated at TG >400 mg/dL to protect against postprandial TG of 1000 mg/dL or greater, which may be associated with an increased risk of pancreatitis).
Blood pressure		
Systolic and diastolic pressure >95th percentile for age, sex, and height percentile	Goals: Systolic and diastolic blood pressure <95th percentile for age, sex, and height	Promote achievement of appropriate weight. Reduce sodium in the diet. Emphasize increased consumption of fruits and vegetables. If BP is persistently above the 95th percentile, consider possible secondary causes (e.g., renal disease, coarctation of the aorta). Consider pharmacologic therapy for individuals above the 95th percentile if lifestyle modification brings no improvement and there is evidence of target organ changes (left ventricular hypertrophy, microalbuminuria, retinal vascular abnormalities). Start blood pressure medication individualized to other patient requirements and characteristics (i.e., age, race, need for drugs with specific benefits)

Weight BMI: >85th percentile is at risk of overweight >90th percentile is overweight	Achieve and maintain BMI <95th percentile for age and sex	Pharmacologic management of hypertension should be accomplished in collaboration with a physician experienced in pediatric hypertension. For children who are at risk of overweight (>85th percentile) or obesity (>95th percentile), a weight management program should be initiated with appropriate energy balance achieved through changes in diet and physical activity. For children of normal height, a secondary cause of obesity is unlikely. Weight management should be directed at all family members who are overweight, using a family-centered, behavioral management approach. Weight management should be done in collaboration with a trained dietitian.
Diabetes	Near normal fasting plasma glucose (<120 mg/dL) Near normal HgA1c (<7%) (goals for fasting glucose and HgA1c should take into consideration age and risk of hypoglycemia)	Management of type 1 and type 2 diabetes in children and adolescents should be accomplished in collaboration with a pediatric endocrinologist. For type 2 diabetes, the first step is weight management with improved diet and exercise. Because of risk for accelerated vascular disease, other risk factors (e.g., blood pressure, lipid abnormalities) should be treated more aggressively in patients with diabetes.
Cigarette smoking	Complete cessation of smoking for children and parents who smoke	Advise every tobacco user (parents and children) to quit and be prepared to provide assistance with this (counseling/referral to develop a plan for quitting using available community resources to help with smoking cessation).

Modified from Kavey RW, Daniels SR, Lauer RM et al: American Heart Association guidelines for primary prevention of atherosclerotic cardiovascular disease beginning in childhood. *Circulation* 107:1562-1566, 2003.

Management of Cardiac Surgical Patients

Mehrdad Salamat, MD, FAAP, FACC

The current trend is to carry out total repair of congenital heart defects (CHDs) at an early age whenever such repair is technically possible. Early total repair may obviate the need for palliative procedures. It may also prevent pulmonary vascular disease or permanent damage to the cardio-vascular system, which is known to develop in certain CHDs. However, recommendations for the timing and type of operation vary from institution to institution. The improved results currently seen with pediatric cardiac surgery are in part attributed to improved operative technique and cardio-pulmonary bypass (CPB) methods. In addition, a coordinated multidisci-plinary approach has contributed to a significant decrease in perioperative morbidity and mortality.

7

Open heart procedures use CPB with some degree of hypothermia and a varying duration of low flow or circulatory arrest. Open procedures are required for repair of intracardiac anomalies (e.g., ventricular septal defect [VSD], tetralogy of Fallot [TOF], transposition of the great arteries [TGA]). Closed procedures do not require CPB; they are performed for repair of extracardiac anomalies (e.g., coarctation of the aorta [COA], patent ductus arteriosus [PDA]) or palliative procedures (e.g., S-P shunt procedures or pulmonary artery [PA] banding). The following sections outline some basic aspects of preoperative and postoperative management of cardiac patients for pediatricians.

I. PREOPERATIVE MANAGEMENT

Good preoperative preparation, including complete delineation of cardiac anatomy and assessment of hemodynamics, is mandatory for a smooth op-erative and postoperative course. Some infants require preoperative stabili-zation with prostaglandin E_1 (continuous IV drip at 0.01 to 0.1 mcg/kg/min) to maintain ductus arteriosus patency while others may need inotro-pic and lusiotropic support. Patients with TGA and restrictive patent fora-men ovale (PFO) may require balloon atrial septostomy.

1. All children should have a careful history and physical examination within a few days before the procedure. This is to gain full understanding of chronic medical problems (e.g., renal dysfunction, asthma) and to uncover acute medical problems (e.g., upper and lower respiratory and urinary tract infections) that would mandate rescheduling of elective surgeries.

2. Laboratory evaluation

a. Complete blood count, urinalysis, serum electrolytes and glucose, blood urea nitrogen (BUN), and serum creatinine of all cardiac patients are routinely obtained.

b. Chest x-ray (CXR) film and ECG of all patients are obtained.

c. Head and renal ultrasound is performed in all neonates with significant congenital heart defects.

d. For open heart procedures, blood coagulation studies—prothrombin time (PT), activated partial thromboplastin time (aPTT), and platelet count—are obtained.

e. If necessary, blood should be collected for chromosome studies (karyotyping and fluorescence in situ hybridization).

3. Patients undergoing CPB whose weight is more than 3.5 kg are cross-matched for four units of packed red blood cells (PRBCs) and those weighing less for two units of whole blood. One to two units of PRBCs are cross-matched for those undergoing closed procedures. In addition, one to four units of platelets are needed for the procedure. Irradiated blood products will be required for immunocompromised patients (e.g., patients with suspected or confirmed chromosome 22 microdeletion).

4. Medications

a. Digoxin is discontinued after the evening dose.

b. Diuretics are discontinued 8 to 12 hours preoperatively (or this may be individualized).

c. Antiarrhythmics are continued at the same dosage until immediately before the surgery.

d. Nonsteroidal antiinflammatory drugs (e.g., aspirin, ibuprofen) and antiplatelet drugs (e.g., dipyridamole) are discontinued 7 to 10 days prior to surgery.

e. Warfarin is discontinued 4 days prior to the planned operation. If the patient is at high risk for thromboembolism, a continuous heparin drip is started 2 days prior to the operation and the infusion rate is adjusted to maintain an aPTT of 60 to 85 seconds.

5. Prevention of infection: Broad-spectrum antibiotics are used to decrease the risk of perioperative infection. These are continued until all chest tubes and intracardiac and vascular monitoring lines are removed.

a. Clindamycin, 10 mg/kg/dose (adolescents/adults: 600 mg/dose) IV every 6 to 8 hours, starting immediately prior to surgery, is the recommended regimen at some institutions.

b. Vancomycin, 10 to 15 mg/kg/dose IV every 6 to 8 hours (maximum dose 4 g/day), and ceftazidime, 40 mg/kg/dose IV every 8 hours (maximum dose 6 g/day), or another third-generation cephalosporin, or gentamicin, 2.5 mg/kg/dose IV every 8 to 12 hours, is used for patients with open chest.

c. A thin layer of mupirocin 2% ointment is applied to both nostrils to prevent methicillin-resistant *Staphylococcus aureus* (MRSA) colonization.

6. For older children the emotional preparation for surgery is as important as the physical preparation.

II. POSTOPERATIVE CARE OF CARDIAC PATIENTS

A high level of vigilance for signs of complications should be maintained during the postoperative period so that appropriate therapy can be initiated early.

A. NORMAL CONVALESCENCE

Physicians should be familiar with the postoperative course of normally recovering patients in order to recognize abnormal convalescence.

1. General care: Successful postoperative management requires accurate monitoring and documentation of the patient's vital signs, medication administration, and laboratory results. Vital signs, including heart rate, arterial or noninvasive blood pressure, oxygen saturation, and respiratory rate, are monitored closely (e.g., every 15 to 60 minutes). Urine and chest tube outputs, end-tidal or transcutaneous CO_2, central venous pressure, and at times, right and left atrial, and pulmonary arterial pressures are recorded meticulously. All administered medications, enteral or parenteral fluids, and blood products are documented. Fluid balance is monitored continuously. Laboratory results and their trends are charted for review.

2. Pulmonary system
a. Arterial blood gases are in the acceptable normal range.
b. CXR films show no evidence of pneumothorax, atelectasis, pleural effusion, or elevation of hemidiaphragm.

3. Cardiovascular system
a. Warm skin, full peripheral pulses with brisk capillary refill, normal blood pressure (BP), and an adequate urine output (at least 1 mL/kg/hr) are clinical evidence of good cardiac output. Decrease in expected systemic venous saturation is a sensitive predictor of low cardiac output. A normal systemic arterial-to-venous oxygen saturation difference of less than 30% is indicative of good cardiac output.
b. Mild arterial hypertension is present in the early postoperative period following CPB (due to increased levels of catecholamines, plasma renin, or angiotensin II).
c. Cardiac rhythm should be sinus and the heart rate relatively high. Ranges of heart rate (beats/min) in normally convalescing postoperative patients are as follows:
   (1) Less than 6 months: 110 to 190
   (2) 6 to 12 months: 100 to 170
   (3) 1 to 3 years: 90 to 160
   (4) Over 3 years: 80 to 150

4. Renal system: Adequate urine output (i.e., above 1 mL/kg/hr) and evidence of adequate solute excretion (e.g., serum K^+ below 5 mEq/L; BUN below 40 mg/dL; creatinine below 1 mg/dL) are signs of normal renal function.

5. Metabolic system

a. Retention of water and sodium and depletion of whole-body potassium are commonly seen following open heart surgery. They result in mild hyponatremia and hypokalemia and a 5% weight gain. In anticipation of fluid overload, mechanical ultrafiltration is performed in selected cases intraoperatively.

b. Mild metabolic acidosis (with a base deficit of -4 mEq/L) associated with mild lactic acidemia is common in the first few hours after CPB and does not usually require treatment.

c. Varying degrees of fever are nearly always present during the first few days, and extensive workup for infection is not indicated. Causes of fever include reaction to CPB, reaction to homologous blood, atelectasis, pleural effusion, low cardiac output, infection, and brainstem damage.

6. Gastrointestinal system: As the splanchnic circulation receives over 25% of total cardiac output, avoidance of low cardiac output syndrome is the principal strategy to prevent gastrointestinal (GI) dysfunction. Feedings are started after the patient becomes hemodynamically stable and are advanced as tolerated. Daily caloric count and its adjustment are crucial. H_2-receptor antagonists (e.g., ranitidine, 1 mg/kg/dose IV every 6 to 8 hours) are initiated for gastric protection.

7. Hematologic system: Clotting studies should be normal, and hemoglobin should be at least 9.5 g/dL or higher depending on the patient's age, cardiac anatomy, and surgical procedure.

8. Neurologic system: The patient should respond appropriately for the level of sedation without evidence of neurologic defects (e.g., hemiplegia, visual field defects) or seizures. Near infrared spectroscopy (NIRS) for transcranial cerebral oximetry is a noninvasive method to monitor frontal lobe oxygen metabolism. Cerebral oxygen saturation, measured by NIRS, is a composite of the oxygen saturation in combined cerebral arterial and venous vascular bed (arterial and venous blood flow ratio of approximately 25:75, with negligible capillary blood). It is a helpful method to detect cerebral hypoxia during low cardiac output states.

B. CARE FOLLOWING AN UNCOMPLICATED OPERATION

Postoperative care in congenital cardiac surgery is extremely unique due to the complexity and heterogeneity of cardiac defects and the wide age range of patient population. Furthermore, the guidelines for postoperative management differ from institution to institution, making this task even more complicated. Although the following recommendations are only one set of these guidelines, one aspect of successful management remains the same: anticipation of possible complications (e.g., decrease of cardiac index 6 to 12 hours postoperatively, pulmonary hypertension in association with particular defects, arrhythmias after specific surgeries, etc.).

1. General care

a. Fluid replacement: Because of the tendency to retain sodium and water, a minimal amount of dextrose in water without sodium ($D_{10}W$

in infants, D_5W in children) or with only a small amount of sodium (D_{10} ¼ NS, D_5 ¼ NS) is administered for approximately 48 hours after surgery. A modest amount of potassium (e.g., KCl, 4 mEq/100 mL IV fluids) is given on the first day of surgery. Recommended fluid volume in the first 24 hours after open procedures is 50% of maintenance volume with a gradual increase over the following postoperative days to 60% and then to 75%.

b. The patient should receive medications for adequate analgesia and sedation. For pain relief, fentanyl (IV drip at 1 to 3 mcg/kg/hr or 1 to 2 mcg/kg/dose IV every 30 to 60 minutes) or morphine sulfate (IV drip at 0.01 to 0.05 mg/kg/hr or 0.1 to 0.2 mg/kg/dose IV every 2 to 4 hours, maximum dose 15 mg/dose) is commonly used. Sedation is achieved by administration of midazolam (0.05 to 0.15 mg/kg/dose IV every 1 to 2 hours or IV drip at 1 to 2 mcg/kg/min) or other benzodiazepams.

2. Pulmonary system

a. Extubated patients should show no signs of respiratory distress (grunting, nasal flaring, and retraction). Good chest expansion and evidence of good air exchange to both lungs should be present. Depending on the hemodynamics or cardiopulmonary pathophysiology, patients may be administered supplemental oxygen via nasal cannula or face mask. Pulmonary physiotherapy (consisting of incentive spirometry, coughing and deep breathing exercise, and chest percussion with postural drainage) is administered as necessary.

b. In intubated patients, CXR films are obtained to check the position of chest tubes and central and arterial lines and to check for evidence of pneumothorax, atelectasis, pleural effusion, or main-stem bronchus intubation. Significant degrees of pneumothorax or pleural effusion may require treatment. Widening of the mediastinal shadow suggests accumulation of blood and requires investigation of the function of the mediastinal chest tube.

(1) In the first postoperative days the goal of ventilation is to maintain adequate arterial partial pressure of oxygen (Pao_2), and mild respiratory alkalosis along with an arterial partial pressure of carbon dioxide ($Paco_2$) between 28 and 35 mm Hg (all to decrease pulmonary vascular resistance [PVR]). Hyperventilation ($Paco_2$ below 28 mm Hg) is corrected by decreasing the ventilator rate, decreasing the tidal volume, and adding dead space (5 to 10 mL at a time) to the airway. Hypoventilation is corrected by the opposite maneuvers. Low Pao_2 is corrected by raising the Fio_2, adding positive-end expiratory pressure (PEEP), or increasing tidal volume. Physiologic PEEP of 3 to 5 cm H_2O is used in children. The use of high mean airway pressure or high levels of PEEP may increase PVR and decrease cardiac output; both should be avoided in a patient who has had a Senning procedure or cavopulmonary anastomosis (e.g., Glenn or Fontan operation).

(2) Tracheal toilet is carried out through the endotracheal tube every 2 hours or more often if necessary. It consists of instillation of 0.5 to 5 mL of saline and suctioning of both main-stem bronchi and bag ventilation for 1 to 2 minutes with oxygen (Fio_2 1) immediately before and after suctioning.

c. Extubation is performed as soon as possible, usually in the operating room in children undergoing closed procedures, within 4 to 8 hours after uncomplicated open heart procedures, and the day after complex open procedures. Criteria for extubation include the following:

  (1) The patient should be awake and alert and should have a favorable nutritional status.

  (2) The patient should be breathing well, with a satisfactory spontaneous respiratory rate for age and no use of accessory respiratory muscles. Ideally, vital capacity should be more than 15 mL/kg. On minimal ventilatory support (Fio_2 no more than 0.4, tidal volume at 8 to 10 mL/kg, and PEEP no more than 5 cm H_2O), there should be adequate Pao_2 and no evidence of acidosis or hypercapnia.

  (3) The patient should be in a reasonable and stable hemodynamic state (normal BP, adequate cardiac output, no significant arrhythmias). There should be no significant pneumothoraces or pleural effusions. The patient should not have important bleeding and should have minimal chest tube drainage.

  (4) Postextubation laryngeal edema is treated with racemic epinephrine (2.25% solution; 0.125 to 0.5 mL diluted with 3 mL of water or normal saline given via nebulizer).

d. Postoperative *pulmonary hypertensive crisis* leads to decreased cardiac output and, if untreated, may be fatal. The best strategy is prevention. Measures to prevent pulmonary hypertensive crisis are important for patients who had severe pulmonary arterial hypertension preoperatively. The following are recommended.

  (1) Adequate analgesia and sedation.

  (2) Paralysis by vecuronium bromide (continuous IV drip at 0.05 to 0.15 mg/kg/hr or intermittent IV infusion of 0.05 to 0.1 mg/kg/dose every 60 minutes) or pancuronium bromide (continuous IV drip at 0.02 to 0.1 mg/kg/hr or intermittent IV infusion of 0.05 to 0.1 mg/kg/dose every 30 to 60 minutes).

  (3) Supplemental oxygen.

  (4) Low PEEP.

  (5) Maintaining alkalotic pH.

  (6) Avoidance of deep and vigorous tracheal aspiration.

  (7) Administration of inhaled nitric oxide (selective pulmonary vasodilator) at 5 to 40 parts per million (usual range 5 to 20 parts per million).

  (8) Intravenous vasodilators (α-adrenergic antagonists, phosphodiesterase inhibitors, nitrovasodilators, and prostaglandins) may be

considered. However, it should be noted that essentially all these agents dilate the systemic vasculature as well, leading to systemic hypotension.

3. Cardiovascular system: Complete correction of the intracardiac defect and adequate intraoperative myocardial protection generally will result in good cardiac function. Signs of reduced cardiac output, abnormal blood pressures, abnormal heart rate, and abnormal rhythm should be monitored continuously.

a. *Low cardiac output syndrome* (LCOS) is the most serious condition of abnormal convalescence. Signs of LCOS include systemic vasoconstriction (poor perfusion, cold extremities, weak pulses), resting tachycardia, oliguria, pulmonary venous congestion (rales, rhonchi), and systemic venous congestion (hepatomegaly, anasarca, ascites). Systemic hypotension may be a late result of LCOS and is an ominous sign. Laboratory findings include metabolic acidosis, lactic acidemia, azotemia, reduced creatinine clearance, rising serum K^+, decreased partial central venous pressure of oxygen (Pvo$_2$) below 30 mm Hg from right atrium (RA) or central venous line, and increased arterial-to-venous oxygen saturation difference of more than 40%. Inadequate cardiac output may be caused by (1) low preload, (2) high afterload, (3) depressed myocardial contractility, (4) cardiac tamponade, (5) arrhythmias, (6) inadequate surgical repair, and (7) pulmonary hypertension. Treatment is directed at the cause.

(1) Low preload may be due to intravascular volume depletion (manifested by decreased RA and left atrium [LA] pressures) or due to diminished blood flow to the left ventricle (LV) (e.g., pulmonary venous obstruction, PA hypertension, pulmonary stenosis [PS], or right ventricle [RV] failure in the absence of adequate intraatrial shunting; evident by elevated RA and decreased LA pressure). In the case of mitral stenosis (MS), which also decreases LV preload, RA and LA pressures are both elevated. Though all these conditions ultimately reduce the LV preload and subsequently the cardiac output, treatment is specific to each condition. Low intravascular volume is treated with IV crystalloid or colloid to increase the intravascular volume to raise central venous pressure to 10 to 15 mm Hg. Other conditions are treated by eliminating the cause.

(2) High afterload (with increased systemic vascular resistance [SVR]) may be caused by hypoxia, acidosis, hypothermia, or pain. In addition to the correction of the cause, the elevated SVR is treated with afterload reduction.

(a) Phosphodiesterase inhibitors (e.g., milrinone, amrinone) play a crucial role in treatment of LCOS. They have not only vasodilatory effects but also lusiotropic and inotropic effects without being arrhythmogenic. These effects occur without an increase in myocardial oxygen consumption. Milrinone is usually initiated in the operating room and is continued as an IV drip at a rate of 0.1 to 1 mcg/kg/min (usual range 0.25 to 0.75 mcg/kg/min) postoperatively.

(b) Nitroprusside (IV drip at 0.3 to 10 mcg/kg/min) or nitroglycerin (IV drip at 0.5 to 6 mcg/kg/min) can be used to further reduce elevated SVR. Both agents have a favorable effect on PVR. In addition, nitroglycerin is a potent coronary vasodilator, which may be beneficial after an arterial switch operation.

(c) Nesiritide, human recombinant form of B-type natriuretic peptide (BNP), promotes not only vasodilation but also diuresis and natriuresis. The experience in children is still limited. A loading dose of 2 mcg/kg IV, followed by infusion of 0.005 to 0.01 mcg/kg/min, has been used in adult trials.

(d) Phenoxybenzamine, a long-acting α-adrenergic blocking agent, is used in selected postoperative patients at some centers.

(3) Depressed myocardial contractility (demonstrated by echo) may be treated by optimizing arterial oxygen saturation, treatment of anemia and acidemia, and administration of inotropic agents. The optimal oxygenation is achieved by maintaining a patent airway with good respiratory care, adjusting Fio_2 if necessary, reducing pulmonary shunting by the use of PEEP, and reducing pulmonary edema by the use of diuretics. The following inotropic agents may be used.

(a) Epinephrine (IV drip at a rate of 0.01 to 0.05 mcg/kg/min; low dose to minimize undesirable α-agonist effects).

(b) Dopamine (continuous IV drip, starting at 2.5 mcg/kg/min and increasing up to 10 mcg/kg/min if necessary).

(c) Isoproterenol or dobutamine may be gradually added if epinephrine and/or dopamine are not effective.

(d) Milrinone (by inhibition of type-III phosphodiesterase, it increases intracellular cAMP, which ultimately augments myocardial contractility) is started with or without a loading dose of 50 mcg/kg and is maintained at an infusion rate of 0.25 to 1 mcg/kg/min.

(4) Cardiac tamponade is treated with urgent decompression of the pericardial space. Early cardiac tamponade results from persistent surgical bleeding not properly drained by the chest tubes; it may even occur when the pericardium is removed or left widely open. It must be suspected when the chest tube drainage abruptly decreases or stops in a patient with previously significant bleeding. Characteristically, the patient is tachycardic and hypotensive with narrowed pulse pressure. Atrial pressures are elevated. Response to volume administration and inotropic agents is minimal. CXR shows widening of the cardiac silhouette. Echo demonstrates pericardial effusion and diastolic collapse of the RA and RV, a sensitive indicator of tamponade. Cardiac tamponade requires prompt pericardiocentesis or surgical exploration for evacuation of the

pericardial hematoma or control of bleeding by urgent opening of the sternotomy, often in the intensive care unit.

(5) Sinus bradycardia or tachycardia may be detrimental in a postoperative patient with limited cardiac reserve.

    (a) Attention to detail is necessary to unmask secondary causes of sinus bradycardia such as medication interaction, hypoxia, hypoglycemia, electrolyte imbalance, increased intracranial pressure, and hypothyroidism. Injury to sinus node or its artery, particularly during Fontan procedure or atrial switch operations (Senning and Mustard), may occur, resulting in persistent sinus bradycardia. If necessary, patients are treated with atrial or ventricular pacing or chronotropic agents. Atrial and ventricular pacing wires are usually placed at the time of open heart procedures and are left postoperatively until desired heart rate and atrioventricular (AV) synchrony are returned and maintained.

    (b) Extreme sinus tachycardia is treated by eliminating causes (e.g., pain, anemia, fever, volume depletion, chronotropic agents). Administration of catecholamines should be minimized, as excessive tachycardia increases myocardial oxygen consumption. Furthermore, tachycardia shortens the diastolic period and consequently reduces coronary blood flow.

    (c) Treatments of other arrhythmias are described in a section to follow.

(6) Revision of surgical repair is occasionally indicated when an inadequate repair (such as a large residual L-R shunt or significant residual COA) is the cause of low cardiac output. Echo and, if necessary, cardiac catheterization may reveal residual defect and its significance.

(7) Pulmonary hypertensive crisis is characterized by an acute rise in PA pressure followed by a reduction in cardiac output and a fall in arterial oxygen saturation. It occurs in neonates and infants who have had CHDs with pulmonary hypertension (e.g., complete endocardial cushion defect [ECD], persistent truncus arteriosus), often after vigorous suctioning of the endotracheal tube. It is difficult to treat and may be fatal; prevention is critically important (see General Care earlier in this chapter). Treatment includes sedation, paralysis, supplemental oxygen, and inhaled nitric oxide.

b. Hypotension and hypertension

    (1) Hypotension, caused by low intravascular volume, recognized by low RA (central venous) and LA pressure, is treated as follows:

        (a) Volume expanders or PRBCs are given as an IV bolus (initially 5 to 10 mL/kg, up to 20 mL/kg). As transfused citrated blood binds ionized calcium, replacement of calcium is necessary to maintain BP and cardiac output.

        (b) Inotropic agents are used if volume expansion fails to raise BP.

      (c) Vasopressin (IV drip at 0.0003 to 0.01 U/kg/min) may be considered in patients with adequate myocardial function but with severe vasodilatory hypotension.

    (2) Severe hypertension is treated with vasodilators (see previous discussion of low cardiac output syndrome earlier in this chapter).

c. Rhythm disorders: Sinus rhythm and maintenance of AV synchrony is optimal. Junctional rhythm may reduce cardiac output by 10% to 15%. In addition to the specific treatment for arrhythmias, possible causes should be investigated and corrected (e.g., oxygenation status, acid-base status, electrolyte imbalance, arrhythmogenic medications). If the patient is hemodynamically unstable, defibrillation or synchronized cardioversion should not be delayed.

    (1) Infrequent and isolated premature atrial contractions (PACs) or premature ventricular contractions (PVCs) are followed without intervention.

    (2) Paroxysmal supraventricular tachycardia (SVT) (AV node and accessory pathway reentry tachycardia) is treated with the drug of choice, adenosine (rapid IV bolus of 0.1 mg/kg/dose followed by rapid saline flush; if unsuccessful, subsequent doses can be increased to 0.2 mg/kg). Intermittent episodes of SVT are treated with IV amiodarone (loading dose: 5 to 10 mg/kg, followed by IV drip at a rate of 5 to 15 mcg/kg/min). Persistent SVT may also be treated with overdrive suppression or synchronized cardioversion. Other medications such as β-receptor blockers, verapamil, procainamide, and digoxin may be used with caution (taking into account myocardial function, BP stability, ventricular preexcitation, etc.).

    (3) Other SVTs (multifocal atrial tachycardia or ectopic atrial tachycardia) are treated by ventricular rate control with medications such as amiodarone, β-receptor blockers, calcium channel blockers, or digoxin.

    (4) Atrial flutter is treated with overdrive atrial pacing (through esophageal or intraoperatively placed temporary atrial leads) or synchronized cardioversion. Procainamide (loading dose: 2 to 6 mg/kg, maximum dose 100 mg/dose followed by IV continuous drip at 20 to 80 mcg/kg/min, maximum 2 g/day) and/or digoxin is the pharmacologic approach for this condition.

    (5) Atrial fibrillation is treated with digoxin or procainamide (in stable patients) or cardioversion (in hemodynamically compromised patients). If unsuccessful, ventricular rate control is the management of choice.

    (6) Postoperative junctional ectopic tachycardia (JET) is a serious and life-threatening arrhythmia. Tachycardia and loss of AV synchrony are responsible for decreasing the cardiac output. Treatment is aimed at both derangements. AV synchrony may be achieved by AV sequential pacing at a rate higher than the JET

rate. However, rate control is more challenging. Lowering the infusion rate of catecholamines (proarrhythmogenic), sedation, fever control, induced hypothermia (34° C to 35° C) using cooling blanket, IV amiodarone, or a combination of IV procainamide and hypothermia are strategies that may be beneficial in ventricular rate control.

(7) Frequent PVCs, if hemodynamically significant, are managed by avoiding arrhythmogenic drugs; optimizing hemodynamic status; or correcting electrolyte imbalance, hypoxia, and acidemia, and they are suppressed with lidocaine (IV bolus 1 mg/kg followed by continuous drip at 20 to 50 mcg/kg/min).

(8) Monomorphic VT with adequate perfusion is treated with amiodarone (loading dose: 5 to 10 mg/kg, followed by IV drip at a rate of 5 to 15 mcg/kg/min), lidocaine (IV bolus of 1 mg/kg, followed by IV drip at 20 to 50 mcg/kg/min), procainamide (loading dose: 2 to 6 mg/kg, maximum dose 100 mg/dose, followed by IV continuous drip at 20 to 80 mcg/kg/min, maximum 2 g/day), esmolol (loading dose of 100 to 500 mcg/kg IV over 1 minute followed by 50 to 500 mcg/kg/min continuous drip), or electrical cardioversion.

(9) Torsades de pointes (uncommon variant of polymorphic VT), which occurs mostly in the setting of prolonged QT, requires a special approach. Amiodarone and procainamide may have a disastrous effect on this type of VT with further prolongation of the QT. Torsades often responds to IV magnesium sulfate (25 to 50 mg/kg, maximum dose 2 g), even when magnesium level is normal. Esmolol and lidocaine may also be effective.

(10) Postoperative advanced second- or third-degree heart block is treated by temporary pacing and/or isoproterenol (IV drip at 0.05 to 2 mcg/kg/min). Permanent pacemaker implantation may be indicated if advanced AV block persists at least 7 days after the surgery.

4. Renal system: Anuria or oliguria (below 1 mL/kg/hr) and evidence of solute accumulation (serum K^+ above 5 mEq/L, BUN above 40 mg/dL, creatinine above 1 mg/dL) indicate acute renal failure. Acute reduction of cardiac output is the most common cause of renal failure. Initial treatment is directed at improving cardiac output and inducing diuresis.

a. Preload and afterload should be optimized.

b. Furosemide, 0.5 to 2 mg/kg/dose every 6 to 12 hours IV or as a continuous IV drip at 0.05 to 0.4 mg/kg/hr, is given if the patient is oliguric.

c. If serum K^+ rises above 6.0 mEq/L, calcium chloride (10 mg/kg/dose, slow central IV push), bicarbonate (1 mEq/kg/dose IV), $D_{25}W$ (2 mL/kg IV; 0.5 g glucose/kg) plus regular insulin (0.1 U/kg IV) solution, and sodium polystyrene sulfonate (Kayexalate®; 1 g/kg PR or NG) are used.

d. Peritoneal dialysis may be necessary if the measures previously outlined are ineffective. Indications for peritoneal dialysis include hypervolemia, azotemia (BUN over 150 mg/dL or lower if rising rapidly), life-threatening hyperkalemia, intractable metabolic acidosis, neurologic complications (secondary to uremia or electrolyte imbalance), calcium-phosphate imbalance, pulmonary compromise, or fluid restrictions limiting caloric intake.

5. Metabolic system

a. Abnormalities of electrolytes and acid-base balance

   (1) Metabolic acidosis is treated if the base deficit is >5 mEq/L. Total extracellular base deficit $\equiv$ Base deficit (mEq/L) $\times$ 0.3 $\times$ BW (kg). The dosage of sodium bicarbonate is half the total extracellular base deficit.

   (2) Lactic acidemia may be caused by low cardiac output syndrome and ensuing poor cerebral and intestinal tissue perfusion. Treatment is directed at improvement of cardiac output.

   (3) Mild hyponatremia does not require treatment except for fluid restriction and diuresis. Serum Na^+ <125 mEq/L requires treatment to elevate sodium levels.

   (4) Hypernatremia with the serum Na^+ >155 mEq/L requires treatment with sodium restriction and liberalization of fluids.

   (5) Hypocalcemia may cause hypotension secondary to decreased myocardial function. It should be followed closely, especially in neonates and patients with DiGeorge syndrome. Ionized calcium level below 1.2 mEq/L should be treated. Central line administration is the ideal route of IV calcium, as extravasation will lead to tissue necrosis.

   (6) Hypomagnesemia may lead to arrhythmia and subsequently to low cardiac output. A magnesium level of more than 0.7 mmol/L (1.4 mEq/L) is desirable.

b. Postoperative hypoglycemia (below 5 mmol/L or 90 mg/dL) or hyperglycemias (above 7.8 mmol/L or 140 mg/dL) have been associated with increased mortality and morbidity. It seems prudent to avoid these conditions. Hypoglycemia is managed with bolus of dextrose or administration of higher concentrated glucose in water. Hyperglycemia is treated with either restriction of glucose and/or infusion of insulin.

c. Postoperative hypothermia could interfere with hemostasis and exacerbate coagulopathy, necessitating gradual rewarming to control hemorrhage. Shivering should be avoided because it increases the oxygen consumption. However, management of junctional ectopic tachycardia may include core temperature cooling. Unlike hypothermia, treatment of postoperative fever (above 38.5° C) is more urgent. Low cardiac output syndrome is one of the causes of postoperative hyperthermia so that management of postoperative fever includes not only antipyretics or cooling but also optimizing cardiac output with afterload reduction.

6. Gastrointestinal system: Adequate caloric intake (120 to 150 kcal/kg/day) is essential in infants recovering from congenital cardiac surgery. Enteral feeding is individualized. When patients are stable hemodynamically, several hours after extubation, oral feeding can be started with clear liquids (e.g., oral rehydration solutions). It is then advanced to an appropriate formula. Nasogastric tube feeding should be used if infants are too weak to suck. Children with prolonged intubation require gavage feeding or total parenteral nutrition. Gastric protection is achieved with H_2-receptor blockade (e.g., ranitidine, 1 mg/kg/dose IV every 6 to 8 hours). Ranitidine dose needs to be adjusted in patients with renal failure, or alternatively protein pump inhibitors (e.g., esomeprazole) could be used. Enterally fed patients should be examined frequently for any signs of intestinal dysfunction. Evidence of abdominal distention, absence of peristalsis, hyperperistalsis, or hematochezia is sought routinely. If one of these develops, enteral feeding is discontinued, nasogastric suction is applied, and parenteral nutrition is considered. GI dysfunction may be caused by LCOS, acute pancreatitis, hepatic or intestinal necrosis, ileus, and others.

7. Hematologic system: Different institutions establish different thresholds for transfusion of PRBCs, fresh frozen plasma, or platelets. Transfusion of blood products depends on hemodynamic status and coagulation status of individual patients.

a. Maintain adequate hemoglobin (Hgb) and a desirable filling pressure (e.g., LA pressure 10 to 15 mm Hg) by infusion of PRBCs or albumin, depending on the patient's Hgb or hematocrit (Hct). Patients with cyanotic congenital heart disease or myocardial dysfunction are given PRBCs to maintain Hct above 40%.

b. Coagulation abnormalities may result from inadequate heparin neutralization (causing prolongation of aPTT), thrombocytopenia (below 50,000 platelets/mm^3), or disseminated intravascular coagulation (DIC; secondary to sepsis, low cardiac output, acidosis, hypoxia, or tissue necrosis or as a reaction to blood transfusion).

   (1) Unneutralized heparin is corrected by administration of additional protamine.

   (2) Thrombocytopenia is treated with slow infusion of platelet concentrates with an infusion pump, given over 20 to 30 minutes; rapid infusion may cause pulmonary hypertension and RV failure.

   (3) DIC (characterized by hemorrhage, tissue necrosis, hemolytic anemia, positive D-dimer test, low platelets and serum fibrinogen, and prolonged PT and aPTT) is managed by prompt and vigorous treatment of the underlying cause. Management may include transfusion of platelets, cryoprecipitates, and/or fresh-frozen plasma, as well as administration of heparin.

c. Excessive postoperative bleeding occurs more frequently in severely cyanotic patients, polycythemic patients, and patients who had a re-operation. Necessity to infuse more than 10 to 15 mL/kg of volume requires investigation for excessive blood loss and for a possible surgical exploration. Surgical exploration is indicated if (1) the chest tube drainage in the absence of clotting abnormalities exceeds 3 mL/kg/hr for 3 hours or (2) there is a sudden marked increase in chest tube drainage of 5 mL/kg/hr in any 1 hour.

d. Long-term anticoagulation with aspirin or warfarin is indicated in selected patients. Patients with cavopulmonary anastomosis (e.g., Glenn or Fontan procedure) or S-P shunts (e.g., modified Blalock-Taussig shunt) are started on aspirin (3 to 5 mg/kg PO once daily) when they are hemodynamically stable and have an adequate platelet count without evidence of active bleeding. Alternatively or additionally, warfarin is given if the patient is in a hypercoagulable state (e.g., factor V Leiden mutation, protein S or C deficiency). Patients with a mechanical valve prosthesis will require warfarin; the dose is adjusted to maintain adequate anticoagulation (INR 2.5 to 3.5).

8. Neurologic system: The incidence of central nervous system anomalies, including brain dysmorphology or neurobehavioral abnormalities, is increased in patients with congenital cardiac defects. These may be multifactorial, isolated findings, or in association with particular genetic defects. In addition, preoperative and perioperative neurologic events complicate establishing the accurate cause of the neurologic insult.

a. Localized neurologic defects such as hemiplegia and visual field defects are abnormal and may be due to air or particulate emboli.

b. Seizures may be caused by hypoxia, metabolic abnormalities, infections, cerebral edema, embolism or hemorrhage, or decreased cerebral perfusion. Early postoperative clinical seizures occur at an incidence rate of 3% to 6%; however, EEG and video monitoring may reveal an incidence of 20% of subclinical seizures. EEG-documented seizures have been associated with worse neurodevelopmental outcome. Management of seizures includes the following:

   (1) Determine arterial blood gases, serum glucose, calcium and electrolytes, cardiac output, and temperature. Correct any abnormalities.

   (2) Anticonvulsant therapy

      (a) Lorazepam, 0.05 to 0.1 mg/kg/dose IV over 2 to 5 minutes (maximum single dose 2 mg; may cause respiratory depression).

      (b) Fosphenytoin, 15 to 20 mg phenytoin equivalent (PE)/kg IV (maximum infusion rate of 150 mg PE/min due to risk of hypotension), followed by a maintenance dose of 5 mg PE/kg/ day IV or IM. Therapeutic levels are 10 to 20 mg/L (free and bound phenytoin) or 1 to 2 mg/L (free phenytoin). Fosphenytoin causes less hypotension than traditional phenytoin; however, both medications are contraindicated in patients with heart block or sinus bradycardia.

      (c) Phenobarbital, 10 to 20 mg/kg IV over 5 to 10 minutes. The full effect may take several hours. Phenobarbital maintenance dose is 5 mg/kg/day given in one or two daily doses.

Therapeutic level is 10 to 40 mg/L. Side effects of phenobarbital include myocardial depression with hypotension, particularly after large and rapid infusion.

c. Choreiform movement and grossly inadequate behavior are major neurologic complications. Pharmacologic control is difficult. These complications usually but not always clear without demonstrable sequelae.

III. SELECTED POSTOPERATIVE COMPLICATIONS

A. PLEURAL EFFUSION

A small amount of fluid is present in the pleural cavity. The reabsorption of this pleural fluid is mainly through the venous system and to some degree through the lymphatic system. Any increase in capillary hydrostatic pressure as a result of disrupted systemic venous hemodynamics (e.g., Fontan surgery, right ventricular failure) may result in accumulation of transudates in the pleural cavity. Trauma to the lymphatic system as caused by cutting large tributaries of the thoracic duct causes buildup of chyle in the pleural space. Both conditions create a management problem.

Duration of *persistent pleural effusion,* as a result of increased systemic venous pressure, which is common after Fontan operation, may be shortened by intraoperative creation of baffle fenestration. Symptoms may include tachycardia, tachypnea, increased work of breathing, and in severe cases, respiratory failure. Diagnosis is usually made by a CXR. Thoracentesis may be necessary for determination of etiology and/or for treatment. Transudates can be differentiated by amount of protein (<3 g/100 mL) and lactate dehyrogenase (<200 IU/L) from exudates (>3 g/100 mL protein and >200 IU/L lactate dehydrogenase), which are caused by increased capillary permeability and may be a sign of infection.

A small amount of pleural effusion can be tolerated well. It usually responds to medical management with diuresis, afterload reduction, and inotropic support. However, a significant amount of pleural effusion will cause cardiorespiratory compromise and will require more aggressive management strategies, including chest tube drainage, pleurodesis with a sclerosing agent (e.g., talc), or even Fontan revision. When the drainage is large, appropriate replacement of fluid, electrolytes, and protein is essential.

Chylothorax, an accumulation of chyle in the pleural cavity, may be caused by trauma to peritracheal lymphatics or transmission of increased systemic venous pressure to the thoracic duct, or a combination of both. It may be seen after operations, such as COA repair, S-P shunt, cavopulmonary anastomosis (e.g., Glenn or Fontan operation), Senning operation or, rarely, after ligation of PDA. Occasionally, chylothorax occurs in combination with chylopericardium.

Chyle may or may not have a creamy appearance, depending on the nutritional status of the patient (consumption of fat results in creamy appearance), but a triglyceride level above 110 mg/dL is highly probable of the diagnosis. The fluid is usually sterile and has abundant lymphocytes (2000 to 20,000/mm^3).

Treatment, apart from the medical management described previously, is directed at drainage of chylothorax (chest tube placement) and reducing the flow of lymph (by limiting physical activity to reduce lymph flow from the extremities).

1. In most cases, chest tube drainage is all that is necessary. If chylothorax develops after chest tube removal, needle aspiration every 3 to 4 days usually constitutes adequate treatment. The drainage slows or stops within 7 days in most cases.

2. Careful attention to the nutrition of the patient is important. Either parenteral hyperalimentation or a diet with medium chain triglycerides as the fat source is called for; medium chain triglycerides are absorbed by the portal system, not the lymphatic system. Serum albumin should be followed closely and replaced if necessary.

3. In some case reports, continuous IV octreotide (0.5 to 5 mcg/kg/hr), a somatostatin analogue, has been used effectively.

4. If the drainage persists, surgical intervention may be considered because continuous loss of chyle results in lymphocyte depletion and subsequent immunocompromise. Indications for the intervention may include (a) average daily loss above 100 mL/age/day for 5 days, (b) the chyle flow not slowing after 2 weeks, or (c) imminent nutritional complications.

5. Thoracic duct ligation with or without chemical pleurodesis has been used successfully. During pleurodesis the introduced chemicals cause inflammation between the parietal and visceral pleura. This reaction causes adhesions between the layers and prevents further fluid accumulation. The procedure may be painful and cause fever.

B. PARALYSIS OF THE DIAPHRAGM

Paralysis or paresis of a hemidiaphragm occurs in about 0.5% to 2% of patients after thoracic surgery, though the incidence may be as high as 10% in young children. It is the result of damage to the phrenic nerve. It may occur after COA repair, PDA ligation, S-P shunt, or open heart surgery and may be due to nerve transection, blunt trauma, stretching during retraction, electrocautery, or hypothermic injury. Infants are more vulnerable to respiratory distress because of their greater dependence on the diaphragm for respiration.

The diagnosis should be suspected if there is persistent unexplained tachypnea, respiratory distress, hypoxia and/or hypercapnia, atelectasis, inability to wean from the ventilator, or persistent elevation of a hemidiaphragm on serial CXR. Fluoroscopy or sonogram that reveals paradoxical motion of the hemidiaphragms is diagnostic if it is done during spontaneous breathing. When paralysis is not caused by transection, return of function usually occurs in 2 weeks to 6 months. In 20% of the cases the paralysis is permanent. Management ranges from conservative to surgical intervention.

1. Some investigators recommend ventilator support only for the initial 2 to 6 weeks.

2. Continuous positive airway pressure (CPAP) may be useful in management, as well as in identifying patients who may benefit from plication.
3. If respiratory insufficiency persists, surgical plication should be considered. Plication of the diaphragm usually is not necessary as long as the patient can be extubated without developing respiratory insufficiency.

C.   POSTPERICARDIOTOMY SYNDROME

Postpericardiotomy syndrome (PPS), a febrile illness with pericardial and pleural reactions, develops after surgery involving pericardiotomy. This occurs in about 25% to 30% of patients who undergo pericardiotomy. The etiology remains speculative. Though questioned in more recent studies, an autoimmune response to cardiac antibodies in association with a recent or remote viral infection was postulated in the 1970s. Studied patients who developed PPS had a high titer of antiheart antibodies along with high antibody titers against adenovirus, coxsackievirus B1–6, and cytomegalovirus.

Onset is a few weeks to a few months (median 4 weeks) after pericardiotomy. PPS is characterized by fever (sustained low grade or spiking up to 40° C), chest pain, irritability, malaise, joint pain, decreased appetite, nausea, and vomiting. Chest pain, which may be severe, is caused by both pericarditis and pleuritis. It may be worse in the supine position or with deep inspiration. It is rare in children younger than 2 years of age. Physical examination may reveal pericardial and pleural friction rubs and hepatomegaly. Tachycardia, tachypnea, rising venous pressure, falling arterial pressure, and narrow pulse pressure with a paradoxical pulse are signs of cardiac tamponade. Blood laboratory findings include leukocytosis with left shift. Erythrocyte sedimentation rate (ESR) and C-reactive protein (CRP) are usually elevated. CXR film shows enlarged cardiac silhouette and pleural effusion. ECG shows persistent ST segment elevation and flat or inverted T waves in the limb and left precordial leads. Echo is a reliable test in confirming the presence and amount of pericardial effusion and in evaluating evidence of cardiac tamponade. Although the disease is self-limited, its duration is highly variable; the median duration is 2 to 3 weeks. About 20% of patients have recurrences.

Bed rest is all that is needed for a mild case. A nonsteroidal antiinflammatory agent such as oral aspirin (80 to 100 mg/kg/day divided in three or four doses) or ibuprofen (20 to 40 mg/kg/day divided in three or four doses) is effective in most cases. In severe cases, corticosteroids (prednisone, 2 mg/kg/day up to 60 mg/day) tapered over 3 to 4 weeks may be indicated if the diagnosis is secure and infection has been ruled out. Emergency pericardiocentesis or creation of a pericardial window may be required if signs of cardiac tamponade are present. Diuretics may be used for pleural effusion.

D.   POSTCOARCTECTOMY HYPERTENSION

Paradoxical hypertension following repair of coarctation of aorta is quite common, particularly in older children. This condition is usually biphasic with mostly systolic hypertension developing within 24 to 48 hours of the procedure, followed by a more delayed phase. The mechanism is believed to be multifactorial, including intraoperative stimulation of sympathetic nerve fibers, postoperative altered baroreceptor activity, and derangement of the renin-angiotensin system. The first phase of hypertension is believed to be the result of increased catecholamine levels and an altered baroreceptor response. Elevated levels of renin and angiotensin are believed to be responsible for the later phase of hypertension, which is more pronounced in diastole.

Systemic hypertension needs to be treated promptly because it could increase the risk of postoperative hemorrhage. In addition to pain management and sedation, short-acting intravenous β-receptor blocker administration (e.g., esmolol; loading dose of 100 to 500 mcg/kg IV over 1 minute followed by 50 to 500 mcg/kg/min continuous drip) can be used to control the first phase of postcoarctectomy hypertension. Other medications that have successfully been used include longer-acting β-receptor blockers (e.g., propranolol, nadolol), combined α- and β-receptor blockers (e.g., labetalol), and vasodilators (nitroprusside, hydralazine). Long-term management of paradoxical hypertension is achieved with angiotensin-converting enzyme (ACE) inhibitors (e.g., enalapril, captopril).

Postcoarctectomy syndrome is a well-described but rare complication of repair of COA. Occurring in up to 5% to 10% of older children, it is characterized by severe, intermittent abdominal pain beginning 2 to 4 days after surgery with accompanying fever, leukocytosis, and vomiting. In severe cases, ascites, ileus, melena, ischemic bowel, and even death have been reported. Persistent paradoxical hypertension may be present. Abdominal findings are believed to be caused by acute inflammatory changes in mesenteric arteries resulting from a sudden increase in pulsatile pressures in arteries distal to the coarctation.

Because of mesenteric arteritis, feeding of solid foods is delayed; some centers advocate NPO status for the first 48 hours following the repair. Treatment includes bowel decompression and treatment of the accompanying hypertension.

E. HEMOLYTIC ANEMIA

Hemolytic anemia may follow cardiac surgery, especially repair of congenital heart defects using synthetic patch material or aortic or mitral prosthetic valve implantation. Hemolysis secondary to red cell trauma is caused by unusual intracardiac turbulence such as periprosthetic leakage.

The onset is 1 to 2 weeks after surgery with placement or insertion of synthetic or prosthetic materials. It is characterized by low-grade fever, anemia, jaundice, dark urine, hepatomegaly, and reticulocytosis. Iron deficiency anemia may develop because of excessive loss of iron in urine in chronic disease. Peripheral smears reveal abnormal crenated and fragmented red blood cells and reticulocytosis. Hemoglobinemia, methemalbuminemia, and hemosiderinuria are also present.

Anemia is treated with either iron replacement therapy or blood transfusion. Most patients respond to oral iron therapy. Some patients are treated with β-receptor blockade to allow healing of the rough surface responsible for hemolysis. Surgical correction of turbulence is indicated if the anemia is severe and the correction is technically possible.

F.   PROTEIN-LOSING ENTEROPATHY

Protein-losing enteropathy (PLE) is a condition characterized by excessive loss of plasma protein through the intestinal mucosa. Although it can be a primary gastrointestinal disorder with intestinal lymphangiectasia and associated peripheral edema, PLE occurs most frequently as a complication of Fontan procedure. It is believed to be caused by chronically elevated central venous pressure secondary to unfavorable PA anatomy, increased PVR, decreased cardiac output, or loss of electrical AV synchrony. PLE in association with Fontan-type operation has a cumulative 10-year occurrence risk of 13% and a poor 5-year survival rate of about 50%.

Children may present a few weeks, months, or even years after the surgery with symptoms of abdominal pain and distention, diarrhea, emesis, and poor weight gain. Patients may be tachycardic if sinus node function is preserved. Tachypnea may be a clue to concurrent pleural effusion. Hepatomegaly is seen frequently. Signs of fluid retention, including ascites and anasarca, may be found on examination.

Serum albumin, immunoglobulins, and total protein are decreased, and fecal $\alpha 1$-antitrypsin clearance is increased. Technetium-99m dextran scintigraphy may be performed to assess the extent or possibly the location of intestinal protein loss. Electrolyte imbalance is seen, which may be iatrogenic secondary to diuretic therapy. ECG needs to be obtained to rule out any arrhythmia such as sinus node dysfunction. CXR may reveal cardiomegaly and/or pleural effusion. Echo is performed to evaluate ventricular function or Fontan baffle obstruction. Cardiac catheterization may be needed as a diagnostic but also as a therapeutic tool.

Treatment includes a protein-rich diet, diuretics, digitalis, and ACE inhibitors, as well as administration of heparin, corticosteroids, or octreotide. More invasive management apart from interventional cardiac catheterization may include pacemaker insertion, repair of residual defects (e.g., repair of AV valve, repair of residual COA), Fontan revision, or cardiac transplantation.

MISCELLANEOUS

TABLE A-1

RECURRENCE RISKS GIVEN ONE SIBLING WHO HAS A CARDIOVASCULAR
ANOMALY

ANOMALY	SUGGESTED RISK (%)
Ventricular septal defect	3.0
Patent ductus arteriosus	3.0
Atrial septal defect	2.5
Tetralogy of Fallot	2.5
Pulmonary stenosis	2.0
Coarctation of the aorta	2.0
Aortic stenosis	2.0
Transposition of the great arteries	1.5
AV canal (complete endocardial cushion defect)	2.0
Endocardial fibroelastosis	4.0
Tricuspid atresia	1.0
Ebstein anomaly	1.0
Persistent truncus arteriosus	1.0
Pulmonary atresia	1.0
Hypoplastic left heart syndrome	2.0

Adapted from Nora JJ, Nora AH: The evaluation of specific genetic and environmental counseling in congenital heart diseases, *Circulation* 57:205-213, 1978.

TABLE A-2

AFFECTED OFFSPRING, GIVEN ONE PARENT WITH A CONGENITAL
HEART DEFECT

DEFECT	MOTHER AFFECTED (%)	FATHER AFFECTED (%)
Aortic stenosis	13-18	3
Atrial septal defect	4-4.5	1.5
AV canal (complete ECD)	14	1
Coarctation of the aorta	4	2
Patent ductus arteriosus	3.5-4	2.5
Pulmonary stenosis	4-6.5	2
Tetralogy of Fallot	6-10	1.5
Ventricular septal defect	6	2

From Nora JJ, Nora AH: Maternal transmission of congenital heart diseases: new recurrence risk figures and the questions of cytoplasmic inheritance and vulnerability to teratogens, *Am J Cardiol* 59:459-463, 1987.
ECD, endocardial cushion defect.

TABLE A-3

CLASSIFICATION OF ANTIARRHYTHMIC DRUGS ACCORDING TO THEIR MECHANISM OF ACTION

CLASS	ACTION	DRUGS
I	Sodium channel blockade	
A	Moderate phase 0 depression and slow conduction (2+)*; prolonged repolarization	Quinidine, procainamide, disopyramide
B	Minimal phase 0 depression and slow conduction (0 to 1+); shortened repolarization	Lidocaine, phenytoin, tocainide, mexiletine
C	Marked phase 0 depression and slow conduction (4+); little effect on repolarization	Encainide, lorcainide, flecainide
II	β-Adrenergic blockade	Propranolol, others
III	Prolonged repolarization	Amiodarone, bretylium
IV	Calcium channel blockade	Diltiazem, verapamil

Adapted from Gilman AG, Goodman LS, Rall TW et al, eds: *Goodman and Gilman's the pharmacological basis of therapeutics*, ed 7, New York, 1985, Macmillan.
*Relative magnitude of effect on conduction velocity is indicated on a scale of 1+ to 4+.

TABLE A-4

NEW YORK HEART ASSOCIATION FUNCTIONAL CLASSIFICATION

CLASS	IMPAIRMENT
I	The patient has the disease, but the condition is asymptomatic.
II	The patient experiences symptoms with moderate activity.
III	The patient has symptoms with mild activity.
IV	The patient's condition is symptomatic at rest.

This is a classification of functional impairment in exercise capacity based on symptoms of dyspnea and fatigue. It is simple and useful in the evaluation of cardiac patients.

TABLE A-5
OXYGEN CONSUMPTION PER BODY SURFACE AREA (ML/MIN/M²) BY SEX, AGE, AND HEART RATE

	HEART RATE (BEATS/MIN)												
AGE (YR)	50	60	70	80	90	100	110	120	130	140	150	160	170
Male Patients													
3				155	159	163	167	171	175	178	182	186	190
4			149	152	156	160	163	168	171	175	179	182	186
6		141	144	148	151	155	159	162	167	171	174	178	181
8		136	141	145	148	152	156	159	163	167	171	175	178
10	130	134	139	142	146	149	153	157	160	165	169	172	176
12	128	132	136	140	144	147	151	155	158	162	167	170	174
14	127	130	134	137	142	146	149	153	157	160	165	169	172
16	125	129	132	136	141	144	148	152	155	159	162	167	
18	124	127	131	135	139	143	147	150	154	157	161	166	
20	123	126	130	134	137	142	145	149	153	156	160	165	
25	120	124	127	131	135	139	143	147	150	154	157		
30	118	122	125	129	133	136	141	145	148	152	155		
35	116	120	124	127	131	135	139	143	147	150			
40	115	119	122	126	130	133	137	141	145	149			

cont'd

TABLE A-5

OXYGEN CONSUMPTION PER BODY SURFACE AREA (ML/MIN/M²) BY SEX, AGE, AND HEART RATE—cont'd

AGE (YR)	HEART RATE (BEATS/MIN)												
	50	60	70	80	90	100	110	120	130	140	150	160	170
Female Patients													
3				150	153	157	161	165	169	172	176	180	183
4			141	145	149	152	156	159	163	168	171	175	179
6		130	134	137	142	146	149	153	156	160	165	168	172
8		125	129	133	136	141	144	148	152	155	159	163	167
10	118	122	125	129	133	136	141	144	148	152	155	159	163
12	115	119	122	126	130	133	137	141	145	149	152	156	160
14	112	116	120	123	127	131	134	138	143	146	150	153	157
16	109	114	118	121	125	128	132	136	140	144	148	151	
18	107	111	116	119	123	127	130	134	137	142	146	149	
20	106	109	114	118	121	125	128	132	136	140	144	148	
25	102	106	109	114	118	121	125	128	132	136	140		
30	99	103	106	110	115	118	122	125	129	133	136		
35	97	100	104	107	111	116	119	123	127	130			
50	94	98	102	105	109	112	117	121	124	128			

From LaFarge CG, Miettinen OS: The estimation of oxygen consumption. *Cardiovasc Res* 4:23-30, 1970.

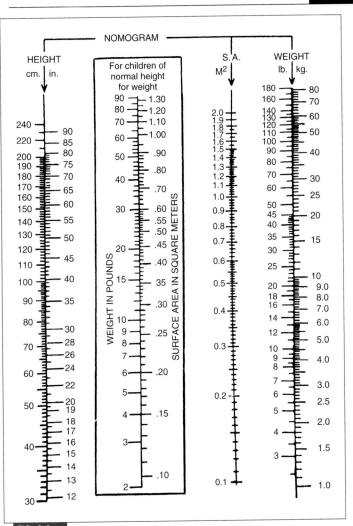

FIG. A-1

Body surface area nomogram.

APPENDIX B:
BLOOD PRESSURE STANDARDS

TABLE B-1

BP LEVELS FOR BOYS BY AGE AND HEIGHT PERCENTILE (NHBPEP*)

AGE	BP PERCENTILE	SYSTOLIC BP (MM HG) PERCENTILE OF HEIGHT							DIASTOLIC BP (MM HG) PERCENTILE OF HEIGHT						
		5TH	10TH	25TH	50TH	75TH	90TH	95TH	5TH	10TH	25TH	50TH	75TH	90TH	95TH
1	50th	80	81	83	85	87	88	89	34	35	36	37	38	39	39
	90th	94	95	97	99	100	102	103	49	50	51	52	53	53	54
	95th	98	99	101	103	104	106	106	54	54	55	56	57	58	58
	99th	105	106	108	110	112	113	114	61	62	63	64	65	66	66
2	50th	84	85	87	88	90	92	92	39	40	41	42	43	44	44
	90th	97	99	100	102	104	105	106	54	55	56	57	58	58	59
	95th	101	102	104	106	108	109	110	59	59	60	61	62	63	63
	99th	109	110	111	113	115	117	117	66	67	68	69	70	71	71
3	50th	86	87	89	91	93	94	95	44	44	45	46	47	48	48
	90th	100	101	103	105	107	108	109	59	59	60	61	62	63	63
	95th	104	105	107	109	110	112	113	63	63	64	65	66	67	67
	99th	111	112	114	116	118	119	120	71	71	72	73	74	75	75
4	50th	88	89	91	93	95	96	97	47	48	49	50	51	51	52
	90th	102	103	105	107	109	110	111	62	63	64	65	66	66	67
	95th	106	107	109	111	112	114	115	66	67	68	69	70	71	71
	99th	113	114	116	118	120	121	122	74	75	76	77	78	79	79
5	50th	90	91	93	95	96	98	98	50	51	52	53	54	55	55
	90th	104	105	106	108	110	111	112	65	66	67	68	69	69	70
	95th	108	109	110	112	114	115	116	69	70	71	72	73	74	74
	99th	115	116	118	120	121	123	123	77	78	79	80	81	81	82

cont'd

TABLE B-1—cont'd
BP LEVELS FOR BOYS BY AGE AND HEIGHT PERCENTILE (NHBPEP*)

AGE	BP PERCENTILE	SYSTOLIC BP (MM HG) PERCENTILE OF HEIGHT							DIASTOLIC BP (MM HG) PERCENTILE OF HEIGHT						
		5TH	10TH	25TH	50TH	75TH	90TH	95TH	5TH	10TH	25TH	50TH	75TH	90TH	95TH
6	50th	91	92	94	96	98	99	100	53	53	54	55	56	57	57
	90th	105	106	108	110	111	113	113	68	68	69	70	71	72	72
	95th	109	110	112	114	115	117	117	72	72	73	74	75	76	76
	99th	116	117	119	121	123	124	125	80	80	81	82	83	84	84
7	50th	92	94	95	97	99	100	101	55	55	56	57	58	59	59
	90th	106	107	109	111	113	114	115	70	70	71	72	73	74	74
	95th	110	111	113	115	117	118	119	74	74	75	76	77	78	78
	99th	117	118	120	122	124	125	126	82	82	83	84	85	86	86
8	50th	94	95	97	99	100	102	102	56	57	58	59	60	60	61
	90th	107	109	110	112	114	115	116	71	72	72	73	74	75	76
	95th	111	112	114	116	118	119	120	75	76	77	78	79	79	80
	99th	119	120	122	123	125	127	127	83	84	85	86	87	87	88
9	50th	95	96	98	100	102	103	104	57	58	58	59	60	61	62
	90th	109	110	112	114	115	117	118	72	73	74	75	76	76	77
	95th	113	114	116	118	119	121	121	76	77	78	79	80	81	81
	99th	120	121	123	125	127	128	129	84	85	86	87	88	88	89
10	50th	97	98	100	102	103	105	106	58	59	60	61	61	62	63
	90th	111	112	114	115	117	119	119	73	73	74	75	76	77	78
	95th	115	116	117	119	121	122	123	77	77	78	79	80	81	81
	99th	122	123	125	127	128	130	130	85	86	86	88	88	89	90
11	50th	99	100	102	104	105	107	107	59	59	60	61	62	63	63
	90th	113	114	115	117	119	120	121	74	74	75	76	77	78	78

Age	BP Percentile	SBP							DBP						
	95th	117	118	119	121	123	124	125	78	78	79	80	81	82	82
	99th	124	125	127	129	130	132	132	86	86	87	88	89	90	90
12	50th	101	102	104	106	108	109	110	59	60	61	62	63	63	64
	90th	115	116	118	120	121	123	123	74	75	75	76	77	78	79
	95th	119	120	122	123	125	127	127	78	79	80	81	82	82	83
	99th	126	127	129	131	133	134	135	86	87	88	89	90	90	91
13	50th	104	105	106	108	110	111	112	60	60	61	62	63	64	64
	90th	117	118	120	122	124	125	126	75	75	76	77	78	79	79
	95th	121	122	124	126	128	129	130	79	79	80	81	82	83	83
	99th	128	130	131	133	135	136	137	87	87	88	89	90	91	91
14	50th	106	107	109	111	113	114	115	60	61	62	63	64	65	65
	90th	120	121	123	125	126	128	128	75	76	77	78	79	79	80
	95th	124	125	127	128	130	132	132	80	80	81	82	83	84	84
	99th	131	132	134	136	138	139	140	87	88	89	90	91	92	92
15	50th	109	110	112	113	115	117	117	61	62	63	64	65	66	66
	90th	122	124	125	127	129	130	131	76	77	78	79	80	80	81
	95th	126	127	129	131	133	134	135	81	81	82	83	84	85	85
	99th	134	135	136	138	140	142	142	88	89	90	91	92	93	93
16	50th	111	112	114	116	118	119	120	63	63	64	65	66	67	67
	90th	125	126	128	130	131	133	134	78	78	79	80	81	82	82
	95th	129	130	132	134	135	137	137	82	83	83	84	85	86	87
	99th	136	137	139	141	143	144	145	90	90	91	92	93	94	94
17	50th	114	115	116	118	120	121	122	65	66	66	67	68	69	70
	90th	127	128	130	132	134	135	136	80	80	81	82	83	84	84
	95th	131	132	134	136	138	139	140	84	85	86	87	87	88	89
	99th	139	140	141	143	145	146	147	92	93	93	94	95	96	97

From the Fourth Report on the Diagnosis, Evaluation, and Treatment of High Blood Pressure in Children and Adolescents, National High Blood Pressure Education Program Working Group on High Blood Pressure in Children and Adolescents, *Pediatrics* 114:555–576, 2004.

* National High Blood Pressure Education Program.

TABLE B-2

BP LEVELS FOR GIRLS BY AGE AND HEIGHT PERCENTILE (NHBPEP*)

AGE	BP PERCENTILE	SYSTOLIC BP (MM HG) PERCENTILE OF HEIGHT							DIASTOLIC BP (MM HG) PERCENTILE OF HEIGHT						
		5TH	10TH	25TH	50TH	75TH	90TH	95TH	5TH	10TH	25TH	50TH	75TH	90TH	95TH
1	50th	83	84	85	86	88	89	90	38	39	39	40	41	41	42
	90th	97	97	98	100	101	102	103	52	53	53	54	55	55	56
	95th	100	101	102	104	105	106	107	56	56	57	58	59	59	60
	99th	108	108	109	111	112	113	114	64	64	65	65	66	67	67
2	50th	85	85	87	88	89	91	91	43	44	44	45	46	46	47
	90th	98	99	100	101	103	104	105	57	58	58	59	60	61	61
	95th	102	103	104	105	107	108	109	61	62	62	63	64	65	65
	99th	109	110	111	112	114	115	116	69	69	70	70	71	72	72
3	50th	86	87	88	89	91	92	93	47	48	48	49	50	50	51
	90th	100	100	102	103	104	106	106	61	62	62	63	64	64	65
	95th	104	104	105	107	108	109	110	65	66	66	67	68	68	69
	99th	111	111	113	114	115	116	117	73	73	74	74	75	76	76
4	50th	88	88	90	91	92	94	94	50	50	51	52	52	53	54
	90th	101	102	103	104	106	107	108	64	64	65	66	67	67	68
	95th	105	106	107	108	110	111	112	68	68	69	70	71	71	72
	99th	112	113	114	115	117	118	119	76	76	76	77	78	79	79
5	50th	89	90	91	93	94	95	96	52	53	53	54	55	55	56
	90th	103	103	105	106	107	109	109	66	67	67	68	69	69	70
	95th	107	107	108	110	111	112	113	70	71	71	72	73	73	74
	99th	114	114	116	117	118	120	120	78	78	79	79	80	81	81
6	50th	91	92	93	94	96	97	98	54	54	55	56	56	57	58
	90th	104	105	106	108	109	110	111	68	68	69	70	70	71	72

cont'd

Age	BP %ile	SBP 5th	SBP 10th	SBP 25th	SBP 50th	SBP 75th	SBP 90th	SBP 95th	DBP 5th	DBP 10th	DBP 25th	DBP 50th	DBP 75th	DBP 90th	DBP 95th
7	95th	108	109	110	111	113	114	115	72	72	73	74	74	75	76
	99th	115	116	117	119	120	121	122	80	80	80	81	82	83	83
8	50th	93	93	95	96	97	99	99	55	56	56	57	58	58	59
	90th	106	107	108	109	111	112	113	69	70	70	71	72	72	73
	95th	110	111	112	113	115	116	116	73	74	74	75	76	76	77
	99th	117	118	119	120	122	123	124	81	81	82	82	83	84	84
9	50th	95	95	96	98	99	100	101	57	57	57	58	59	60	60
	90th	108	109	110	111	113	114	114	71	71	71	72	73	74	74
	95th	112	112	114	115	116	118	118	75	75	75	76	77	78	78
	99th	119	120	121	122	123	125	125	82	82	83	83	84	85	86
10	50th	96	97	98	100	101	102	103	58	58	58	59	60	61	61
	90th	110	110	112	113	114	116	116	72	72	72	73	74	75	75
	95th	114	114	115	117	118	119	120	76	76	76	77	78	79	79
	99th	121	121	123	124	125	127	127	83	83	84	84	85	86	87
11	50th	98	99	100	102	103	104	105	59	59	59	60	61	62	62
	90th	112	112	114	115	116	118	118	73	73	73	74	75	76	76
	95th	116	116	117	119	120	121	122	77	77	77	78	79	80	80
	99th	123	123	125	126	127	129	129	84	84	85	86	86	87	88
12	50th	100	101	102	103	105	106	107	60	60	60	61	62	63	63
	90th	114	114	116	117	118	119	120	74	74	74	75	76	77	77
	95th	118	118	119	121	122	123	124	78	78	78	79	80	81	81
	99th	125	125	126	128	129	130	131	85	85	86	87	87	88	89
13	50th	102	103	104	105	107	108	109	61	61	61	62	63	64	64
	90th	116	116	117	119	120	121	122	75	75	75	76	77	78	78
	95th	119	120	121	123	124	125	126	79	79	79	80	81	82	82
	99th	127	127	128	130	131	132	133	86	86	87	88	88	89	90
14	50th	104	105	106	107	109	110	110	62	62	62	63	64	65	65
	90th	117	118	119	121	122	123	124	76	76	76	77	78	79	79
	95th	121	122	123	124	126	127	128	80	80	80	81	82	83	83

TABLE B-2—cont'd

BP LEVELS FOR GIRLS BY AGE AND HEIGHT PERCENTILE (NHBPEP*)

AGE	BP PERCENTILE	SYSTOLIC BP (MM HG) PERCENTILE OF HEIGHT							DIASTOLIC BP (MM HG) PERCENTILE OF HEIGHT						
		5TH	10TH	25TH	50TH	75TH	90TH	95TH	5TH	10TH	25TH	50TH	75TH	90TH	95TH
	99th	128	129	130	132	133	134	135	87	87	88	89	89	90	91
14	50th	106	106	107	109	110	111	112	63	63	63	64	65	66	66
	90th	119	120	121	122	124	125	125	77	77	77	78	79	80	80
	95th	123	123	125	126	127	129	129	81	81	81	82	82	84	84
	99th	130	131	132	133	135	136	136	88	88	89	90	90	91	92
15	50th	107	108	109	110	111	113	113	64	64	64	65	66	67	67
	90th	120	121	122	123	125	126	127	78	78	78	79	80	81	81
	95th	124	125	126	127	129	130	131	82	82	82	83	83	85	85
	99th	131	132	133	134	136	137	138	89	89	90	91	91	93	93
16	50th	108	108	110	111	112	114	114	64	64	65	66	66	67	68
	90th	121	122	123	124	126	127	128	78	78	79	80	81	81	82
	95th	125	126	127	128	130	131	132	82	82	83	84	85	85	86
	99th	132	133	134	135	137	138	139	90	90	90	91	91	93	93
17	50th	108	109	110	111	113	114	115	64	65	65	66	67	67	68
	90th	122	122	123	125	126	127	128	78	79	79	80	81	81	82
	95th	125	126	127	129	130	131	132	82	83	83	84	85	85	86
	99th	133	133	134	136	137	138	139	90	90	91	91	92	93	93

From the Fourth Report on the Diagnosis, Evaluation, and Treatment of High Blood Pressure in Children and Adolescents, National High Blood Pressure Education Program Working Group on High Blood Pressure in Children and Adolescents, *Pediatrics* 114:555-576, 2004.
* National High Blood Pressure Education Program.

TABLE B-3

AUSCULTATORY BLOOD PRESSURE VALUES FOR BOYS 5 TO 17 YEARS OLD
(SAN ANTONIO CHILDREN'S BLOOD PRESSURE STUDY)

				PERCENTILES				
AGE (YR)	**5TH**	**10TH**	**25TH**	**MEAN**	**75TH**	**90TH**	**95TH**	**99TH***
Systolic Pressure								
5	78	81	87	92	98	103	106	112
6	81	84	89	95	100	105	108	114
7	82	85	90	96	102	107	110	116
8	83	86	92	97	103	108	111	117
9	85	88	93	99	104	109	113	118
10	86	89	95	100	106	111	114	120
11	88	91	97	102	108	113	116	122
12	91	94	99	105	111	116	119	125
13	94	97	102	108	113	118	122	127
14	96	99	105	110	116	121	122	130
15	99	102	107	113	118	124	127	132
16	100	103	108	114	120	125	128	134
17	100	103	109	114	120	125	128	134
Diastolic Pressure (K5)								
5	34	37	43	49	55	60	63	70
6	38	41	47	53	59	64	67	73
7	40	44	49	55	61	66	70	76
8	42	45	50	56	62	68	71	77
9	42	45	51	57	63	68	71	77
10	42	45	51	57	63	68	71	77
11	42	45	51	57	63	68	71	77
12	42	45	50	56	62	68	71	77
13	42	45	51	56	62	68	71	77
14	42	45	51	57	63	68	71	77
15	43	46	51	57	63	69	72	78
16	45	48	53	59	65	71	74	80
17	47	51	56	62	68	73	77	83

Data from Park MK, Menard SW, Yuan C: Comparison of blood pressure in children from three
ethnic groups, *Am J Cardiol* 87:1305-1308, 2001.
*The 99th percentile values were added after publication.

TABLE B-4

AUSCULTATORY BLOOD PRESSURE VALUES FOR GIRLS 5 TO 17 YEARS OLD
(SAN ANTONIO CHILDREN'S BLOOD PRESSURE STUDY)

AGE (YR)	*PERCENTILES*							
	5TH	**10TH**	**25TH**	**MEAN**	**75TH**	**90TH**	**95TH**	**99TH***
Systolic Pressure								
5	79	82	87	92	97	102	105	110
6	80	83	88	93	98	103	106	111
7	81	84	89	94	99	104	107	112
8	83	86	91	96	101	106	109	114
9	85	88	93	98	103	108	111	116
10	87	90	95	100	105	110	113	118
11	89	92	97	102	107	112	115	120
12	91	94	98	104	109	113	116	122
13	92	95	100	105	110	115	118	123
14	93	96	101	106	111	116	119	124
15	94	97	101	107	112	117	119	125
16	94	97	102	107	112	117	120	125
17	95	98	103	108	113	118	121	126
Diastolic Pressure (K5)								
5	35	38	44	49	55	60	63	69
6	38	41	47	52	58	63	66	72
7	40	41	49	54	60	65	68	74
8	42	45	50	56	61	67	70	75
9	43	46	51	56	62	67	70	76
10	43	46	51	57	63	68	71	77
11	43	46	51	57	63	68	71	77
12	43	46	52	57	63	68	71	77
13	43	47	52	57	63	68	71	77
14	44	47	52	58	63	68	72	77
15	44	47	52	58	64	69	72	78
16	45	48	53	59	64	69	73	78
17	46	49	54	59	65	70	73	79

Data from Park MK, Menard SW, Yuan C: Comparison of blood pressure in children from three ethnic groups, *Am J Cardiol* 87:1305-1308, 2001.
*The 99th percentile values were added after publication.

TABLE B-5

DINAMAP (MODEL 8100) BLOOD PRESSURE VALUES FOR BOYS 5 TO 17 YEARS
OLD (SAN ANTONIO CHILDREN'S BLOOD PRESSURE STUDY)

AGE	*PERCENTILES*							
(YR)	5TH	10TH	25TH	MEAN	75TH	90TH	95TH	99TH*
Systolic Pressure								
5	90	93	98	104	110	115	118	124
6	92	95	100	106	112	117	120	126
7	93	96	102	107	113	118	121	127
8	94	97	103	108	114	119	123	128
9	95	99	104	110	115	121	124	130
10	97	100	105	110	117	122	125	131
11	99	102	107	113	119	124	127	133
12	101	104	109	115	121	126	129	135
13	104	107	112	118	123	129	132	138
14	106	109	114	120	126	131	134	140
15	108	111	116	122	128	133	136	141
16	109	112	117	123	128	134	137	143
17	109	112	117	123	129	134	137	143
Diastolic Pressure								
5	46	49	53	58	63	68	71	76
6	47	49	54	59	64	68	71	76
7	47	50	54	59	64	69	72	77
8	48	51	55	60	65	70	72	78
9	49	51	56	61	66	70	73	78
10	49	52	56	61	66	71	74	79
11	49	52	57	62	67	71	74	79
12	50	52	57	62	67	71	74	79
13	50	52	57	62	67	71	74	79
14	50	52	57	62	67	72	74	79
15	50	52	57	62	67	72	74	79
16	50	53	57	62	67	72	74	80
17	50	53	57	62	67	72	75	80

From Park MK, Menard SW, Schoolfield J: Oscillometric blood pressure standards for children, *Pediatr Cardiol* 26(5):601-607, 2005.
*The 99th percentile values were added after submission of the manuscript.

TABLE B-6

DINAMAP (MODEL 8100) BLOOD PRESSURE VALUES FOR GIRLS 5 TO 17 YEARS OLD (SAN ANTONIO CHILDREN'S BLOOD PRESSURE STUDY)

AGE (YR)	PERCENTILES							
	5TH	10TH	25TH	MEAN	75TH	90TH	95TH	99TH*
Systolic Pressure								
5	90	93	98	103	109	114	117	122
6	91	94	99	1043	110	115	118	123
7	92	95	100	106	111	116	119	125
8	94	97	102	107	113	118	121	126
9	95	98	103	109	114	119	122	128
10	97	100	105	110	116	121	124	129
11	98	101	106	112	117	122	125	131
12	100	103	107	113	118	123	126	132
13	101	104	109	114	120	125	128	133
14	102	104	109	115	120	125	128	134
15	102	105	110	115	121	126	129	134
16	102	105	110	115	121	126	129	134
17	102	105	110	115	121	126	129	134
Diastolic Pressure								
5	46	48	53	59	64	68	71	76
6	47	49	54	59	64	68	71	76
7	47	50	54	60	65	69	72	77
8	48	50	55	60	65	70	73	78
9	49	51	55	61	66	70	73	78
10	49	51	56	61	66	71	74	79
11	49	52	56	62	67	71	74	79
12	50	52	57	62	67	71	74	79
13	50	53	57	62	67	71	74	79
14	50	53	58	62	67	72	74	79
15	50	54	58	62	67	72	74	79
16	50	54	58	62	67	72	74	80
17	50	54	58	62	67	72	75	80

From Park MK, Menard SW, Schoolfield J: Oscillometric blood pressure standards for children, *Pediatr Cardiol* 26(5):601-607, 2005.

*The 99th percentile values were added after submission of the manuscript.

APPENDIX C:
CARDIOVASCULAR RISK FACTORS

TABLE C-1
SERUM LIPID AND LIPOPROTEIN LEVELS IN U.S. CHILDREN AND ADOLESCENTS (MG/DL)

	SEX	AGE (YR)	5TH	25TH	50TH	75TH	90TH	95TH
						PERCENTILE VALUES		
TOTAL CHOLESTEROL	BOYS	0-4	117	141	156	176	192	209
		5-9	125	147	164	180	197	209
		10-14	123	144	160	178	196	208
		15-19	116	136	150	170	188	203
	GIRLS	0-4	115	143	161	177	195	206
		5-9	130	150	168	184	201	211
		10-14	128	148	163	179	196	207
		15-19	124	144	160	177	197	209
LDL CHOLESTEROL	BOYS	5-9	65	82	93	106	121	133
		10-14	66	83	97	112	126	136
		15-19	64	82	96	112	127	134
	GIRLS	5-9	70	91	101	118	129	144
		10-14	70	83	97	113	130	140
		15-19	61	80	96	114	133	141
HDL CHOLESTEROL	BOYS	5-9	39	50	56	65	72	76
		10-14	38	47	57	63	73	76
		15-19	31	40	47	54	61	65
	GIRLS	5-9	37	48	54	63	69	75
		10-14	38	46	54	60	66	72
		15-19	36	44	53	63	70	76

cont'd

TABLE C-1—cont'd
SERUM LIPID AND LIPOPROTEIN LEVELS IN U.S. CHILDREN AND ADOLESCENTS (MG/DL)

							PERCENTILE VALUES	
SEX	AGE (YR)	5TH	25TH	50TH	75TH	90TH	95TH
TRIGLYCERIDE	**BOYS**	0-4	30	46	53	69	87	102
		5-9	31	45	53	67	88	104
		10-14	33	56	61	80	105	129
		15-19	38	55	71	94	124	152
	GIRLS	0-4	35	46	61	79	99	115
		5-9	33	45	57	73	93	108
		10-14	38	56	72	93	117	135
		15-19	40	55	70	90	117	136

From Report of the Expert Panel on Blood Cholesterol Levels in Children and Adolescents, National Cholesterol Education Program, U.S. Department of Health and Human Services, National Institute of Health, NIH Publication 91-2732, September 1991.
HDL, high-density lipoprotein; LDL, low-density lipoprotein.

TABLE C-2
ESTIMATED VALUE FOR PERCENTILE REGRESSION OF WAIST CIRCUMFERENCE FOR EUROPEAN-AMERICAN CHILDREN AND ADOLESCENTS ACCORDING TO SEX*

AGE (YR)	PERCENTILE FOR BOYS					PERCENTILE FOR GIRLS				
	10TH	25TH	50TH	75TH	90TH	10TH	25TH	50TH	75TH	90TH
2	42.9	46.9	47.1	48.6	50.6	43.1	45.1	47.4	49.6	52.5
3	44.7	48.8	49.2	51.2	54.0	44.7	46.8	49.3	51.9	55.4
4	46.5	50.6	51.3	53.8	57.4	46.3	48.5	51.2	54.2	58.2
5	48.3	52.5	53.3	56.5	60.8	47.9	50.2	53.1	56.5	61.1
6	50.1	54.3	55.4	59.1	64.2	49.5	51.8	55.0	58.8	64.0
7	46.5	50.6	51.3	53.8	57.4	46.3	48.5	51.2	54.2	58.2
8	48.3	52.5	53.3	56.5	60.8	47.9	50.2	53.1	56.5	61.1
9	50.1	54.3	55.4	59.1	64.2	49.5	51.8	55.0	58.8	64.0
10	46.5	50.6	51.3	53.8	57.4	46.3	48.5	51.2	54.2	58.2
11	59.1	63.6	65.8	72.2	81.1	57.5	60.2	64.4	70.3	78.3
12	60.9	65.5	67.9	74.9	84.5	59.1	61.9	66.3	72.6	81.2
13	62.7	67.4	70.0	77.5	87.9	60.7	63.6	68.2	74.9	84.1
14	64.5	69.2	72.1	80.1	91.3	62.3	65.3	70.1	77.2	86.9
15	66.3	71.1	74.1	82.8	94.7	63.9	67.0	72.0	79.5	89.8
16	68.1	72.9	76.2	85.4	98.1	65.5	68.6	73.9	81.8	92.7
17	69.9	74.8	78.3	88.0	101.5	67.1	70.3	75.8	84.1	95.5
18	71.7	76.7	80.4	90.6	104.9	68.7	72.0	77.7	86.4	98.4

From Fernandez JR, Redden DT, Pietrobelli A et al: Waist circumference percentiles in nationally representative samples of African-American, European-American, and Mexican-American children and adolescents, *J Pediatr* 145:439-444, 2004.

* Waist circumference was measured with a tape at just above the uppermost lateral border of the right ileum at the end of normal expiration.

TABLE C-3
ESTIMATED VALUE FOR PERCENTILE REGRESSION OF WAIST CIRCUMFERENCE FOR AFRICAN-AMERICAN CHILDREN AND ADOLESCENTS ACCORDING TO SEX*

	PERCENTILE FOR BOYS					PERCENTILE FOR GIRLS				
AGE (YR)	10TH	25TH	50TH	75TH	90TH	10TH	25TH	50TH	75TH	90TH
2	43.2	44.6	46.4	48.5	50.0	43.0	44.6	46.0	47.7	50.1
3	44.8	46.3	48.3	50.7	53.2	44.6	46.3	48.1	50.6	53.8
4	46.3	48.0	50.1	52.9	56.4	46.1	48.0	50.2	53.4	57.5
5	47.9	49.7	52.0	55.1	59.6	47.7	49.7	52.3	56.2	61.1
6	49.4	51.4	53.9	57.3	62.8	49.2	51.4	54.5	59.0	64.8
7	51.0	53.1	55.7	59.5	66.1	50.8	53.2	56.6	61.8	68.5
8	52.5	54.8	57.6	61.7	69.3	52.4	54.9	58.7	64.7	72.2
9	54.1	56.4	59.4	63.9	72.5	53.9	56.6	60.9	67.5	75.8
10	55.6	58.1	61.3	66.1	75.7	55.5	58.3	63.0	70.3	79.5
11	57.2	59.8	63.2	68.3	78.9	57.0	60.0	65.1	73.1	83.2
12	58.7	61.5	65.0	70.5	82.1	58.6	61.7	67.3	75.9	86.9
13	60.3	63.2	66.9	72.7	85.3	60.2	63.4	69.4	78.8	90.5
14	61.8	64.9	68.7	74.9	88.5	61.7	65.1	71.5	81.6	94.2
15	63.4	66.6	70.6	77.1	91.7	63.3	66.8	73.6	84.4	97.9
16	64.9	68.3	72.5	79.3	94.9	64.8	68.5	75.8	87.2	101.6
17	66.5	70.0	74.3	81.5	98.2	66.4	70.3	77.9	90.0	105.2
18	68.0	71.7	76.2	83.7	101.4	68.0	72.0	80.0	92.9	108.9

From Fernandez JR, Redden DT, Pietrobelli A et al: Waist circumference percentiles in nationally representative samples of African-American, European-American, and Mexican-American children and adolescents, *J Pediatr* 145:439-444, 2004.

* Waist circumference was measured with a tape at just above the uppermost lateral border of the right ileum at the end of normal expiration.

TABLE C-4

ESTIMATED VALUE FOR PERCENTILE REGRESSION OF WAIST CIRCUMFERENCE FOR MEXICAN-AMERICAN CHILDREN AND ADOLESCENTS ACCORDING TO SEX*

AGE (YR)	PERCENTILE FOR BOYS					PERCENTILE FOR GIRLS				
	10TH	25TH	50TH	75TH	90TH	10TH	25TH	50TH	75TH	90TH
2	44.4	45.6	47.6	49.8	53.2	44.5	45.7	48.0	50.0	53.5
3	46.1	47.5	49.8	52.5	56.7	46.0	47.4	50.1	52.6	56.7
4	47.8	49.4	52.0	55.3	60.2	47.5	49.2	52.2	55.2	59.9
5	49.5	51.3	54.2	58.0	63.6	49.0	51.0	54.2	57.8	63.0
6	51.2	53.2	56.3	60.7	67.1	50.5	52.7	56.3	60.4	66.2
7	52.9	55.1	58.5	63.4	70.6	52.0	54.5	58.4	63.0	69.4
8	54.6	57.0	60.7	66.2	74.1	53.5	56.3	60.4	65.6	72.6
9	56.3	58.9	62.9	68.9	77.6	55.0	58.0	62.5	68.2	75.8
10	58.0	60.8	65.1	71.6	81.0	56.5	59.8	64.6	70.8	78.9
11	59.7	62.7	67.2	74.4	84.5	58.1	61.6	66.6	73.4	82.1
12	61.4	64.6	69.4	77.1	88.0	59.6	63.4	68.7	76.0	85.3
13	63.1	66.5	71.6	79.8	91.5	61.1	65.1	70.8	78.6	88.5
14	64.8	68.4	73.8	82.6	95.0	62.6	66.9	72.9	81.2	91.7
15	66.5	70.3	76.0	85.3	98.4	64.1	68.7	74.9	83.8	94.8
16	68.2	72.2	78.1	88.0	101.9	65.6	70.4	77.0	86.4	98.0
17	69.9	74.1	80.3	90.7	105.4	67.1	72.2	79.1	89.0	101.2
18	71.6	76.0	82.5	93.5	108.9	68.6	74.0	81.1	91.6	104.4

From Fernandez JR, Redden DT, Pietrobelli A et al: Waist circumference percentiles in nationally representative samples of African-American, European-American, and Mexican-American children and adolescents, *J Pediatr* 145:439-444, 2004.

* Waist circumference was measured with a tape at just above the uppermost lateral border of the right ileum at the end of normal expiration.

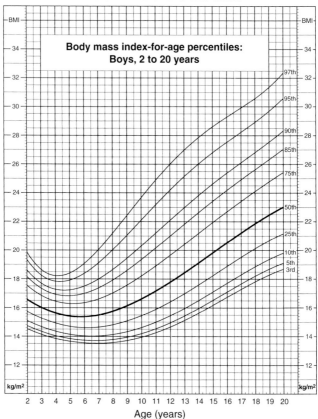

CDC Growth Charts: United States

**Body mass index-for-age percentiles:
Boys, 2 to 20 years**

Age (years)

Published May 30, 2000.

Source: Developed by the National Center for Health Statistics in collaboration with
the National Center for Chronic Disease Prevention and Health Promotion (2000).

FIG. C-1

Body mass index-for-age percentile for boys 2 to 20 years old. *(From Kuczmarski RJ,
Ogden CL, Grummer-Strawn LM et al: CDC growth charts: United States. Advance
data from vital and health statistics; no 314, Hyattsville, Maryland, 2000, National
Center for Health Statistics.)*

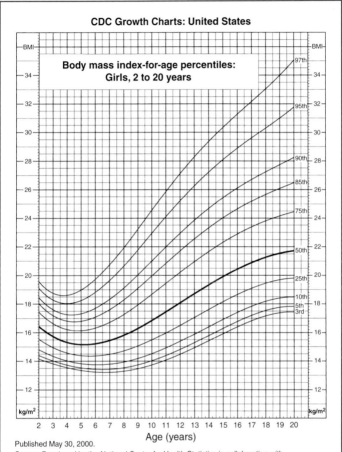

CDC Growth Charts: United States

Body mass index-for-age percentiles:
Girls, 2 to 20 years

Published May 30, 2000.
Source: Developed by the National Center for Health Statistics in collaboration with
the National Center for Chronic Disease Prevention and Health Promotion (2000).

FIG. C-2

Body mass index-for-age percentile for girls 2 to 20 years old. *(From Kuczmarski RJ, Ogden CL, Grummer-Strawn LM et al: CDC growth charts: United States. Advance data from vital and health statistics; no 314, Hyattsville, Maryland, 2000, National Center for Health Statistics.)*

APPENDIX D:
NORMAL ECHOCARDIOGRAPHY VALUES

TABLE D-1

STAND-ALONE M-MODE ECHO MEASUREMENTS. LA, RV, AND LV SIZE AND THICKNESS OF LV WALL BY BODY SURFACE AREA: MEAN (90% TOLERANCE LIMITS) (IN MM)

BSA (m²)	0.25	0.3	0.4	0.5	0.6	0.7	0.8	0.9	1.0	1.2	1.4	1.6	1.8	2.0
BW (kg)*	3	4	7	10	13	16	19	23	28	37	46	55	70	80
AO														
Dimension†	11	12	13	14	15	16	17	18	19	21	22	23	24	24
	(7-15)	(7.5-16)	(9-17.5)	(9.5-19)	(10.5-21)	(11.5-22)	(12.5-24)	(13-24.5)	(13.5-25)	(14.5-27)	(15.5-29)	(16-30.5)	(16-32)	(16-33)
LA														
Dimension‡	15	16	18	19	20	22	23	24	26	27	28	29	29	30
	(7-22)	(8-23)	(9-25)	(11-27)	(12-29)	(13-31)	(14-33)	(15-34)	(16-35)	(17-38)	(17-40)	(18-42)	(18-43)	(18-44)
RV														
Dimension†	8	9.5	10	10	11	12	13	14	14	16	18	20	22	23
	(-16)	(-17)	(-17)	(2.5-18)	(3-19)	(3.5-21)	(4-22)	(4.5-23)	(5-24)	(6-26)	(6.5-29)	(7-32)	(7.5-35)	(8-42)
LV														
Dimension†	20	22	25	27	30	33	35	37	39	42	43	45	45	46
	(11-29)	(13-30)	(16-33)	(18-37)	(21-40)	(23-43)	(25-45)	(27-47)	(28-50)	(30-53)	(31-56)	(32-58)	(32-61)	(32-62)
LV														
Dimension‡	12	13	15	17	19	20	22	23	24	26	27	28	28	28
	(7-17)	(8-19)	(9-21)	(11-23)	(12-25)	(14-27)	(15-28)	(16-30)	(17-31)	(18-34)	(19-36)	(10-37)	(19-38)	(19-39)
IVS														
Thickness†	3.5	3.5	4	4	4.5	5	5	5.5	5.5	6	7	7.5	8	8.5
	(1.5-5.5)	(1.5-5.5)	(1.5-6)	(2-6.5)	(2-7)	(2-7)	(2.5-7.5)	(2.5-8)	(3-8.5)	(3-9)	(3.5-10)	(4-11)	(4-12)	(4.5-13)
LVPW	3.5	3.5	4	4	4.5	5	5	5	5.5	6	7	7.5	8	8.5
Thickness†	(1.5-5.5)	(1.5-5.5)	(2-6)	(2-6.5)	(2-7)	(2.5-7.5)	(2.5-7.5)	(3-8)	(3-8.5)	(3-9.5)	(3.5-10)	(4-11)	(4-12)	(4.5-13)

* Approximate weight for average-size individual.
† Diastolic
‡ Systolic

AO, aorta; BSA, body surface area; BW, body weight; IVS, interventricular septum; LA, left atrium; LV, left ventricle; LVPW, left ventricular posterior wall; RV, right ventricle.

TABLE D-2

TWO-D ECHO-DERIVED M-MODE MEASUREMENTS: AORTIC ANNULUS, LA, AND
LV DIMENSIONS BY AGE: MEAN (95% CONFIDENCE LIMIT) (IN MM)

AGE (YR)	AORTIC ANNULUS (PL)	LA DIAMETER (PL)	LV DIAMETER (PL)
1	10 (7-13)	17 (12-22)	24 (17-32)
2	11 (8.5-4)	18 (13-23)	27 (19-33)
3	12 (9.5-15)	20 (15-25)	28 (22-36)
4	13 (10-16)	21 (16-26)	31 (24-38)
5	14 (11-17)	22 (17-27)	33 (26-39)
6	15 (12-18)	23 (18-28)	34 (28-41)
7	15 (13-19)	24 (19-29)	36 (29-43)
8	16 (14-19)	25 (20-30)	37 (31-44)
9	17 (14-20)	26 (21-31)	38 (32-45)
10	17 (15-20)	27 (22-32)	40 (33-47)
11	18 (15-21)	27 (22-32)	41 (34-48)
12	18 (16-21)	28 (23-33)	42 (35-49)
13	19 (16-21)	29 (23-34)	43 (37-51)
14	19 (16-22)	29 (23-34)	43 (36-50)
15	19 (16-22)	29 (24-34)	43 (37-51)
16	19 (17-22)	29 (24-34)	44 (38-52)
17	19 (17-22)	29 (24-34)	44 (38-52)
18	19 (17-22)	29 (24-34)	45 (38-52)

Values have been derived from graphic data of Nidorf SM, Picard MH, Triulzi MO et al: New perspectives in the assessment of cardiac chamber dimensions during development and adulthood,
J Am Coll Cardiol 19:983-988, 1992.

Values rounded off to the nearest 0.5 mm for measurements <10 mm and to the nearest 1 mm for
measurements ≥10 mm.

PL, parasternal long-axis view.

TABLE D-3

M-MODE ECHO MEASUREMENTS: LA AND LV DIMENSIONS BY HEIGHT (IN MM): MEAN (95% CONFIDENCE LIMIT)

Height (cm)	40	50	60	70	80	90	100	110	120	130	140	150	160	170	180	190	200
LA Diameter (PL)	12 (7-18)	14 (8.5-19)	15 (10-20)	17 (11-22)	18 (13-23)	19 (14-24)	20 (15-26)	22 (17-27)	23 (18-28)	24 (19-30)	26 (21-31)	27 (22-32)	28 (23-33)	30 (24-35)	31 (26-36)	32 (27-38)	33 (28-39)
LV Diameter (PL)	17 (10-24)	19 (13-26)	22 (14-28)	24 (17-31)	26 (19-33)	28 (21-35)	30 (23-37)	32 (25-40)	35 (27-42)	37 (30-45)	39 (32-47)	42 (34-49)	44 (37-51)	46 (39-53)	48 (41-55)	50 (43-57)	52 (45-59)

Values have been derived from graphic data of Nidorf SM, Picard MH, Triulzi MO et al: New perspectives in the assessment of cardiac chamber dimensions during development and adulthood, *J Am Coll Cardiol* 19:983-988, 1992.

Values rounded off to the nearest 0.5 mm for measurements <10 mm and to the nearest 1 mm for measurements ≥10 mm.

PL, parasternal long-axis view.

TABLE D-4
DIMENSIONS OF AORTA AND PULMONARY ARTERIES BY TWO-DIMENSIONAL ECHO*†

ECHO VIEWS		BSA (m²)	0.25	0.3	0.4	0.5	0.6	0.7	0.8	1.0	1.2	1.4	1.6	1.8	2.0
		Approx. BW (Kg)	3	4	7	10	13	16	19	28	37	46	55	70	80
	AA		10 (7-13)†	11 (7.5-15)	13 (9-16)	14 (10-18)	15 (11-19)	16 (12-20)	17 (12-21)	18 (14-23)	20 (15-25)	22 (16-27)	23 (18-29)	25 (19-31)	26 (20-32)
	MPA		9 (5-12)	10 (6-13)	11 (7-14)	12 (8-16)	13 (9-17)	14 (9-18)	15 (11-19)	16 (12-21)	17 (13-23)	19 (14-24)	21 (14-26)	22 (14-28)	23 (15-29)
	RPA		5.5 (3.5-8)	6 (4-8.5)	6.5 (4.5-9)	7.5 (5-10)	8 (5.5-10)	8.5 (6-11)	9 (7-11)	10 (7-12)	10 (8-14)	11 (8-15)	12 (8.5-16)	13 (9-16)	13 (9-17)
	AA		7.5 (4-10)	8 (4.5-11)	9 (6-12)	10 (6.5-13)	11 (7.5-14)	12 (8.5-15)	12 (9-16)	14 (11-18)	15 (12-19)	17 (14-21)	18 (13-23)	19 (14-24)	20 (15-25)
	TA		6 (4-8.5)	7 (4.5-9)	8 (5.5-11)	9 (6.5-11)	10 (7.5-12)	11 (8-13)	11 (8.5-14)	13 (10-16)	15 (11-17)	15 (12-18)	17 (13-19)	18 (14-21)	19 (15-22)
	RPA		6 (4-8)	6.5 (4.5-9)	7.5 (5-10)	8.5 (6-11)	9 (6.5-11)	9.5 (7-12)	10 (8-13)	12 (9-15)	13 (10-16)	14 (11-17)	15 (11-18)	16 (12-19)	16 (13-20)
	TA		9 (6-11)	10 (7-12.5)	11 (8-14)	12 (9.5-15)	13 (10.5-16)	14 (11-17)	15 (13-18)	17 (14-20)	19 (15-22)	20 (17-24)	22 (18-27)	24 (19-28)	25 (20-30)
	RPA		6 (4-8)	6.5 (4.5-9)	7 (5-10)	8 (6-10)	9 (6.5-11)	9.5 (7.5-11)	10 (8-12)	11 (9-14)	12 (10-15)	13 (11-16)	15 (11-18)	16 (12-19)	16 (13-20)

Values have been derived from graphic data of Snider AR, Enderlein MA, Teitel DJ et al: Two-dimensional echocardiographic determination of aortic and pulmonary artery sizes from infancy to adulthood in normal subjects. *Am J Cardiol* 53:218-224, 1984.

*Values are rounded off to the nearest 0.5 mm for measurements <10 mm and to the nearest 1 mm for measurements ≥10 mm. Measurements are made at the end of diastole (the Q wave), using a leading-edge technique.

† Figures in parentheses are the tolerance limits weighted for body surface area for prediction of normal values for 80% of the future population with 50% confidence.

AA, ascending aorta; AO, aorta; BSA, body surface area; BW, body weight; LA, left atrium; MPA, main pulmonary artery; RA, right atrium; RPA, right pulmonary artery; RV, right ventricle; SVC, superior vena cava; TA, transverse aorta.

TABLE D-5

AORTIC ROOT DIMENSION BY 2D ECHO: MEAN (95% CL)*

Height (cm)	50	60	70	80	90	100	110
Aortic Annulus	7 (4-10)	8 (5.5-11.5)	9.5 (6.5-13)	10.5 (7-13.5)	12 (8.5-14.5)	13 (9.5-16)	14 (11-17)
Sinus of Valsalva	9 (5-13.5)	11 (7-15)	13 (8-17)	14 (10-18.5)	15.5 (12-20)	17.5 (13.5-22)	19 (15-23.5)
Supraaortic Ridge	7 (4-10)	8.5 (5.5-11.5)	10 (7-13)	11.5 (8-14)	12.5 (9-15.5)	14 (10.5-17)	15 (12-18.5)
Ascending Aorta	7.5 (3-11.5)	9 (5-12.5)	10.5 (6.5-14)	12 (8-15.5)	13.5 (9.5-17)	15 (11-18.5)	16.5 (12.5-20)

SOV/ Aortic Annulus	1.37 (95% CL, 1.18-1.56)
SAR/Aortic Annulus	1.11 (95% CL, 0.95-1.28)
AAO/Aortic Annulus	1.16 (95% CL, 0.97-1.35)

Values are derived from graphic data of Sheil ML, Jenkins O, Sholler GF: Echocardiographic assessment of aortic root dimensions in normal children based on measurement of a new ratio of aortic size independent of growth, *Am J Cardiol* 75:711-715, 1995.

*Measurements were obtained in the parasternal long-axis view, perpendicular to the long axis, using a leading-edge technique, during systole. Values are rounded off to the nearest 0.5 mm.

AAO, ascending aorta; SAR, supraaortic ridge; SOV, sinus of Valsalva.

120	130	140	150	160	170	180	190
15	16.5	17	18.5	19	20.5	21.5	23
(12-18)	(13.5-19)	(14-20)	(15.5-21.5)	(16.5-23)	(17.5-24)	(18.5-24.5)	(19.5-25.5)
20.5	22.5	24	26	27.5	29	30	32
(16.5-25)	(18-26.5)	(20-27.5)	(21.5-29.5)	(23-31.5)	(25-33)	(26-34.5)	(28-36)
16.5	18	19	20	21.5	23	24	25.5
(13.5-19.5)	(14.5-20.5)	(16-22)	(17.5-23.5)	(18.5-25)	(20-26)	(21.5-27.5)	(22.5-28.5)
18	19	20.5	21.5	23	24	26	27.5
(14-21.5)	(15-22.5)	(17-24)	(18-25.5)	(19.5-27)	(21-28)	(22-30)	(23.5-32)

TABLE D-6

MITRAL AND TRICUSPID VALVE ANNULUS DIAMETER BY 2D ECHO: MEAN (95% CL)

BSA (m²)	0.2	0.25	0.3	0.4	0.5	0.6	0.7	0.8	0.9	1.0	1.2	1.4
BW (kg)[†]	2	3	4	7	10	13	16	19	23	28	37	46
Mitral Valve (PL)	10	12	13	16	18	19	21	22	23	24	25	26
	(7-13)	(9-15)	(10-16)	(13-19)	(15-21)	(16-23)	(18-24)	(18-26)	(19-26)	(20-27)	(22-28)	(23-30)
Mitral Valve (A4C, S4C)*	12	15	17	20	23	25	27	29	31	32	35	36
	(7-17)	(10-20)	(12-22)	(16-25)	(18-28)	(20-31)	(22-32)	(23-35)	(25-36)	(26-37)	(28-40)	(31-42)
Tricuspid Valve (A4C, S4C)*	12	15	17	21	23	26	27	29	31	32	34	36
	(8-17)	(10-19)	(12-22)	(16-26)	(18-29)	(20-31)	(22-33)	(33-36)	(24-37)	(25-38)	(25-42)	(28-44)

Adapted from data presented in graphic form by King DH, Smith EO, Huhta LC et al: Mitral and tricuspid valve annular diameter in normal children determined by two-dimensional echocardiography, *Am J Cardiol* 55:787-789, 1985.

* Measurements greater of two projections A4C and S4C.

[†] Approximate weight for average-size individuals.

Measurements made at onset of R waves on ECG, using inner edge to inner edge method.

A4C, apical four-chamber view; S4C, subcostal four-chamber view; PL, parasternal long-axis view.

TABLE D-7
SELECTED 2-D ECHO MEASUREMENTS OF VALVE ANNULI IN NEONATES: 95% PREDICTION INTERVAL (MM)*

Body Weight (kg)	0.5	1.0	1.5	2.0	2.5	3.0	3.5	4.0	4.5	5.0
Aortic valve annulus (PL)	4-5.5	4.5-6	4.5-6.5	5-7	5.5-7.5	6-8	6.5-8.5	7-9	7.5-9	8-9.5
Pulmonary valve annulus (PL)	4-7.5	4.5-8	5.5-9	6-9.5	6.5-10	7.5-11	8-11.5	8.5-12	9.5-13	10-13.5
Mitral valve annulus (PL)	5.5-9.5	6-10	6.5-11	7-11.5	8-12	8.5-13	9-13.5	9.5-14	10-14.5	11-15.5
Mitral valve annulus (apical view)	6-9.5	6.5-10	7.5-11	8-11.5	8.5-12	9-12.5	9.5-13	10.5-14	11-14.5	11.5-15
Tricuspid valve annulus (apical view)	6.5-9.5	7-10.5	8-11	8.5-12	9.5-12.5	10-13.5	11-14	11.5-15	12-15.5	13-16

Data are derived from graphic presentation by Tacy TA, Vermillion RP, Ludomirsky A: Range of normal valve annulus size in neonates, *Am J Cardiol* 75:541-543, 1995.
* Values rounded off to the nearest 0.5 mm.
PL, parasternal long-axis view.

TABLE D-8
NORMAL DIMENSIONS OF MAJOR CORONARY ARTERIES (MEAN PLUS 2 AND 3 STANDARD DEVIATIONS)*

	BSA (M²)	0.2	0.3	0.4	0.5	0.6	0.7	0.8	1.0	1.2	1.4	1.6	1.8	2.0
LAD[†]	Mean	1.2	1.4	1.6	1.8	1.9	2.0	2.2	2.3	2.5	2.7	2.8	2.9	3.0
	Mean + 2SD	1.5	1.8	2.1	2.3	2.5	2.7	2.8	3.0	3.3	3.5	3.7	4.0	4.2
	Mean + 3SD	1.7	2.0	2.3	2.5	2.8	3.0	3.2	3.4	3.8	4.0	4.3	4.5	4.7
RCA	Mean	1.3	1.4	1.6	1.7	1.8	2.0	2.1	2.3	2.5	2.7	2.8	3.0	3.2
	Mean + 2SD	1.9	2.1	2.3	2.4	2.6	2.7	2.8	3.1	3.4	3.6	3.8	4.0	4.3
	Mean + 3SD	2.2	2.4	2.6	2.8	3.0	3.1	3.3	3.5	3.8	4.1	4.3	4.5	4.8
LMCA	Mean	1.7	1.9	2.1	2.3	2.4	2.5	2.7	2.9	3.1	3.3	3.4	3.6	3.7
	Mean + 2SD	2.3	2.6	2.8	3.0	3.3	3.4	3.6	3.9	4.2	4.4	4.6	4.8	5.1
	Mean + 3SD	2.7	3.0	3.2	3.4	3.7	3.9	4.0	4.3	4.7	4.9	5.2	5.5	5.8

Values are from graphic data of Kurotobi S, Nagai T, Kawakami N et al: Coronary diameter in normal infants, children and patients with Kawasaki disease, *Pediatr Int* 44:1-4, 2002.

* Measurements are made from inner edge to inner edge. Values are rounded off to the nearest 0.1 mm.

† The dimension of LMCA should not be measured at orifice and immediate vicinity.

LAD, left anterior descending; LMCA, left main coronary artery; RCA, right coronary artery.

DOSAGES OF DRUGS USED IN PEDIATRIC CARDIOLOGY

TABLE E-1
DOSAGES OF DRUGS USED IN PEDIATRIC CARDIOLOGY

DRUG	ROUTE AND DOSAGE	TOXICITY OR SIDE EFFECTS	HOW SUPPLIED
Acetazolamide (Diamox) (Carbonic anhydrase inhibitor, diuretic)	*Children:* IV, PO: 5 mg/kg/dose, QD-QOD *Adults:* IV, PO: 250-375 mg/dose, QD-QOD	GI irritation, paresthesia, sedation, hypokalemia, acidosis, reduced urate secretion, aplastic anemia, polyuria, renal calculi Contraindications: hepatic failure, severe renal failure, sulfonamide hypersensitivity	Tab: 125, 250 mg Susp: 25, 50 mg/mL Caps, sustained release: 500 mg Inj: 500 mg/mL
Acetylsalicylic acid (Aspirin)	*Children and adults:* **Antiplatelet therapy:** PO: 3-5 mg/kg, QD **Antipyretic/analgesic:** PO, PR: 10-15 mg/kg/dose, q4-6 hr (max 4g/24 hr) **Antiinflammatory:** PO: 80-100 mg/kg/24 hr, TID-QID	Rash, nausea, hepatotoxicity, GI bleeding, bronchospasm, GI distress, tinnitus Contraindications: hepatic failure, bleeding disorder, hypersensitivity, children <16 yr old with chickenpox or flu symptoms (due to the association with Reye syndrome)	Tab: 325, 500 mg Tab, enteric-coated: 81,165, 325, 500, 650 mg Tab, chewable: 81 mg Supp: 60, 80, 120, 125, 200, 300, 325, 600, 650 mg, and 1.2 g
Adenosine (Adenocard) (Antiarrhythmic)	*Children and adults:* **For SVT:** IV: 100-200 mcg/kg; repeat q1-2 min, with increment of 50 mcg/kg, to maximum of 250 mcg/kg (max single dose 12 mg)	Bronchospasm, chest pain, transient asystole, bradycardia and tachycardia Transient AV block in atrial flutter/fibrillation (±)	Inj: 3 mg/mL (2, 4 mL)

cont'd

TABLE E-1—cont'd

DOSAGES OF DRUGS USED IN PEDIATRIC CARDIOLOGY

DRUG	ROUTE AND DOSAGE	TOXICITY OR SIDE EFFECTS	HOW SUPPLIED
Amiodarone (Cordarone) (Class III antiarrhythmic)	*Children:* IV (in emergency situation): *Loading:* 5 mg/kg, slow infusion over 30 min, followed by infusion of 7 mcg/kg/min (which is calculated to deliver 10 mg/kg/24 hr) Switch to oral maintenance dose as soon as clinical condition permits PO: 10-20 mg/kg/24 hr (*infants*) or 10 mg/kg/24 hr (*children and adolescents*) in 2 doses for 5 to 14 days, followed by maintenance dose of 5-7 mg/kg once a day [*Therapeutic level:* 0.5-2.5 mg/L] *Adults:* PO: *Loading:* 800-1600 mg QD for 1-3 wk, then reduce to 600-800 mg QD for 1 mo *Maintenance:* 200-400 mg QD	Progressive dyspnea and cough (pulmonary fibrosis), worsening of arrhythmias, hepatotoxicity, nausea and vomiting, corneal microdeposits, hypotension, heart block, ataxia, hypothyroidism or hyperthyroidism, photosensitivity Contraindications: AV block, sinus node dysfunction, sinus bradycardia	Tab: 200, 400 mg Susp: 5 mg/mL Inj: 50 mg/mL

Drug	Dosage	Toxicity or Side Effects	How Supplied
Amlopidine (Norvasc) (Calcium channel blocker, antihypertensive)	**For hypertension:** *Children:* PO: Initial 0.1 mg/kg/dose QD-BID; may be increased gradually to a max of 0.6 mg/kg/24 hr *Adults:* PO: 5-10 mg/dose QD (max 10 mg/24 hr)	Edema, dizziness, flushing, palpitation, headache, fatigue, nausea, abdominal pain, somnolence	Tab: 2.5, 5, 10 mg Susp: 1 mg/mL
Atenolol (Tenormin) (β_1-adrenoceptor blocker, antihypertensive, antiarrhythmic)	*Children:* PO: 1-2 mg/kg/dose, QD *Adults:* PO: 25-100 mg/dose, QD for 1-2 wk (alone or with diuretic for hypertension); may increase to 200 mg QD	CNS symptoms (dizziness, tiredness, depression), bradycardia, postural hypotension, nausea and vomiting, rash, blood dyscrasias (agranulocytosis, purpura)	Tab: 25, 50, 100 mg Susp: 2 mg/mL Inj: 0.5 mg/mL (10 mL)
Atorvastatin (Lipitor) (Antilipemic, "statin," HMG-CoA reductase inhibitor)	*Children:* PO: Starting dose 10 mg QD for 4-6 wk; increase to 20 mg QD and 40 mg QD as needed (Adult max dose: 80 mg/24 hr)	Headache, constipation, diarrhea, elevated liver enzymes, rhabdomyolysis, myopathy	Tab: 10, 20, 40, 80 mg
Azathioprine (Imuran, Azasan) (Immunosuppressant)	*Children:* IV, PO: *Initial:* 3-5 mg/kg/24 hr, QD *Maintenance:* 1-3 mg/kg/24 hr (to produce WBC count around 5000/mm³); may be reduced if WBC count falls below 4000/mm³	Bone marrow suppression (leukopenia, thrombocytopenia, anemia), GI symptoms (nausea and vomiting)	Tab: 25, 50, 75, 100 mg Susp: 50 mg/mL Inj: 100 mg powder for reconst

cont'd

TABLE E-1—cont'd
DOSAGES OF DRUGS USED IN PEDIATRIC CARDIOLOGY

DRUG	ROUTE AND DOSAGE	TOXICITY OR SIDE EFFECTS	HOW SUPPLIED
Bosentan (Tracleer) (Nonselective endothelin receptor blocker)	*For pulmonary hypertension:* *Children:* PO: *<20 kg:* 31.25 mg BID *20-40 kg:* 62.5 mg BID *>40 kg:* 125 mg BID *Adults:* PO: 125 mg BID	Liver dysfunction, decrease in hemoglobin, fluid retention, heart failure, headache	Tab: 62.5, 125 mg
Bumetanide (Bumex) (Loop diuretic)	*Children:* PO, IM, IV: >6 mo: 0.015-0.1 mg/kg/dose, QD-QOD *Adults:* PO: 0.5-2 mg/dose, QD-BID IV: 0.5-1 mg over 1-2 min, q2-3 hr PRN (max 10 mg/24 hr)	Hypotension, cramps, dizziness, headache, electrolyte losses (hypokalemia, hypocalcemia, hyponatremia, hypochloremia), metabolic alkalosis	Tab: 0.5, 1, 2 mg Inj: 0.25 mg/mL
Calcium glubionate (Neo-Calglucon 6.4% elemental calcium) (Calcium supplement)	*For neonatal hypocalcemia:* PO: 1200 mg/kg/24 hr, q4-6 hr *Maintenance:* *Infants and children:* PO: 600-2000 mg/kg/24 hr, QID (max 9 g/24 hr) *Adults:* PO: 6-18 g/24 hr, QID	GI irritation, diarrhea, dizziness, headache Best absorbed when given before meals	Syrup: 1.8 g/5 mL (480 mL) (1.2 mEq Ca/mL)

Drug	Dosage	Adverse effects	Supplied
Captopril (Capoten) (ACE inhibitor, antihypertensive, vasodilator)	*Neonates:* PO: 0.1-0.4 mg/kg/24 hr, TID-QID *Infants:* PO: Initially 0.15-0.3 mg/kg/dose, QD-QID; titrate upward if needed (max 6 mg/kg/24 hr) *Children:* PO: Initially 0.3-0.5 mg/kg/dose, TID; titrate upward if needed (max 6 mg/kg/24 hr, BID-QID) *Adolescents and adults:* PO: Initially 12.5-25 mg/dose, BID-TID; increase weekly if needed by 25 mg/dose to max dose 450 mg/24 hr (Adjust dose with renal failure)	Neutropenia/agranulocytosis, proteinuria, hypotension and tachycardia, rash, taste impairment, hyperkalemia Evidence of fetal risk if given during 2nd and 3rd trimesters (same with all other ACE inhibitors)	Tab: 12.5, 25, 50, 100 mg Susp: 0.75, 1 mg/mL
Carnitine (Carnitor)	*Children:* PO: 50-100 mg/kg/24 hr, BID-TID; increase slowly as needed (max 3 g/24 hr) *Adults:* PO: 330 mg-1 g/dose, BID-TID IV (*child and adult*): 50 mg/kg as loading dose, then 50 mg/kg/24 hr, q4-6 hr	Nausea and vomiting, abdominal cramps, diarrhea, seizure	Tab: 330, 500 mg Caps: 250 mg Oral sol: 100 mg/mL (118 ml) Inj: 200 mg/mL (5 mL)

cont'd

TABLE E-1—cont'd
DOSAGES OF DRUGS USED IN PEDIATRIC CARDIOLOGY

DRUG	ROUTE AND DOSAGE	TOXICITY OR SIDE EFFECTS	HOW SUPPLIED
Carvedilol (Coreg, Coreg CR) (Nonselective α- and β-adrenergic blocker)	*Children:* PO: Initial 0.09 mg/kg/dose, BID; increase gradually to 0.36 and 0.75 mg/kg as tolerated to adult max dose of 50 mg/24 hr *Adults:* PO: 3.125 mg, BID for 2 wk; increase slowly to a max dose of 25 mg BID as needed (for heart failure) (max 25 mg BID for <85kg; 50 mg BID for >85 kg)	Dizziness, hypotension, headache, diarrhea, rarely AV block	Tab: 3.125, 6.125, 12.5, 25 mg Tab, extended release: 10, 20, 40, 80 mg
Chloral hydrate (Noctec, Aquachloral) (Sedative, hypnotic)	*As sedative:* *Children:* PO, PR: 25-50 mg/kg/dose q6-8 hr Sedation for procedures: 25-100 mg (max dose 2g) *Adults:* PO, PR: 250 mg/dose q8 hr *As hypnotic:* *Adults:* PO, PR: 500-2000 mg/dose	Mucous membrane irritation (laryngospasm if aspirated), GI irritation, excitement/delirium, hypotension Contraindicated in hepatic and renal impairment	Caps: 500 mg Syrup: 250, 500 mg/5 mL Supp: 324, 500, 648 mg

Drug	Dosage	Side effects	How supplied
Chlorothiazide (Diuril) (Diuretic)	*Children:* PO: 20-40 mg/kg/24 hr, BID IV: 2-8 mg/kg/24 hr, BID *Adults:* PO, IV: 250-2000 mg/dose QD-BID	Hypercalcemia, hyperbilirubinemia, hyperglycemia, hyperuricemia, hypochloremic alkalosis, hypokalemia, hyponatremia, prerenal azotemia, hyperlipidemia, rarely pancreatitis, blood dyscrasias, allergic reactions	Tab: 250, 500 mg Susp: 250 mg/5 mL (237 mL) Inj: 500 mg powder for reconst with 18 mL sterile water
Cholestyramine (Questran, Prevalite) (Antilipemic, bile acid sequestrant)	*Children:* PO: 250-1500 mg/kg/24 hr, BID-QID *Adults:* PO: *Starting:* 1 packet (or scoopful) of Questran powder or Questran Light 1-2 times/day *Maintenance:* 2-4 packets or scoopfuls/24 hr in 2 doses (or 1-6 doses) (max 6 packets/24 hr)	Constipation and other GI symptoms, bleeding, hyperchloremic acidosis	Packet of 9-g Questran powder or 5-g Questran Light, each packet containing 4 g anhydrous cholestyramine resin
Clofibrate (Atromid-S) (Antilipemic, triglyceride-lowering agent)	*Children:* PO: 0.5-1.5 mg/24 hr, BID-TID *Adults:* PO: *Initial and maintenance:* 2 g/24 hr, BID-TID	Nausea and other GI symptoms (vomiting, diarrhea, flatulence), headache, dizziness, fatigue, rash, blood dyscrasias, myalgia, arthralgia, hepatic dysfunction	Caps: 500 mg

cont'd

TABLE E-1—cont'd

DOSAGES OF DRUGS USED IN PEDIATRIC CARDIOLOGY

DRUG	ROUTE AND DOSAGE	TOXICITY OR SIDE EFFECTS	HOW SUPPLIED
Clopidogrel (Plavix) (Antiplatelet)	*Children:* PO: 1 mg/kg/24 hr to max (adult dose) of 75 mg/24 hr *Adults:* PO: 75 mg/dose, QD	Bleeding, especially when used with aspirin, neutropenia or agranulocytosis, abdominal pain constipation, rash, syncope, palpitation	Tab: 75 mg
Colestipol (Colestid) (Antilipemic, bile acid sequestrant)	*Children:* PO: 300-1500 mg/24 hr in 2-4 doses *Adults:* PO: *Starting dose:* 5 g 1-2 times/24 hr; increment of 5 g q1-2 mo *Maintenance:* 5-30 g/24 hr, BID-QID (mix with 3-6 oz water or another fluid)	Constipation and other GI symptoms (abdominal distention, flatulence, nausea and vomiting, diarrhea), rarely rash, muscle and joint pain, headache, dizziness	Packet: 5 g

Cyclosporine, Cyclosporine microemulsion (Sandimmune, Gengraf, Neoral) (Immunosuppressant)	*Children:* PO: 15 mg/kg as a single dose given 4-12 hr pretransplant; give same daily dose for 1-2 wk posttransplant, then reduce by 5% per wk to 5-10 mg/kg/24 hr, QD-BID [*Therapeutic level:* 100-300 ng/mL] IV: 5-6 mg/kg as a single dose given 4-12 hr pretransplant; administer over 2-6 hr; give same dose posttransplant until patient able to tolerate oral form	Nephrotoxicity, tremor, hypertension, less commonly hepatotoxicity, hyperlipidemia, hirsutism, gum hypertrophy, rarely lymphoma, hypomagnesemia	Oral sol: 100 mg/mL (50 mL) Neoral sol: 100 mg/mL (50 mL) Caps: 25, 50, 100 mg Neoral caps: 25, 100 mg Inj: 50 mg/mL
Diazoxide (Hyperstat IV, Proglycem) (Antihypertensive, peripheral vasodilator)	**For hypertensive crisis:** *Children and adults:* IV: 1-3 mg/kg (max 150 mg single dose); repeat q5-15 min; titrate to desired effect	Hypotension, transient hyperglycemia, nausea and vomiting, sodium retention (CHF±)	Inj: 15 mg/mL

cont'd

TABLE E-1—cont'd
DOSAGES OF DRUGS USED IN PEDIATRIC CARDIOLOGY

DRUG	ROUTE AND DOSAGE	TOXICITY OR SIDE EFFECTS	HOW SUPPLIED
Digoxin (Lanoxin, Digitek) (Cardiac glycoside, antiarrhythmic, inotrope)	*Children:* PO: *Total digitalizing dose:* Premature infant: 20 mcg/kg; Full-term newborn: 30 mcg/kg; Child 1 mo-2 yr: 40-50 mcg/kg; Child >2-10 yr: 30-40 mcg/kg; >10 yr and <100 kg: 10-15 mcg/kg PO: *Maintenance:* 25%-30% of TDD/24 hr BID IV: 75%-80% of PO dose *Adults:* PO: *Loading:* 8-12 mcg/kg *Maintenance:* 0.10-0.25 mg/24 hr [*Therapeutic level:* 0.8-2 ng/mL]	AV conduction disturbances, arrhythmias, nausea and vomiting (see Box 6-3 for ECG changes)	Elixir: 50 mcg/mL (60 mL) Tab: 125, 250, mcg Caps: 50, 100, 200 mcg. Inj: 100, 250 mcg/mL
Digoxin immune Fab (Digibind), Digifab) (Antidigoxin antibody)	*Infants and children:* IV: 1 vial (40 mg) dissolved in 4 mL H₂O, over 30 min *Adults:* IV: 4 vials (240 mg)	Allergic reaction (rare), hypokalemia, rapid AV conduction in atrial flutter	Inj: 38, 40 mg powder for reconst

| Diltiazem (Cardizem, Cardizem SR, Cardizem CD, Dilacor XR, Tiazac) (Calcium channel blocker, antihypertensive) | *Children:* PO: 1.5-2 mg/kg/24 hr, TID-QID (max 3.5 mg/kg/24 hr) *Adolescents:* Immediate release: PO: 30-120 mg/dose, TID-QID; usual range 180-360 mg/24 hr Extended release: PO: 120-300 mg/24 hr QD-BID (BID dosing with Cardizem SR; QD dosing with Cardizem CD, Dilacor XR, and Tiazac) | Dizziness, headache, edema, nausea and vomiting, heart block, and arrhythmias Contraindicated in second- and third-degree AV block, sinus node dysfunction, acute MI with pulmonary congestion Maximum antihypertensive effect seen within 2 weeks | Tab: 30, 60, 90, 120 mg Tab, extended-release: 120, 180, 240, 300, 360, 420 mg Caps extended-release: 60, 90, 120, 180, 240, 300, 360, 420 mg Inj: 5 mg/mL (5, 10 mL) |
| Dipyridamole (Persantine) (Antiplatelet) | *Children:* PO: 2-6 mg/kg/24 hr, TID *Adults:* PO: 75-100 mg QID (as an adjunct to warfarin therapy; not to use with aspirin) | Vasodilation, rarely dizziness, angina | Tab: 25, 50, 75 mg |

cont'd

TABLE E-1—cont'd

DOSAGES OF DRUGS USED IN PEDIATRIC CARDIOLOGY

DRUG	ROUTE AND DOSAGE	TOXICITY OR SIDE EFFECTS	HOW SUPPLIED
Disopyramide (Norpace) (Class IA antiarrhythmic)	*Children:* PO: <1 yr: 10-30 mg/kg/24 hr, q6 hr; 1-4 yr: 10-20 mg/kg/24 hr, q6 hr; 4-12 yr: 10-15 mg/kg/24 hr, q6 hr; 12-18 yr: 6-15 mg/kg/24 hr, q6 hr (q4 hr dosing when using regular caps) *Adults:* PO: 150 mg/dose q6 hr or 300 mg (extended release) q12 hr (max 1.6 g/24 hr) *[Therapeutic level: 3-7 mg/L]*	Heart failure or hypotension, anticholinergic effects (urinary retention, dry mouth, constipation), nausea and vomiting, hypoglycemia	Caps: 100, 150 mg Caps, CR: 100, 150 mg Susp: 1 mg/mL, 10 mg/mL
Dobutamine (Dobutrex) (β-adrenergic stimulator)	*Children:* IV infusion: 2.5-15 mcg/kg/min in D₅W or NS (incompatible with alkali solution) (max 40 mcg/kg/min) *Adults:* IV infusion: 2.5-10 mcg/kg/min (max 40 mcg/kg/min)	Tachyarrhythmias, hypertension, nausea and vomiting, headache Contraindicated in HOCM and atrial flutter/ fibrillation)	Inj: 12.5 mg/mL (20 mL)

Drug	Dosage	Adverse effects/notes	Formulation
Dopamine (Intropin, Dopastat) (Natural catecholamine inotropic agent)	*Children:* IV: Effects are dose dependent: 2-5 mcg/kg/min—increases RBF and urine output (minimum effects on heart rate and cardiac output) 5-15 mcg/kg/min—increases heart rate, cardiac contractility and cardiac output >20 mcg/kg/min—α-adrenergic effects with decreased RBF ($\pm$) (Incompatible with alkali solution)	Tachyarrhythmias, nausea and vomiting, hypotension or hypertension, extravasation (tissue necrosis [treat with local infiltration of phentolamine])	Inj: 40, 80, 160 mg/mL (5, 10, 20 mL)
Enalapril, Enalaprilat (Vasotec) (ACE inhibitor, vasodilator)	*Children:* PO: 0.1 mg/kg/dose QD or BID; increase PRN over 2 wks (max 0.5 mg/kg/24 hr) *Adults:* **For CHF:** PO: Start with 2.5 mg, QD or BID (usual range 5-20 mg/24 hr) **For hypertension:** PO: Start with 5 mg, QD (usual dose 10-40 mg/24 hr)	Hypotension, dizziness, fatigue, headache, rash, diminishing taste, neutropenia, hyperkalemia, chronic cough Evidence of fetal risk if given during 2nd and 3rd trimesters (same with all other ACE inhibitors)	Tab: 2.5, 5, 10, 20 mg (Enalapril) Oral susp: 1 mg/mL Inj: 1.25 mg/mL (Enalaprilat)

cont'd

TABLE E-1—cont'd
DOSAGES OF DRUGS USED IN PEDIATRIC CARDIOLOGY

DRUG	ROUTE AND DOSAGE	TOXICITY OR SIDE EFFECTS	HOW SUPPLIED
Enoxaparin (Lovenox) (Low-molecular-weight heparin, anticoagulant)	***For DVT treatment:*** *Infants <2 months:* SC: 1.5 mg/kg/dose, q12 hr *Infants ≥2 months to adults:* SC: 1 mg/kg/dose, q12 hr (Adjust dose to achieve target antifactor Xa levels of 0.5-1 units/mL) ***For DVT prophylaxis:*** *Infants <2 months:* SC: 1 mg/kg/dose, q12 hr *Infants ≥2 mo up to 18 yr:* SC: 0.5 mg/kg/dose, q12 hr *Adults:* SC: 30 mg, BID for 7-10 days	Bleeding Contraindicated in major bleeding and drug-induced thrombocytopenia Protamine sulfate is the antidote; 1 mg protamine sulfate neutralizes 1 mg enoxaparin	Inj: 100 mg/mL (3 mL)
Epinephrine (Adrenalin) (α-, β_1-, and β_2-adrenergic stimulator)	***For asystole and bradycardia:*** *Children:* IV/ET: 0.1-0.3 mL/kg of 1:10,000 sol (or 0.01-0.03 mg/kg) q3-5 min ***For circulatory shock or heart failure:*** *Children:* IV: 0.1-1 mcg/kg/min; titrate to effect	Tachyarrhythmias, hypertension, nausea and vomiting, headache, tissue necrosis (±)	Inj: 0.1 mg/mL (1:10,000 sol), 10 mL prefilled syringe) 1 mg/mL (1:1000 sol, 1, 30 mL)

Esmolol (Brevibloc) (β₁-selective adrenergic blocking agent, antihypertensive, class II antiarrhythmic)	*Children:* *Loading:* IV: 100-500 mcg/kg over 1 min *Maintenance:* IV: 25-100 mcg/kg/min; increase by 25-50 mcg/kg to a maximum of 300 mcg/kg/min (usual maintenance dose 50-500 mcg/kg/min)	Bronchospasm, CHF, hypotension, nausea and vomiting	Inj: 10, 20, 250 mg/mL
Ethacrynic acid (Edecrin) (Loop diuretic)	*Children:* PO: 1 mg/kg/dose, QD-TID (max 3 mg/kg/24 hr) IV: 1 mg/kg/dose *Adults:* PO: 50-100 mg, QD (max 400 mg) IV: 0.5-1 mg/kg/dose or 50 mg/dose	Dehydration, hypokalemia, prerenal azotemia, hyperuricemia, eighth cranial nerve damage (deafness), abnormal LFT, agranulocytosis or thrombocytopenia, GI irritation, rash	Tab: 25mg Inj: 50 mg vial for reconst with 50 mL D₅W
Flecainide (Tambocor) (Class IC antiarrhythmic)	*For sustained VT:* *Children:* PO: Initial 1-3 mg/kg/24 hr, q8 hr (usual range: 3-6 g/kg/24 hr, q8 hr); monitor serum level to adjust dose if needed *Adults:* PO: 100 mg/dose BID; may increase by 50 mg q12 hr every 4 days to max dose of 600 mg/24 hr [*Therapeutic level:* 0.2-1 mg/L]	Worsening of HF, bradycardia, AV block, dizziness, blurred vision, dyspnea, nausea, headache, increased PR and QRS duration	Tab: 50, 100, 150 mg Susp: 5, 20 mg/mL

cont'd

TABLE E-1—cont'd

DOSAGES OF DRUGS USED IN PEDIATRIC CARDIOLOGY

DRUG	ROUTE AND DOSAGE	TOXICITY OR SIDE EFFECTS	HOW SUPPLIED
Fludrocortisone acetate (Florinef) (Fluohydrisone) (Corticosteroid)	*For syncopal episodes:* *Children:* PO: 0.1 mg/dose, QD *Adults:* PO: 0.2 mg/dose, QD	Hypertension, hypokalemia, acne, rash, bruising, headache, GI ulcers, and growth suppression Weight gain (1-2 kg in 2-3 wk)	Tab: 0.1 mg
Furosemide (Lasix, Furomide) (Loop diuretic)	*Children:* IV: 0.5-2 mg/kg/dose, BID-QID PO: 1-2 mg/kg/dose, QD-TID (max 6 mg/kg/dose) *Adults:* IV, PO: 20-80 mg/24 hr, BID-QID	Hypokalemia, hyperuricemia, prerenal azotemia, ototoxicity, rarely bloody dyscrasias, rash	Oral liquid: 10 mg/mL, 40 mg/5 mL Tab: 20, 40, 80 mg Inj: 10 mg/mL
Heparin (Anticoagulant)	*Infants and children:* IV: *Initial:* 50 U/kg IV bolus *Maintenance:* 10-25 U/kg/hr or 50-100 U/kg q4 hr (Adjust dose to give APTT 1.5-2.5 times control, 6-8 hr after IV infusion (or 3.5-4 hr after intermittent injection))	Bleeding Antidote: protamine sulfate (1 mg per 100 U heparin in previous 4 hr)	Inj: 1000, 2000, 2500, 5000, 7500, 10,000, 20,000, 40,000 U/mL

Drug	Dosage	Toxicity/side effects	How supplied
	Adults: IV: *Initial:* 10,000 U IV injection *Maintenance:* 5000-10,000 U q4-6 hr IV drip: *Initial dose:* 5000 U followed by 20,000-40,000 U/24 hr		
Hydralazine (Apresoline) (Peripheral vasodilator, antihypertensive)	*For hypertensive crisis:* *Children:* IM, IV: 0.15-0.2 mg/kg/dose; may be repeated q4-6 hr (max 20 mg/dose) *Adults:* IM, IV: 20-40 mg/dose; repeat q4-6 hr PRN *For chronic hypertension:* *Children:* PO: 0.75-3 mg/kg/24 hr, BID-QID *Adults:* PO: Start with 10 mg 4 times/24 hr for 3-4 days; increase to 25 mg/dose QID for 3-4 days; then up to 50 mg QID	Hypotension, tachycardia and palpitation, lupus-like syndrome with prolonged use (fever, arthralgia, splenomegaly and positive LE-cell preparation), blood dyscrasias	Tab: 10, 25, 50, 100 mg Oral liquid: 1.25, 2, 4 mg/mL Inj: 20 mg/mL
Hydrochlorothiazide (HydroDIURIL, Esidrix, Hydro-Par, Oretic) (Thiazide diuretic)	*Children:* PO: 2-4 mg/kg/24 hr, BID (max 100 mg/24 hr) *Adults:* PO: 25-100 mg/24 hr, QD-BID (max 200 mg/24 hr)	Same as for chlorothiazide	Tab: 25, 50, 100 mg Caps: 12.5 mg Sol: 10 mg/mL (500 mL)

cont'd

TABLE E-1—cont'd
DOSAGES OF DRUGS USED IN PEDIATRIC CARDIOLOGY

DRUG	ROUTE AND DOSAGE	TOXICITY OR SIDE EFFECTS	HOW SUPPLIED
Ibuprofen (NeoProfen) (Nonsteroidal antiinflammatory)	**For PDA closure in premature infants:** *Neonates ≤32 weeks (500-1500 g):* IV: Initial dose 10 mg/kg, followed by two doses of 5 mg/kg after 24 and 48 hours (hold 2nd and 3rd dose if urine output is <0.6 mL/kg/hr)	Sepsis, anemia, interventricular hemorrhage, apnea, GI disorders, renal impairment Contraindicated in interventricular hemorrhage, thrombocytopenia, necrotizing enterocolitis, significant renal dysfunction	Inj: 17.1 mg/mL ibuprofen lysine equivalent to 10 mg/mL of ibuprofen (2 mL)
Inamrinone (Inocor) (Phosphodiesterase type-III inhibitor)	*Children:* IV: *Loading:* 0.75 mg/kg over 2-3 min *Maintenance:* 5-10 mcg/kg/min *Adults:* IV: *Loading:* 0.75 mg/kg over 2-3 min *Maintenance:* 5-10 mcg/kg/min	Thrombocytopenia, hypotension, tachyarrhythmias, hepatotoxicity, nausea and vomiting, fever	Inj: 5 mg/mL (20 mL)
Indomethacin (Indocin) (Nonsteroidal antiinflammatory, antipyretic agent, PG synthesis inhibitor)	**For PDA closure in premature infants:** IV: *<48 hr:* 0.2, 01, and 0.1 mg/kg/ dose, q12-24 hr *2-7 days:* 0.2, 0.2, and 0.2 mg/kg/ dose, q12-24 hr *>7 days:* 0.2, 0.25, and 0.25 mg/ kg/dose, q12-24 hr	GI or other bleeding, GI disturbances, renal impairment, electrolyte disturbances (↓ Na, ↑ K levels)	Vial: 1 mg

Drug	Dosage	Comments	Supplied
Isoproterenol (Isuprel) (β_1- and β_2-adrenergic stimulator)	*Children:* IV: 0.1-2 mcg/kg/min, titrated to desired effect *Adults* IV: 2-20 mcg/min, titrated to desired effect (incompatible with alkali solution)	Similar to epinephrine	Inj: 0.2 mg/mL (1:5000 sol: 1, 5 mL)
Ketamine (Ketalar) (General anesthetic)	**For cyanotic spells:** *Infants:* IM: 2-3 mg/kg; repeat smaller doses q30 min PRN IV: 1-3 mg/kg/dose over 60 sec; repeat smaller doses q30 min PRN	Hypertension/tachycardia, respiratory depression or apnea, CNS symptoms (dreamlike state, confusion, agitation)	Inj: 10, 50, 100 mg/mL
Ketorolac (Toradol) (Nonsteroidal antiinflammatory agent)	*Children:* IV, IM: 0.5 mg/kg/dose q6 hr (max single dose 30 mg) *Adults:* IV, IM: 30 mg/dose q6 hr PO *(adult and child >50 kg):* 10 mg PRN q6 hr	GI bleeding, nausea, dyspepsia, decreased platelet function, interstitial nephritis Consider adding acid blocker with systemic use Contraindicated in patients with hepatic or renal failure	Tab: 10 mg Inj: 15 mg/mL (1 mL), 30 mg/mL (1, 2 mL)
Labetalol (Normodyne, Trandate) (α- and β-adrenergic antagonist)	*Children:* PO: Initial 4 mg/kg/24 hr, BID (max 40 mg/kg/24 hr) IV (for hypertensive emergency): Initial 0.2-1 mg/kg/dose q10 min PRN (max 20 mg/dose)	Orthostatic hypotension, edema, CHF, bradycardia Contraindicated in asthma	Tab: 100, 200, 300 mg Susp: 10, 40 mg/mL Inj: 5 mg/mL (20, 40 mL)

cont'd

TABLE E-1—cont'd
DOSAGES OF DRUGS USED IN PEDIATRIC CARDIOLOGY

DRUG	ROUTE AND DOSAGE	TOXICITY OR SIDE EFFECTS	HOW SUPPLIED
Lidocaine (Xylocaine) (Class IB antiarrhythmic)	*Children:* IV: *Loading:* 1 mg/kg/dose slow IV, q5-10 min PRN *Maintenance:* 30 mcg/kg/min (Range 20-50 mcg/kg/min) *Adults:* IV: *Loading:* 1 mg/kg/dose q5 min *Maintenance:* 1-4 mg/min [*Therapeutic level:* 1.5-5 mg/L]	Seizure, respiratory depression, CNS symptoms (anxiety, euphoria or drowsiness), arrhythmias, hypotension or shock	Inj: 0.5%, 1%, 1.5%, 2%, 4%, 10%, 20% (1% ≡ 10 mg/mL)
Lisinopril (Zestril, Prinivil) (ACE inhibitor, antihypertensive)	*For hypertension:* *Children ≥6 yr:* PO: Initial 0.07 mg/kg/24 hr; (max initial dose is 5 mg/24 hr), increase dose at 1-2 week intervals (max 0.6 mg/kg/day or 40 mg/24 hr) *Adults:* PO: Initial 10 mg QD; may increase upward as needed to max dose 80 mg/24 hr	Dry nonproductive cough, rash, hypotension, hyperkalemia, angioedema, rarely bone marrow depression Evidence of fetal risk if given during 2nd and 3rd trimesters (same with all other ACE inhibitors)	Tab: 2.5, 5, 10, 20, 30, 40 mg

Losartan (Cozaar) (Angiotensin II-receptor blocker)	**For hypertension:** *Children ≥6 yr:* PO: 0.7 mg/kg/24 hr, QD-BID (max 50 mg/24 hr) *Adults:* PO: Initial dose 50 mg, QD (max 100 mg QD)	Hypotension, dizziness, nasal congestion, muscle cramps Evidence of fetal risk if given during 2nd and 3rd trimesters	Tab: 25, 50, 100 mg
Lovastatin (Mevacor) (Antilipemic, HMG-CoA reductase inhibitor)	*Adolescents:* PO: Starting dose 10 mg/24 hr QD for 6-8 wk; increase to 20 mg/24 hr for 8 wk, and then increase to 40 mg/24 hr for 8 wk *Adults:* PO: Starting dose 20 mg/day, QD-BID (range 40-80 mg/24 hr) (max dose with concurrent amiodarone or verapamil use is 40 mg/24 hr)	Mild GI symptoms, myositis syndrome, elevated transaminase levels, increased CK levels	Tab: 10, 20, 40 mg

cont'd

TABLE E-1—cont'd

DOSAGES OF DRUGS USED IN PEDIATRIC CARDIOLOGY

DRUG	ROUTE AND DOSAGE	TOXICITY OR SIDE EFFECTS	HOW SUPPLIED
Methyldopa (Aldomet) (Antihypertensive)	**For hypertensive crisis:** *Children:* IV: Start at 2-4 mg/kg/dose q6-8 hr (max dose 65 mg/kg/24 hr or 3 g/24 hr, whichever is less) *Adults:* IV: 250-500 mg q6 hr (max 1 g q6 hr) **For hypertension:** *Children:* PO: 10 mg/kg/24 hr, BID-QID; may be increased or decreased (max dose 65 mg/kg/24 hr or 3 g/24 hr, whichever is less) *Adults:* PO: 250 mg/dose, BID-TID for 2 days; may be increased or decreased q2 days (usual dose: 0.5-2 g/24 hr, BID-QID) (max 3 g/24 hr)	Sedation, orthostatic hypotension and brady-cardia, lupus-like syndrome, Coombs (+) hemolytic anemia and leukopenia, hepatitis or cirrhosis, colitis, impotence	Inj: 50 mg/mL (5mL) Susp: 50 mg/mL Tab: 250, 500 mg

Metoprolol (Lopressor) (β-adrenoceptor blocker)	*Children >2 yr:* PO: Initially 0.1-0.2 mg/kg/dose, BID; gradually increase to 1-3 mg/kg/24 hr *Adults:* PO: Initially 100 mg/24 hr, QD-TID; may increase to 450 mg/24 hr, BID-TID (usual dose 100-450 mg/24 hr) (Usually used with hydrochlorothi-azide 25-100 mg/24 hr)	CNS symptoms (dizziness, tiredness, depression), bronchospasm, bradycardia, diarrhea, nausea and vomiting, abdominal pain	Tab: 25, 50, 100 mg Tab, extended release: 25, 50, 100, 200 mg
Metolazone (Zaroxolyn, Diulo, Mykrox) (Thiazide-like diuretic)	*Children:* PO: 0.2-0.4 mg/kg/24 hr, QD-BID *Adults:* PO: For hypertension: 2.5-5 mg QD For edema: 5-20 mg, QD	Electrolyte imbalance, GI disturbance, hyper-glycemia, bone marrow depression, chills, hyperuricemia, hepatitis, rash May be more effective than thiazide diuretics in impaired renal function	Tab: 0.5 (Mykrox), 2.5, 5, 10 mg Susp: 1 mg/mL
Mexiletine (Mexitil) (Class IB an-tiarrhythmic)	*Children:* PO: 6-8 mg/kg/24 hr, BID-TID for 2-3 days; then 2-5 mg/kg/dose q6-8 hr Increase 1-2 mg/kg/dose q2-3 days until desired effect achieved (with food or antacid) *Adults:* PO: 200 mg q8 hr for 2-3 days; increase to 300-400 mg q8 hr (usual dose 200-300 mg q8 hr) [*Therapeutic level:* 0.75-2 mcg/mL]	Nausea and vomiting, CNS symptoms (head-ache, dizziness, tremor, paresthesia, mood changes), rash, hepatic dysfunction (±)	Caps: 150, 200, 250 mg

cont'd

TABLE E-1—cont'd

DOSAGES OF DRUGS USED IN PEDIATRIC CARDIOLOGY

DRUG	ROUTE AND DOSAGE	TOXICITY OR SIDE EFFECTS	HOW SUPPLIED
Milrinone (Primacor) (Phosphodiesterase type-III inhibitor)	*Children:* IV: *Loading:* 10-50 mcg/kg over 10 min; then 0.1-1 mcg/kg/min *Adults:* IV: *Loading:* 50 mcg/kg over 10 min 0.5 mcg/kg/min (range 0.375-0.75 mcg/kg/min)	Arrhythmias, hypotension, hypokalemia, thrombocytopenia	Inj: 1 mg/mL (5, 10, 20 mL) Inj, premixed in D$_5$W: 200 mcg/mL (100, 200 mL)
Minoxidil (Loniten) (Peripheral vasodilator)	*Children <12 yr:* PO: 0.2 mg/kg/24 hr, QD-BID initially; increase 0.1-0.2 mg/kg/24 hr q3 days until desired effect achieved (usual dose 0.25-1 mg/kg/24 hr, QD-BID; max 50 mg/24 hr) *Children >12 yr and adults:* PO: 5 mg/dose, QD initially; may be increased to 10, 20, 40 mg, QD-BID q3-day interval (usual dose 10-40 mg/24 hr, QD-BID; max 100 mg/24 hr)	Reflex tachycardia and fluid retention (used with a β-blocker and diuretic), pericardial effusion, hypertrichosis, rarely blood dyscrasias (leukopenia, thrombocytopenia)	Tab: 2.5, 10 mg

Morphine sulfate (Narcotic, analgesic)	*Children:* SC, IM, IV: 0.1-0.2 mg/kg/dose q2-4 hr (max 15 mg/dose) *Adults:* SC, IM, IV: 2.5-20 mg/dose q2-6 hr PRN	CNS depression, respiratory depression, nausea and vomiting, hypotension, bradycardia	Inj: 0.5, 1, 2, 4, 5, 8, 10, 15, 25, 50 mg/mL
Mycophenolate mofetil (CellCept) (Immunosuppressant)	*Children:* PO: 600 mg/m^2/dose, BID (max 2000 mg/24 hr) [*Therapeutic level:* 5-7 ng/mL] *Adults:* PO/IV: 2000-3000 g/24 hr, BID	Headache, GI symptoms, hypertension, bone marrow suppression (anemia), fever, increased risk of developing lymphomas or other malignancies	Tab: 500 mg Caps: 250 mg Oral susp: 200 mg/mL Inj: 500 mg
Nifedipine (Procardia, Adalat) (Calcium channel blocker)	*For hypertrophic cardiomyopathy:* *Children:* PO: 0.5-0.9 mg/kg/24 hr, TID-QID *For hypertension:* *Children:* PO: 0.25-0.5 mg/kg/24 hr, QD-BID (max 3 mg/kg/24 hr up to 120 mg/24 hr) *Adults:* PO: Initially 10 mg/dose, TID; titrate up to 20 to 30 mg/dose, TID-QID over 7-14 days (usual dose 10-20 mg TID; max dose 180 mg/24 hr)	Hypotension, peripheral edema, CNS symptoms (headache, dizziness, weakness), nausea	Caps: 10, 20 mg Tab, sustained release (Adalat CC, Procardia XL): 30, 60, 90 mg

cont'd

TABLE E-1—cont'd
DOSAGES OF DRUGS USED IN PEDIATRIC CARDIOLOGY

DRUG	ROUTE AND DOSAGE	TOXICITY OR SIDE EFFECTS	HOW SUPPLIED
Nitroglycerin (Nitro-Bid, Tridil, Nitrostat) (Peripheral vasodilator)	*Children:* IV: 0.5-1 mcg/kg/min Increase 1 mcg/kg/min q20 min to titrate to effect (max 6 mcg/kg/min) (Dilute in D$_5$W or NS with final concentration <400 mcg/mL; light sensitive) *Adults:* IV: Initial dose: 5 mcg/min through infusion pump Increase 5 mcg/min q3-5 min until desired effect achieved	Hypotension, tachycardia, headache, nausea and vomiting	Inj: 0.5, 5 mg/mL Inj, premixed in D$_5$W: 100, 200, 400 mcg/mL
Nitroprusside (Nipride) (Peripheral vasodilator)	*Children:* IV: 0.3-0.5 mcg/kg/min, titrate to effect with BP monitoring (usual dose 3-4 mcg/kg/min; max dose 10 mcg/kg/min) (Dilute stock solution [50 mg] in 250-2000 mL D$_5$W; light sensitive)	Hypotension, palpitation, and cyanide toxicity (metabolic acidosis earliest and most reliable evidence) Monitor thiocyanate level when used >48 hr and in patients with renal or hepatic dysfunction; thiocyanate level should be <50 mg/L; cyanate levels >2 mcg/mL are toxic levels	Inj: 25 mg/mL (2 mL) Inj: 50 mg for reconst with 2-3 mL D$_5$W)

| Norepinephrine (Levophed, levarterenol) (α_1- and β_1-adrenoceptor stimulant) | *Children:* IV: 0.1 mcg/kg/min IV infusion initially; increase dose to attain desired effect (max 2 mcg/kg/min) *Adults:* IV: Start at 4 mcg/min IV infusion; titrate to effect (usual dose range 8-12 mcg/min) | Hypertension, bradycardia (reflex), arrhythmias, tissue necrosis (treat with phentolamine infiltration) | Inj: 1 mg/mL (4 mL) |
| Phentolamine (Regitine) (α-adrenoceptor blocker) | **For diagnosis of pheochromocytoma:** *Children:* IM, IV: 0.05-0.1 mg/kg/dose; repeat q5 min until hypertension is controlled; then q2-4 hr PRN *Adults:* IM, IV: 2.5-5 mg/dose; repeat q5 min until hypertension is controlled; then q2-4 hr PRN **For treatment of extravasated α-adrenergic drugs:** SC: Make a solution of 0.5-1 mcg/mL with NS. Inject 1-5 mL (in 5 divided doses) around the site of extravasation (max 0.1-0.5 mg/kg or 5 mg total) | Hypotension, tachycardia or arrhythmias, nausea and vomiting | Inj: 5 mg powder for reconst |

cont'd

TABLE E-1—cont'd
DOSAGES OF DRUGS USED IN PEDIATRIC CARDIOLOGY

DRUG	ROUTE AND DOSAGE	TOXICITY OR SIDE EFFECTS	HOW SUPPLIED
Phenylephrine (Neo-Synephrine) (α_1-adrenoceptor stimulant)	**For hypotension:** *Children:* IM, SC: 0.1 mg/kg/dose q1-2 hr PRN (max dose 5 mg) IV: 5-10 mcg/kg/dose IV bolus q10-15 min or 0.1-0.5 mcg/kg/min *Adults:* IM, SC: 2-5 mg/dose q1-2 hr PRN (max dose 5 mg) IV: 0.1-0.5 mg/dose IV bolus q10-15 min PRN; start IV drip at 100-180 mcg/min (usual maintain dose 40-60 mcg/min)	Arrhythmias, hypertension, angina	Inj: 10 mg/mL
Phenytoin (Dilantin) (Class IB antiarrhythmic, anticonvulsant)	*Children:* IV: 2-4 mg/kg/dose over 5-10 min followed by PO dose PO: 2-5 mg/kg/24 hr, BID-TID [*Therapeutic level:* 5-18 mcg/mL for arrhythmias, 10-20 mcg/mL for seizures] *Adults:* IV: 100 mg q5 min (total 500 mg) PO: 250 mg QID for 1 day, 250 mg/dose BID for 2 days, and 300-400 mg/24 hr, QD-QID	Rash, Stevens-Johnson syndrome, CNS symptoms (ataxia, dysarthria), lupus-like syndrome, blood dyscrasias, peripheral neuropathy, gingival hypertrophy	Susp: 125 mg/5 mL (240 mL) Tab, chewable: 50 mg (Infatab) Caps: 100 mg Caps, extended release: 30, 100, 200, 300 mg Inj: 50 mg/mL

Potassium chloride	**Supplement in diuretic therapy:** *Children:* PO: 1-2 mEq/kg/24 hr, TID-QID (or 0.8-1.5 mL 10% potassium chloride/kg/24 hr, or 0.4-0.7 mL 20% potassium chloride/kg/24 hr, TID-QID	GI disturbances, ulcerations, hyperkalemia	Oral sol: 10% (1.3 mEq/mL), 20% (2.7 mEq/mL) Caps, sustained release: 8, 10 mEq Tabs, sustained release: 8, 10, 15, 20 mEq
Potassium gluconate	**Supplement in diuretic therapy:** *Children:* PO: 1-2 mEq/kg/24 hr TID-QID, or 0.8-1.5 mL/kg/24 hr TID-QID	Same as for potassium chloride	Elixir: 1.3 mEq/mL
Pravastatin (Pravachol) (Antilipemic, HMG-CoA reductase inhibitor)	*Children (8-13 yr):* PO: Starting dose 10 mg QD for 4-6 wk; increase to 20 QD as needed *Adolescents (14-18 yr):* PO: 40 mg QD (adult max dose 40 mg/day)	Headache, constipation, diarrhea, elevated liver enzymes, rhabdomyolysis, myopathy	Tabs: 10, 20, 40, 80 mg
Prazosin (Minipress) (Postsynaptic α_1-adrenergic blocker, antihypertensive)	*Children:* PO: 5 mcg/kg as a test dose; then increase to 20 mg/24 hr, BID-QID initially; increase to 20 mg/24 hr, BID-QID (usual dose 6-15 mg/24 hr)	CNS symptoms (dizziness, headache, drowsiness), palpitation, nausea	Caps: 1, 2, 5 mg

cont'd

TABLE E-1—cont'd
DOSAGES OF DRUGS USED IN PEDIATRIC CARDIOLOGY

DRUG	ROUTE AND DOSAGE	TOXICITY OR SIDE EFFECTS	HOW SUPPLIED
Procainamide (Procanbid, Pronestyl) (Class IA antiarrhythmic)	*Children:* IV: *Loading:* 2-6 mg/kg/dose over 5 min repeated q10-30 min (max 100 mg) *Maintenance:* 20-80 mcg/kg/min (max 2 g/24 hr) PO: 15-50 mg/kg/24 hr q3-6 hr (max 4 g/24 hr) *Adults:* IV: *Loading:* 50-100 mg/dose q5 min PRN *Maintenance:* 1-6 mg/min PO: immediate release 250-500 mg/ dose q3-6 hr (sustained release 500-1000 mg/dose q6 hr) *[Therapeutic level:* 4-10 mcg/mL]*	Nausea and vomiting, blood dyscrasias, rash, lupus-like syndrome, hypotension, confusion or disorientation	Tab, sustained release: 250, 500, 750, 1000 mg Caps: 250, 375, 500 mg Susp: 5, 50, 100 mg/mL Inj: 100, 500 mg/mL
Propranolol (Inderal) (β-adrenoceptor blocker, class II antiarrhythmic)	*For hypertension:* *Children:* PO: 0.5-1 mg/kg/24 hr, BID-QID; may increase q 3-5 days (usual dose 2-4 mg/kg/24 hr; max dose 8 mg/kg/24 hr)	Hypotension, syncope, bronchospasm, nausea and vomiting, hypoglycemia, lethargy or depression, heart block	Tab: 10, 20, 40, 60, 80, 90 mg Caps, extended release: 60, 80, 120, 160 mg Oral sol: 20, 40 mg/5 mL Concentrated sol: 80 mg/mL Inj: 1 mg/mL

For arrhythmias:

Children:

IV: 0.01-0.15 mg/kg/dose over 10 min; repeat q6-8 hr PRN (max 1 mg/dose for infants; 3 mg/dose for children)

PO: Start at 0.5-1 mg/kg/24 hr, TID-QID; increase dose q3-5 days PRN (usual dose 2-4 mg/kg/24 hr; max dose 16 mg/kg/24 hr)

Adults:

IV: 1 mg/dose q5 min (max 5 mg)

PO: 10-20 mg/dose TID-QID; increase PRN (usual dose 40-320 mg/24 hr, TID-QID)

Prostaglandin E₁ or alprostadil (Prostin VR, PGE₁) (Vasodilator)

For patency of ductus arteriosus:

IV:

Begin infusion at 0.05-0.1 mcg/kg/min.

When desired effect achieved, reduce to 0.05, 0.025, and 0.01 mcg/kg/min.

If unresponsive, dose may be increased to 0.4 mcg/kg/min.

Apnea, flushing, bradycardia, hypotension, fever

Inj: 500 mcg/mL

cont'd

TABLE E-1—cont'd
DOSAGES OF DRUGS USED IN PEDIATRIC CARDIOLOGY

DRUG	ROUTE AND DOSAGE	TOXICITY OR SIDE EFFECTS	HOW SUPPLIED
Protamine sulfate (Heparin antidote)	**Antidote to heparin over-dose:** IV: Each 1 mg protamine neutralizes approx. 100 U heparin given in preceding 3-4 hr. Slow IV infusion at rate not exceeding 20 mg/min or 50 mg/10 min. (Check APTT)	Hypotension, bradycardia, dyspnea, flushing, coagulation problem	Inj: 10 mg/mL
Quinidine (Cardioquin, Quinidex, Quinaglute) (Class IA antiarrhythmic)	*Children:* Test dose for idiosyncrasy: 2 mg/kg once (PO as sulfate; IM/IV as gluconate) Therapeutic dose: IV (as gluconate): 2-10 mg/kg/dose, q3-6 hr PRN PO (as sulfate): 15-60 mg/kg/24 hr, q6 hr *Adults:* Test dose: 200 mg once PO/IM Therapeutic dose: PO (as sulfate, immediate release): 100-600 mg/dose q4-6 hr. Begin at 200 mg/dose and titrate to desired effect, or PO (sulfate, sustained release): 300-600 mg/dose q8-12 hr.	Nausea and vomiting, ventricular arrhythmias, prolonged QRS complex, depressed myocardial contractility, blood dyscrasias, symptoms of cinchonism	*Gluconate* (62% quinidine): Tab, slow-release: 324 mg Inj: 80 mg/mL *Sulfate* (83% quinidine): Tabs: 200, 300 mg Tab, slow-release: 300 mg Susp: 10 mg/mL

	PO (as gluconate): 324-972 mg q8-12 hr IM (as gluconate): 400 mg/dose q4-6 hr IV (as gluconate): 200-400 mg/dose, infused at a rate of ≤10 mg/min [*Therapeutic level:* 3-7 mg/L]	
Sildenafil (Revatio, Viagra) (Phosphodiesterase type-V inhibitor)	***For pulmonary hypertension:*** *Neonates:* PO: 0.25-1 mg/kg/dose, BID-QID *Infants and children:* PO: 0.25-1 mg/kg/dose, q4-6 hr *Adults:* PO: 20 mg TID	Hypotension, tachycardia, flushing, head-ache, rash, nausea, diarrhea, priapism, platelet dysfunction, myalgia, paresthesia, blurred vision, epistaxis, dyspnea Contraindicated in concurrent use of organic nitrates	Tab: 20, 25, 50, 100 mg
Simvastatin (Zocor) (Antilipemic, HMG-CoA reductase inhibitor)	*Children:* PO: Starting dose 10 mg QD Increment of 10 mg q6-8 wk to max dose of 40 mg QD as needed (Adult max 80 mg/24 hr)	Headache, constipation, diarrhea, elevated liver enzymes, rhabdomyolysis, myopathy	Tab: 5, 10, 20, 40, 80 mg

cont'd

TABLE E-1—cont'd
DOSAGES OF DRUGS USED IN PEDIATRIC CARDIOLOGY

DRUG	ROUTE AND DOSAGE	TOXICITY OR SIDE EFFECTS	HOW SUPPLIED
Sirolimus (Rapamune) (Immunosuppressant)	*Children:* PO: *Loading:* 3 mg/m^2 *Maintenance:* 1 mg/m^2/day QD *Adults:* PO: *Loading:* 6 mg *Maintenance:* 2 mg/day QD [*Therapeutic level:* 6-15 ng/mL]	Hypertension, peripheral edema, chest pain, fever, headache, acne, hirsutism, hypercholesterolemia, neurotoxicity, abdominal pain, anemia, pneumonitis	Tab: 1, 2 mg Oral sol: 1 mg/mL
Sodium polystyrene sulfonate (Kayexalate, Kionex) (Potassium-removing resin)	***For hyperkalemia (slowly effective, taking hours to days):*** *Children:* PO, NG: 1 g/kg/dose, q6 hr PR: 1 g/kg/dose, q2-6 hr *Adults:* PO, NG, PR: 15 g QD-QID (cation-exchange resin with practical exchange rates of 1 mEq potassium per 1 g resin) (NOTE: Delivers 1 mEq sodium for each mEq of potassium removed)	Nausea and vomiting, constipation, severe hypokalemia (muscle weakness, confusion [monitor serum potassium levels, ECG]), hypocalcemia or hypernatremia (edema)	Powder: 454, 480 g Susp: 15 g/60 mL

Sotalol (Betapace) (Class II and III antiarrhythmic)	**For SVT and VT:** PO: 80–120 mg/m^2/24 hr, TID (*infants*) BID (*older children and adults*)	Chest pain, palpitation, hypoglycemia, hypotension, torsades de pointes, nausea and vomiting, abdominal pain, CNS symptoms (depression, weakness, dizziness), bronchospasm, heart block, bradycardia, negative inotropic effects, QT prolongation (Discontinue if QTc >550 ms)	Tab: 80, 120, 160, 240 mg Syrup: 5 mg/mL
Spironolactone (Aldactone) (Potassium-sparing diuretic, aldosterone antagonist)	*Children:* PO: 3 mg/kg/24 hr, BID-TID *Adults:* PO: 50–100 mg/24 hr, TID-QID (max 200 mg/24 hr)	Hyperkalemia (when given with potassium supplements and ACE inhibitors), GI distress, rash, gynecomastia, agranulocytosis Contraindicated in renal failure	Tab: 25, 50, 100 mg Susp: 1, 2, 2.5, 5, 25 mg/mL
Streptokinase (Streptase, Kabikinase) (Thrombolytic enzyme)	**For thrombolysis:** (Use in consultation with a hematologist) *Children:* IV: 3500–4000 U/kg over 30 min, followed by 1000-1500 U/kg/hr, or 2000 U/kg load over 30 min followed by 2000 U/kg/hr (Duration of infusion based on response but generally does not exceed 3 days. Obtain tests at baseline and q4 hr: APTT, TT, fibrinogen, PT, hematocrit, platelet count. APTT and TT should be <2 times control.)	Potential for allergic reaction with repeated use; premedicate with acetaminophen and antihistamine, and repeat q4-6 hr	Inj: 250,000, 750,000, 1,500,000 IU powder for reconst

cont'd

TABLE E-1—cont'd

DOSAGES OF DRUGS USED IN PEDIATRIC CARDIOLOGY

DRUG	ROUTE AND DOSAGE	TOXICITY OR SIDE EFFECTS	HOW SUPPLIED
Tacrolimus (Prograf) (Immunosuppressant)	*Children and adults:* PO: 0.15-0.4 mg/kg/day, BID IV: 0.03-0.15 mg/kg/day continuous infusion [*Therapeutic level:* 5-15 ng/mL]	Hypertension, hypotension, peripheral edema, myocardial hypertrophy, chest pain, fever, headache, encephalopathy, pruritus, hypercholesterolemia, electrolyte imbalance, neurotoxicity, nephrotoxicity, diarrhea, anemia, dyspnea	Caps: 0.5, 1, 5 mg Susp: 0.5 mg/mL Inj: 5 mg/mL (1 mL)
Tolazoline (Priscoline) (α-adrenoceptor blocker)	*For neonatal pulmonary hypertension:* IV: *Loading:* 1-2 mg/kg over 10 min *Maintenance:* 1-2 mg/kg/hr	Hypotension and tachycardia, pulmonary hemorrhage, GI bleeding, arrhythmias, thrombocytopenia, leukopenia	Inj: 25 mg/mL
Triamterene (Dyrenium) (Potassium-sparing diuretic)	*Children:* PO: 2-4 mg/kg/24 hr, QD-BID; may increase up to max 6 mg/kg/24 hr or 300 mg/24 hr *Adults:* PO: 50-100 mg/24 hr, QD-BID (max 300 mg/24 hr)	Nausea and vomiting, leg cramps, dizziness, hyperuricemia, rash, prerenal azotemia	Caps: 50, 100 mg

Urokinase
(Abbokinase)
(Thrombolytic
enzyme)

For thrombolysis (in vein thrombosis or pulmonary embolism):
(Should be used in consultation with a hematologist)
Children:
IV:
Loading: 4400 U/kg over 10 min
Maintenance: 4400 U/kg/hr for 6-12 hr. Some patients may require 12-72 hr of therapy.
(Monitor same laboratory tests as for streptokinase)

For occluded IV catheter clearance:
Aspiration method: Use 5000 U/mL concentrate. Instill into the catheter a volume equal to the internal volume of catheter over 1-2 min, leave in place for 1-4 hr, then aspirate. May repeat with 10,000 U/mL if no response. Do not infuse into the patient.
IV infusion method: 150-200 U/kg/ hr in each lumen for 8-48 hr at a rate of at least 20 mL/hr
Adults:
For pulmonary embolism:
IV: Priming dose: 4400 U/kg
IV infusion: 4400 U/kg/hr for 12 hr by infusion pump

Bleeding, allergic reactions, rash, fever and chills, bronchospasm

Inj: 5000 U/mL

cont'd

TABLE E-1—cont'd
DOSAGES OF DRUGS USED IN PEDIATRIC CARDIOLOGY

DRUG	ROUTE AND DOSAGE	TOXICITY OR SIDE EFFECTS	HOW SUPPLIED
Verapamil (Isoptin, Calan) (Calcium channel blocker, class IV antiarrhythmic)	**For dysrhythmia (SVT):** *Children:* IV: 1-15 yr (for SVT): 0.1-0.3 mg/kg over 2 min May repeat same dose in 15 min (max dose 5 mg first dose; 10 mg second dose) *Adults:* IV: 5-10 mg, 10 mg second dose **For hypertension:** *Children:* PO: 4-8 mg/kg/24 hr, TID *Adults:* PO: 240-480 mg/24 hr, TID	Hypotension, bradycardia, cardiac depression	Tab: 40, 80, 120 mg Tab, extended release: 120, 180, 240 mg Caps, extended release: 100, 120, 180, 200, 240, 300, 360 mg Susp: 50 mg/mL Inj: 2.5 mg/mL
Vitamin K₁	**Antidote to dicumarol or warfarin:** PO/IM/SC/IV: 2.5-10 mg/dose in 1 dose for correction of excessive PT from dicumarol or warfarin overdose		Tab: 5 mg Inj: 2, 10 mg/mL

Warfarin (Coumadin, Safarin) (Anticoagulant)	*Children:* PO: *Initial:* 0.1-0.2 mg/kg/dose QD in evening for 2 days (max dose 10 mg/dose) (In liver dysfunction, 0.1 mg/kg/day, max 5 mg/dose) *Maintenance:* 0.1 mg/kg/24H QD (Monitor INR after 5-7 days of new dosage. Keep INR at 2.5-3.5 for mechanical prosthetic valve; 2-3 for prophylaxis of DVT, pulmonary emboli.) (Heparin preferred initially for rapid anticoagulation; warfarin may be started concomitantly with heparin or may be delayed 3-6 days.) *Adults:* PO: *Initial:* 5-15 mg/dose QD for 2-5 days *Maintenance:* 2-10 mg/day (Adjust dosage based on INR)	Bleeding (antidote: vitamin K or fresh-frozen plasma) *Increased PT response:* salicylates, acetaminophen, alcohol, lipid-lowering agents, phenytoin, ibuprofen, some antibiotics *Decreased PT response:* antihistamines, barbiturates, oral contraceptives, vitamin C, diet high in vitamin K Onset of action: 36-72 hr and full effects in 4-5 days Mode of action: inhibits hepatic synthesis of vitamin K-dependent factors (I, VII, IX, X)	Tab: 1, 2, 2.5, 3, 4, 5, 6, 7.5, 10 mg Inj: 5 mg

cont'd
For table footnote, see next page.

ACE, angiotensin-converting enzyme; APTT, activated partial thromboplastin time; AV, atrioventricular; BID, two times a day; BP, blood pressure; Caps, capsule; CHF, congestive heart failure; CK, creatine kinase; CNS, central nervous system; CR, controlled release; D_5W, 5% dextrose in water; DVT, deep vein thrombosis; ECG, electrocardiogram; ET, endotracheal; GI, gastrointestinal; HMG-CoA, 3-hydroxy-3-methylglutaryl coenzyme A; HOCM, hypertrophic obstructive cardiomyopathy; IM, intramuscular; Inj, injection; INR, international normalized ratio; IV, intravenous; LFT, liver function test; max, maximum; NE, norepinephrine; NG, nasogastric; NS, normal saline; PDA, patent ductus arteriosus; PG, prostaglandin; PO, by mouth; PR, per rectum; PRN, as necessary; PT, prothrombin time; q, every; QD, once a day; QID, four times a day; QOD, every other day; RBF, renal blood flow; reconst, reconstitution; SC, subcutaneous; sol, solution; Supp, suppository; Susp, suspension; Tab, tablet; TDD, total digitalizing dose; TID, three times a day; TT, thrombin time; WBC, white blood cell; ($\pm$), may occur.

Index

Page numbers followed by 'b' indicate boxes, 'f' indicate figures, 't' indicate tables